CHILDHOOD TRAUMATIC BRAIN INJURY

CHILDHOOD TRAUMATIC BRAIN INJURY

DIAGNOSIS, ASSESSMENT, AND INTERVENTION

EDITED BY

Erin D. Bigler
Elaine Clark, and
Janet E. Farmer

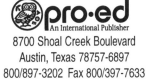

8700 Shoal Creek Boulevard
Austin, Texas 78757-6897
800/897-3202 Fax 800/397-7633
Order online at http://www.proedinc.com

This text has been adapted from material that previously appeared in the *Journal of Learning Disabilities.*

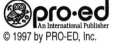

An International Publisher

© 1997 by PRO-ED, Inc.
8700 Shoal Creek Boulevard
Austin, Texas 78757-6897
800/897-3202 Fax 800/397-7633
Order online at http://www.proedinc.com

Library of Congress Cataloging-in-Publication Data

Childhood traumatic brain injury : diagnosis, assessment, and
  intervention / edited by Erin D. Bigler, Elaine Clark, and Janet E.
  Farmer.
        p.   cm.
  Articles reprinted from Journal of learning disabilities.
  Includes bibliographical references and indexes.
  ISBN 0-89079-718-8 (alk. paper)
  1. Brain-damaged children—Rehabilitation.   2. Brain-damaged
children—Education.   3. Brain—Wounds and injuries—Patients—
Rehabilitation.   4. Brain—Wounds and injuries—Patients—
Education.   I. Bigler, Erin D., 1949– .   II. Clark, Elaine.
III. Farmer, Janet E.   IV. Journal of learning disabilities.
  [DNLM: 1. Brain Injuries—in infancy & childhood—collected
works.
  2. Brain Injuries—rehabilitation—collected works.   WS 340 C5363
  1997]
RJ496.B7C48   1997
617.4'810443'083—dc21
DNLM/DLC   97-7468
for Library of Congress   CIP

Printed in the United States of America
   2   3   4   5   6   7   8   10   01   00

Contents

Foreword

It is fitting that in this, the Decade of the Brain, a continuing monograph related to childhood traumatic brain injury (TBI) that focuses on its relationship to the problems of learning and behavior that are often the natural sequelae of such injuries would be forthcoming from a series first appearing in the *Journal of Learning Disabilities.* It is fitting, as well, that the progenitors of such a project would consist of a neuropsychologist (Erin Bigler), a school psychologist and clinical neuropsychologist (Elaine Clark), and a clinical psychologist with a specialty in rehabilitation psychology and neuropsychology (Janet Farmer). Closed-head injury was first recognized as representing a silent epidemic in the 1960s and 1970s. Many children with TBI (and children and adolescents have the highest rate of traumatic brain injury within the population) most often carry no visible scars following a traumatic brain injury. Those close to such individuals note significant changes in their behavior and learning. Neuropsychological changes are the most prominent, with complaints of memory difficulty being the most common following such an injury, followed closely by difficulty with attention and concentration, and alterations in mood. Too often in the past, the victims of traumatic brain injuries who survived were sent home from the acute care setting in the guise of being fully recovered and without additional sequelae. We know these children continue to suffer disorders of learning and behavior that require careful attention and the care of a therapeutic team of individuals. The complexities of brain functions and the management of the sequelae of traumatic injury to the brain require an approach that produces integrative services by the medical, psychological, and educational professionals involved in the child's life. The significant role of the family has also been recognized and is clearly addressed in this monograph.

The many advances in functional neuroanatomy of recent years, many of which are related to advances in the technology of neuroimaging, are described in the opening sections of the monograph by one of the leading researchers in the field, Erin Bigler (also an editor of this monograph). His chapter lays an anatomical foundation for the works to follow, and also provides insight into the interactional utility and synergy of imaging and neuropsychological assessment for understanding the outcomes of TBI in individual patients. These children pose special problems of assessment, especially in the educational environment, but also within acute care settings. Janet Farmer and her colleagues follow Bigler's foundational chapter by outlining the comprehensive, multidisciplinary evaluations that should take place during rehabilitation of children with traumatic brain injury in order to promote their reentry and integration into the school setting. These authors not only detail the physical and cognitive changes that are sometimes evident in such patients, but also denote the necessity of evaluating behavioral and affective changes, which often produce the greatest barriers to successful rehabilitation. The attentional deficits and potential amotivational aspects of TBI in children must be identified, and their functional abilities assessed, to increase the likelihood of obtaining the most positive long-term outcome. The special problems posed by such children when returning to a school setting (from which they have likely lost their peer group) from a period of acute care hospitalization, and subsequent time in a rehabilitation facility, are addressed by Dr. Clark. She provides the reader with an overview of the planning process for such students and specific information on their learning needs, and she highlights these issues via a case history.

Janiece Lord-Maes and John Obrzut follow with a discussion of differ-. ences in age effects on the longer term cognitive sequelae of TBI, with specific detail on the relationship of age and TBI to specific learning disorders. Recent findings with regard to more long-term sequelae are reviewed here, as well. Special management techniques necessary for attending to the memory and attention problems of these children are next reviewed by Catherine Mateer and her colleagues. They review the major approaches to ameliorating the common problems of disturbances of memory, attention, and executive function that occur in these children. They focus not only on direct work with the victim of brain injury, but also on making appropriate alterations in the environment and in teaching strategies, to allow children to compensate for areas in which they have more specific weaknesses.

As noted earlier, victims of traumatic brain injury also exhibit changes in behavior and emotion. The management of the behavioral disturbances in individuals with brain injury requires a more specialized knowledge than does management of more garden-variety behavior problems typically seen by child clinicians. Children with TBI have special deficits that often change their response to traditional behaviorally based interventions. Thomas Kehle and his colleagues review some of these special problems related to managing behavioral disturbances in children with TBI, placing a special emphasis on the cognitive problems that in fact interfere with the effectiveness of interventions.

It is also known that individuals with traumatic brain injury are at higher risk of engaging in alcohol and substance abuse than the general population. These special problems are reviewed by Jeffrey Kreutzer and his colleagues. Their results suggest that although postinjury illicit drug use rates are relatively low, alcohol use remains a significant problem in this population. Because individuals consuming alcohol are also at higher risk for head injury and individuals with a history of head injury are at higher risk of a second head injury, the use of any substance that alters motor function or level of consciousness (e.g., alcohol) requires careful attention on a long-term basis.

The impact of a traumatic brain injury goes beyond the effects felt by the victim of the injury. There are substantial effects for families and other caregivers. Children are most likely to sustain a TBI in a motor vehicle accident. In such a circumstance, it is common for a parent or sibling to also sustain a substantial injury—or even die—in the impact. All of these factors work to compound the insidious effects of the head injury on the long-term cognitive and emotional recovery of brain-injured patients. Shari Wade and her colleagues review the impact of traumatic brain injury on the family and note that parents who were not injured will report increased psychological symptoms when a child suffers a traumatic brain injury as opposed to other traumatic injuries that do not have brain involvement. Jane Conoley and Susan Sheridan take a family-systems approach to this problem, noting the psychological, financial, role, and relationship risks that are experienced by the entire family system, and they review specific strategies that might help families in the recovery and reentry processes. The specific responses of the educational community to such problems are reviewed by Rik D'Amato and Barbara Rothlisberg in the final work of the monograph; they denote suggestions for an integrated approach to intervention that should optimize long-term recovery.

Since the federal government has mandated special educational services for children with TBI, this monograph is one of the first comprehensive treatments of how such services should be derived and integrated for individual children. Educational environments are not particularly well equipped, inherently, to accept and integrate children with long-term sequelae of traumatic brain injury into the school environ. New structures may have to be designed within the existing school systems to allow greater flexibility in the education of these children, who as a group will have tremendously variable needs, perhaps more variable than any other nominally defined group of children. For now, under the guidance of the scholars and practitioners published in this monograph, we begin with focusing on the individual child who has been the victim of a traumatic brain injury. Perhaps what is next is that we advocate for structural change to enhance the accommodations of these highly variable victims within the context of what can at times be a regimented—and perhaps even rigid—system of instruction and discipline.

Cecil R. Reynolds

PART I

Introduction

1. Traumatic Brain Injury: 1990s Update

ERIN D. BIGLER, ELAINE CLARK, AND

JANET E. FARMER

The *Journal of Learning Disabilities* introduced a special series on traumatic brain injury (TBI) in 1987 (Bigler, 1987). The preface to that series, written by J. Lee Wiederholt, reviewed the historical role that TBI has played in the study of learning disabilities. Case in point: The first indications that some disorders of learning were related to neurologic aberrations came from comparing individuals with some form of learning disorder to those with known acquired cerebral trauma (see Wiederholt, 1974). This history clearly demonstrates the theoretical and clinical underpinnings uniting the studies of cerebral trauma and learning disorders or disabilities.

Another facet of brain trauma history needs brief review as well. Prior to the advent of regional trauma centers and the development of modern medical treatments for the acute preservation of trauma victims, patients with moderate to severe traumatic brain injury typically died. With their deaths, not only was the need for any long-term therapy or follow-up obviated, but also the opportunity to study brain–behavior relationships was lost. Even in individuals who did survive a moderate to severe brain injury, the investigation of brain–behavior relationships was severely limited. Prior to the advent of computerized tomography (CT) imaging, circa 1974, no methods existed by which the brain could be visualized in vivo except through neurosurgery. So, with TBI survivors prior to the 1970s, not much could be accomplished to advance our understanding of brain injury and behavior because of the visual inaccessibility of the brain in living individuals.

Obviously, all of this has changed in this, the "Decade of the Brain." We now have a variety of exquisite methods for imaging the brain that yield information both about its distinctive structure, as in CT and magnetic resonance (MR) imaging, and about its physiology and metabolic functioning, such as obtained in positron emission tomography (PET), single photon emission computed tomography (SPECT), magnetoencephalography (MEG), and quantitative electroencephalography (QEEG; see Bigler, 1994). Essentially all major population areas of the industrialized world now have regional trauma centers with specific diagnostic and treatment programs for persons with brain injury, and many areas have organized long-term treatment programs for the survivors of TBI. Accordingly, we have never been in a better position to study brain–behavior relations in humans than we are today or to address the clinical needs of this brain-injury population.

So why study survivors of TBI? TBI remains one of the leading causes of disability induction in adolescents and young adults. All of these individuals have an entire life ahead of them; those in the public school age range have years of public education and, potentially, postsecondary training in store. For those of us who provide services to individuals with TBI, there is a natural drive to study TBI in order to establish the very best circumstances for recovery and adaptation that can be made. Also, by studying survivors of TBI, we may be further enlightened as to the role that the brain plays in learning and behavior. For example, although they did not use the traumatic brain injury model, Galaburda and colleagues employed a similar logic as the basis of their investigations of the neuroanatomic and neurobiologic factors associated with dyslexia. In comparing the "normal" brain with that of an individual with a history of "dyslexia," they discovered a variety of neuroanatomic and neurophysiologic irregularities that likely represent the neurobiologic basis of that particular form of learning disorder (see Galaburda, 1993; Galaburda, Menard, & Rosen, 1994).

The JLD series of 1987 addressed the significant contemporary issues of nearly a decade ago. Much has changed since that review. There have been a variety of significant advances in both clinical and basic neuroscience as well as applied aspects of TBI research and treatment. Because of the continued prevalence of brain injury, individuals with neurological deficits as a result of TBI continue to need the attention of a variety of health and educational specialists. The survivors of TBI affect all levels of society, from individual/family needs to national policies governing health care and rehabilitation. This book has been designed to address those needs by updating and expanding the original series.

There has also been a realization that acute rehabilitation during hospitalization alone is not sufficient to optimize outcomes. Many persons with moderate to severe injuries may require long-term supportive services to achieve a maximal level of independence and quality of life. Rehabilitation professionals have been challenged to provide a continuum of care from the time of injury to the point of full reintegration into the community. Because of the complexity of the problems that can arise following TBI, this requires linkages among treatment providers in the hospital, school, and community.

For children with TBI, one of the most positive changes in the past few years was the passage of the Individuals with Disabilities Education Act (IDEA; P.L. 106-476), which included Traumatic Brain Injury as a special education diagnostic category. This law has increased educators' awareness of TBI and has allowed students greater access to appropriate educational services. However, although IDEA opened the door for improved communication between rehabilitation and school professionals about the needs of children with TBI, approaches to the transition from hospital to school have not yet been fully standardized. This is not surprising, as educators have been faced with the challenge of complying with a law that requires them to provide services to students they feel inadequately prepared to work with. Many educators do not understand what needs these students have, and some are not even aware of what it means to be TBI. Because the definition was quite ambiguous at first, in the 2 years following the time the law passed and the rules were written, a number of states wrote their own guidelines to serve these students. Whereas some decided to interpret TBI more broadly, others decided to take a more conservative stance and limit the definition to head injuries only. Some decided to ignore it altogether. No longer can educators neglect their responsibility to serve these students who are eligible for services under the federal law.

These students represent a large and diverse population. Although their injuries have the potential to disrupt not only learning, but social, emotional, and physical functioning as well, the magnitude of the problem is often underestimated. Further, the services the students receive are often inadequate. Many are discharged from rehabilitation programs prematurely—if they receive services at all. Left with minimal support, the students and their families turn to the schools for answers and assistance. Because funds to pay for outside services are limited, yet recovery can go on for years, the school system plays a crucial role in the rehabilitation process. Unless health care reform takes a dramatic, and unexpected, turn, schools will continue to be the largest service provider for children with traumatic brain injuries.

Obviously, schools cannot be expected to provide all the services these students need. They can, however, be expected to assist the students and their families in obtaining resources. To do this, educators must work in conjunction with other agencies and community programs. Thoughtful, timely planning will also help to prevent service gas and ensure continuity in programming.

The chapters in this book identify important aspects of this collaboration. Farmer, Clippard, Luehr-Wiemann, Wright, and Owings's chapter is written from the perspective of hospital-based professionals, and chapter 11 by Clark describes transition concerns from an educational viewpoint. These chpters demonstrate the need to integrate acute and rehabilitation hospital care and school services. The authors of each chapter place a similar emphasis on having a solid foundation of knowledge about the typical consequences of brain injury, as well as on individualized assessment of child and family needs. Having such common goals across hospital and school settings can only improve the potential for a positive child outcome following TBI.

Because of the increasing scope of treatments, rehabilitation, and various services for the survivor of TBI, this book comprises a broad spectrum of topics. We refer the reader back to the original series and the compilation of articles in the edited text by Bigler (1990). The basic issues of TBI will not be fully reiterated in this book, and the editor recommends that the readers review the previous published works as a supplement to it.

Chapter 2, by Bigler, will provide an update on brain imaging in TBI. A considerable improvement in imaging capabilities has led to a much more refined understanding of the role of trauma in altering brain structure and the relationship of altered brain structure to behavior. As mentioned, the chapters by Farmer et al. and by Clark address new developments aimed at improving hospital- and community-based treatment services for individuals with TBI and their transition to school. Rehabilitation specialists have focused on refining their ability to identify and treat impairments resulting from brain injury. Increasing knowledge about the natural course of recovery from TBI has made it possible to anticipate barriers to recovery and provide early intervention to prevent unnecessary disability. The trend is toward using a multidisciplinary-team approach that includes the patient and the family in decision making about treatment goals.

2. Brain Imaging and Behavioral Outcome in Traumatic Brain Injury

ERIN D. BIGLER

In 1987 a special series on traumatic brain injury (TBI) was initiated by the *Journal of Learning Disabilities,* followed by the publication of the textbook titled *Traumatic Brain Injury: Mechanisms of Damage, Assessment, Intervention, and Outcome (*Bigler, 1990). At that point in time, magnetic resonance imaging had just been clinically released (circa 1985), some detailed histopathological (microscopic analysis of damaged cells) studies recently had been published, and the first large-scale multicenter traumatic brain injury (TBI) research protocols were under way (see Levin, Grafman, & Eisenberg, 1987; Levin, Gary, & Eisenberg, 1990). However, since that time, an absolute explosion of basic and clinical neuroscience research on the neuropathology of TBI has occurred. The task of this review is to update the reader on these topical areas. The basic issues of TBI previously reviewed (see Bigler, 1987, 1990, 1994a, 1994b) will not be reiterated. Accordingly, the present review will assume that the reader is familiar with this previous work or can refer to it for background.

CELLULAR-LEVEL PATHOLOGY IN TBI

Figure 2.1 displays a standard schematic of a neuron with the major divisions labeled, along with a view of the brain depicting the three major anatomic

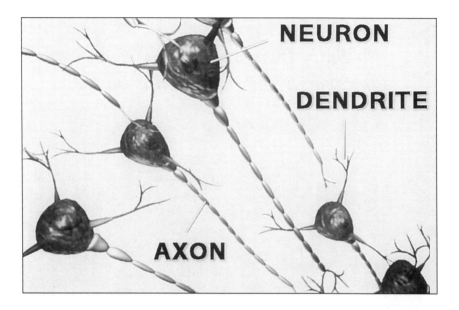

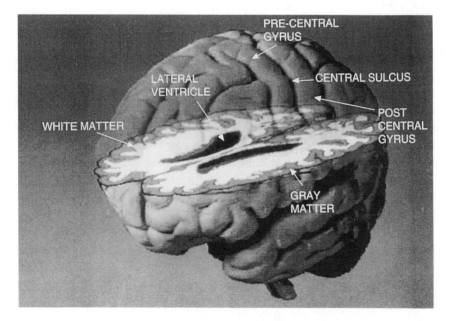

Figure 2.1. **(A)** Neuron schematic. This illustration depicts a schematic outline of several neurons. The irregular shape of the axon is due to the myelin coating. The myelin coating is what gives the appearance of white matter and thereby, white matter represents pathways of interconnections between neurons. This illustration is greatly oversimplified, as each cell has thousands of dendritic branches and numerous terminal branches as well as collateral branches at the terminus of the axon. **(B)** Brain schematic showing the relationship between white and gray matter and the lateral ventricles.

divisions—gray matter (where neuron cell bodies reside); white matter (axon element of the neuron coated with a fatty sheath called myelin, which gives "white" appearance to white matter); and spaces, or cavities, filled with cerebrospinal fluid (CSF, the water-like fluid that surrounds the outer surface of the brain and that is contained in the inner cavities, the ventricles, of the brain).

Past research on TBI has focused on shear/strain effects at the level of the axon and the axon's response to tensile effect (see Bigler, 1987, 1990; Salazar, 1992). These concepts are rather straightforward. Any structure can withstand only so much tensile strength when stretched lengthwise. Because of the deformation characteristics that may occur during trauma, there may be tissue compression and stretching that exceeds the boundaries of normal tissue extension capabilities, particularly along the axon. This in turn leads to a tear or rupture of the axon. Once damaged, the axon may retract and degenerate back to the cell body, which may also lead to cell death. This is referred to as *retrograde* degeneration of the axon. At the point distal (meaning away from the cell body) to the tear or rupture from the cell body, the axon fiber will degenerate. This degeneration is called *anterograde,* meaning forward of, in front of, or downstream from the actual lesion site. If there is sufficient anterograde degeneration, the postsynaptic neuron next in line may be deactivated, or what is referred to as "deafferented." This may lead to metabolic change in the cell, and, in some cases, to cell death. At the time of publication of the 1987 JLD TBI series, the shear/strain factors in injury were thought to be most responsible for diffuse axonal injury (DAI). However, as will be discussed later in this chapter, a variety of other factors may contribute significantly to DAI as well.

As a consequence of rotational effects, a twisting force may be exerted at the level of the axon. This twisting action can literally tear the axon, resulting in the same degenerative effects described above. This shearing action also may result in hemorrhagic lesions (bleeding) involving the rupture of capillaries in the brain. The shearing effect may be greatest at the boundaries between white and gray matter and most frequently occurs in the frontal and temporal lobe regions of the brain (Kurth, Bigler, & Blatter, 1994). Thus, on magnetic resonance (MR) scanning, the residual effects of shearing are often seen at gray matter/white matter junctions. This is depicted in Figure 2.2.

Until recently, these predominantly white matter shear/strain effects were the focus of research. However, more current research has begun to examine cellular metabolic factors, the role of excitatory neurotransmitters that may actually damage the cell or render it metabolically dysfunctional, and electron-microscope–identified changes in cellular microstructure (Landis, 1994; Povlishock, 1992; see Figures 2.3 and 2.4). Also, mechanical deformation of the cell as a consequence of trauma may set into motion a variety of physiological and structural deficits. These factors will be discussed next.

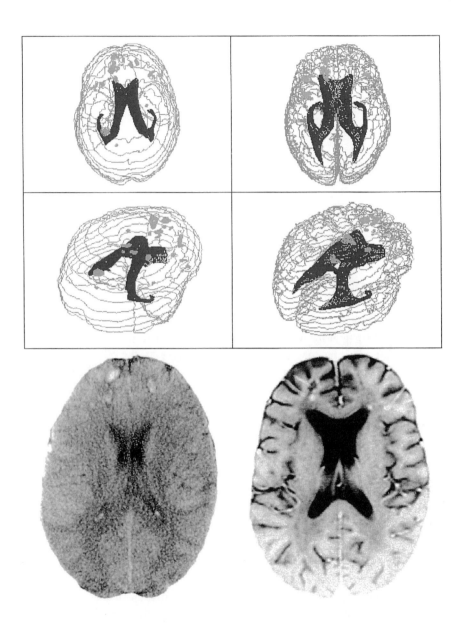

Figure 2.2.   (left column) At the bottom is a day-of-injury (DOI) CT scan, with 3-D representations above (middle—left posterior oblique; top—dorsal view). Note the location of acute petechial hemorrhagic lesions often at the juncture of gray matter/white matter boundary. Compare to Figure 2.1B and it is apparent that many of the hemorrhages are right at the border between white and gray matter. **(right column)** Follow-up MRI scan depicting the location of chronic lesions corresponding to acute injury and, again, at the gray matter/white matter juncture. Also, note the ventricular expansion. (See Bigler, 1992, for details on the 3-D imaging technique.)

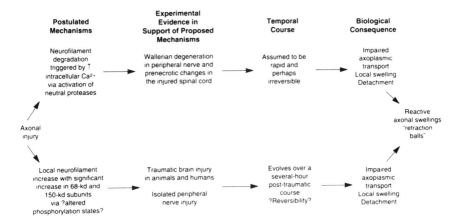

| Postulated Mechanisms | Experimental Evidence in Support of Proposed Mechanisms | Temporal Course | Biological Consequence |

Figure 2.3. Some contemporary thoughts on the pathobiology of various forms of axonal injury. **Upper panel:** the more traditional belief that virtually all axonal injury is triggered by an increase in extracellular calcium with an activation of neutral proteases that result in neurofilament degradation. Included are examples of conditions in which the calcium-mediated damage has been demonstrated, together with their reported temporal course and ultimate consequence. **Lower panel:** Premise regarding the pathobiology of traumatically induced axonal injury is detailed. In contrast to the concept of neurofilament degradation, Povlishock's (1992) studies suggest an increase in several neurofilament subunits, particularly the 68-kd subunit, a specialized unit of the axon involved in axoplasmic transport. In addition, Povlishock's (1993) more recent studies in which this neurofilamentous change has been demonstrated, together with their temporal course and their ultimate biological consequence, further support this hypothesis. (*Note.* Figures 2.3. and 2.4 from "Pathobiology of traumatically induced axonal injury in animals and man" by J. T. Povlishock, 1992, *Annals of Emergency Medicine, 22,* pp. 982, 984. Copyright © 1992 by Mosby-Year Book, Inc. Reproduced with permission.)

A variety of animal models have been developed to study the pathophysiology of TBI (see reviews by Adams, Doyle, Ford, Graham, & McLellan, 1989; Hayes & Ellison, 1989; Povlishock, 1992, 1993; Steward, 1989). However, the early models utilized a method wherein direct brain impact occurred, which is not the case in most traumatic human brain injuries. In 1987, Dixon, Lyeth, and Povlishock developed a "fluid percussion model," wherein a saline solution focused by a canula (a small tube) and released under pressure produces a much more reproducible injury that approximates what occurs with the typical high-velocity–impact head injury (seen, e.g., in motor vehicle or auto/pedestrian accidents). Once such an injury is induced, typically in a rodent or feline model, then the effects of that injury can be studied over time in terms of anatomic and physiological changes.

For example, Schmidt and Grady (1993) demonstrated a breakdown of the blood–brain barrier (BBB)—a physiological (chemical) "barrier" in the central nervous system that protects the brain from invasion of foreign substances (Neuwelt, 1989a, 1989b) at several common sites, regardless of the

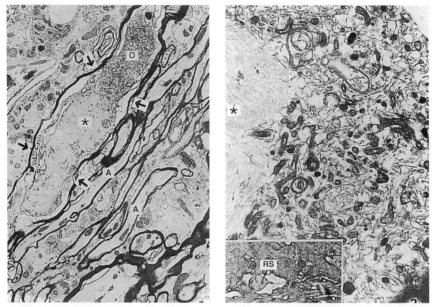

Figure 2.4. **(left)** An electron micrograph several hours after injury showing the onset of reactive axonal change. Within the axon, an accumulation of organelles (o) surrounds a neurofilamentous mass (*). Note that the entire reactive axonal segment is compressed by an intact myelin sheath (arrows). Also note that despite these dramatic intra-axonal reactive axonal change, numerous axons (A) coursing the field show no evidence of change. Original magnification x 6,000. **(right)** Electron micrograph of fully developed reactive axonal swelling 24 hours after injury. Inset: A light micrograph of a thick plastic section reveals a fully developed reactive swelling (RS). When this reactive swelling is visualized at the electron-microscopic level, it is easily seen that it is composed of a neurofilamentous core (*) encompassed by a sea of organelles delivered by continued anterograde transport. Original magnification: Inset x 500; electron micrograph, x 22,000.

point of impact. In Schmidt and Grady's study, the cortex (outer surface of the brain that houses cell bodies) immediately adjacent to the point of impact demonstrated BBB breakdown, along with the hippocampus and several other subcortical structures (dorsal thalamus, septal area, pontine tegmentum, periaqueductal gray, substantia nigra, and a narrow rim adjacent to ventricular and cisternal spaces). Published at the same time was a separate study by Hicks, Smith, Lowenstein, Saint Marie, and McIntosh (1993) that also demonstrated the selective vulnerability of the hippocampus to trauma, again implicating a breakdown of the BBB as a major contributing factor. This breakdown in the BBB may lead to neurotoxic and/or excitotoxic damaging effects at the level of the hippocampus.

Of particular importance with the Schmidt and Grady (1993) and Hicks et al. (1993) research is that the hippocampal formation, the most critical limbic system structure for memory function, appeared to be the most sensitive to damage, regardless of the point of impact or severity of injury. Povlishock (1992) demonstrated conspicuous axonal injury in the parahippocampal gyrus region in addition to traditional areas of white-matter axonal injury (corpus callosum, dorsal lateral quadrant of the brain stem, and subcortical white matter) in a postmortem human study. These findings are most intriguing because one of the most common symptoms exhibited by patients who experience TBI is a disturbance in memory function. Because, as indicated above, the hippocampus is one of the key limbic structures involved in memory function, it may be that its selective vulnerability is the primary factor in the prominence of this symptom. Clinically, on MR imaging the hippocampal formation often will be smaller in size (Bigler, Blatter, et al., in press; Bigler, Johnson, et al., in press; see Figure 2.5).

Other physiological factors may provide a basis for hippocampal involvement as well. Katayama et al. (1990) demonstrated that with the fluid percussion model of brain injury, an excessive release of potassium (an ion critical for neural transmission and typically residing as part of the intracellular fluid) and glutamate (an excitatory neurotransmitter) occurs throughout the brain. Additionally, the disruption of any ions (K+, Na+, Cl-) critical to neurological function will also be disruptive to cellular activity. Excessive release of excitatory neurotransmitters may lead to a condition called *excitotoxicity* (prolonged over-excitation impairs metabolical cell function), which in turn may lead to cell death or disruption of normal function (Salazar, 1992). Additionally, there are a variety of local immune responses that may alter neuronal integrity (Povlishock, 1992).

Returning to the Schmidt and Grady (1993) study, there is another intriguing element to their findings: Several of the other structures that were commonly affected by concussion were what are referred to as *central midline structures*—pontine tegmentum, periaqueductal gray, substantia nigra, and thalamus. These structures are critical for certain neuroregulatory functions and likewise play a key role in the sleep–wakefulness–arousal cycle. Another common sequela of head injury is some disruption of attention and concentration (Bigler, 1990). It may be that damage/dysfunction at this level has something to do with the consistent clinical expression of these symptoms.

Research recently has demonstrated an additional mechanism of cellular damage: cell deformation. Murphy and Horrocks (1993) demonstrated that mechanical deformation, such as in trauma, may produce membrane perturbations that are irreversible. Such damage can render the cell dysfunctional but not necessarily dead. Altered membrane integrity may influence neural transmission; slowed or altered neural transmission may significantly disrupt normal neurologic function.

Another area of research has focused on axon cytoskeletal and microtubule structure, or its internal architecture (P. S. Fishman & Mattu, 1993;

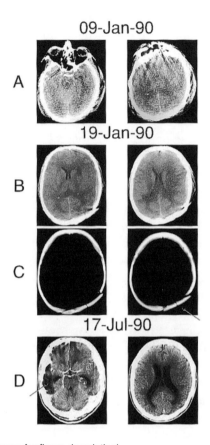

09-Jan-90

A

19-Jan-90

B

C

17-Jul-90

D

Figure 2.5. (see next page for figure description)

Povlishock, 1993). Brain trauma may disrupt microtubule structure and other aspects of cytoskeletal status, particularly at the level of the axon, and some of this may be related to tensile strength and shear/strain aspects of the injury, as previously discussed. Regardless of the etiologic factors, the disruption of the microtubule structure of an axon, though perhaps not resulting in cell death, can still render the axon dysfunctional or nonfunctional. Cytoskeletal failure leads to impairment of axoplasmic transport, which in turn results in axonal swelling and ultimate disconnection; disconnection from the dendritic field of the postsynaptic cell alters functioning in that target cell. In fact, Povlishock's (1992, 1993) research suggests that these cytoskeletal changes are the factors most responsible for the pathogenesis of DAI. Lastly, there is a growing body of research demonstrating that damage to glial tissue (which plays supportive and regulatory roles in maintaining the

Normal

Patient

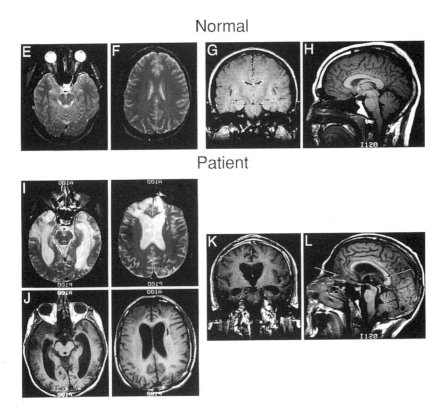

Figure 2.5. Typical neuroimaging sequence in TBI. **(A)** Day-of-injury CT scan depicting a swollen brain in that the ventricular system and cisternal spaces are ill-defined. The CT scan levels that follow below are matched to be somewhat the same. **(B)** CT scan 10 days postinjury depicting better definition of the ventricular system, a sign of decreasing cerebral edema. Note that the ventricular system remains shifted to the left, an indication of greater edema in the right hemisphere. **(C)** CT scan with bone window depicting area of skull fracture (arrow). This was an industrial accident wherein the patient fell approximately 30 feet, striking the back of his head, resulting in a skull fracture. It should be noted in the CT and MR (see I, J, & L) studies that follow, that areas of greatest damage were in the anterior frontal and temporal regions (see text for explanation). **(D)** CT studies 7 months postinjury depicting left temporal lobe encephalomalacia (arrow), scattered bifrontal encephalomalacia (areas of darkness and uneven intensity), and ventricular dilation. Note the prominence of the temporal horns (white arrowhead is pointing to the right hippocampus temporal horn region). **(I–L)** MRI studies 1 year postinjury compared to noninjured control in the same patient. **(I and J)** Note the extensive bilateral frontal-temporal lobe wasting and ventricular expansion when compared to the noninjured brain above. I and J are at identical levels but differ in the "weighting" of the MR image. I is a "T-2" weighted MR scan, whereas J is based on a "T-1" weighting. Both are in the horizontal (or axial—top down) plane. **(K)** Coronal section through the temporal horns of the lateral ventricle. Note the dilation and shrinkage of the hippocampal formation (arrow) when compared to a similarly matched normal comparison in G. **(L)** Sagittal view depicting corpus callosum atrophy (arrow) with a tear in the posterior aspect of the corpus callosum, along with inferior-frontal encephalomalacia (arrow) and generalized atrophy as depicted by the enlargement of cortical sulci and size of the ventricular system (compared to normal scans above).

composition of extracellular fluids), in addition to the axon damage, may contribute to the pathophysiology of TBI (Landis, 1994). Povlishock's (1992, 1993) research also demonstrates, as would be expected, that under normal circumstances, the degree of DAI is related to the severity of injury. In the human postmortem brain, he has demonstrated that the distribution of damaged axons per x 100 microscopic field was approximately 15 with high-speed motor vehicle accidents. In contrast, patients who succumb following a fall had only 5 per x 100 microscopic fields. However, in this important study there was one exception—an elderly gentleman who had a history of alcohol abuse had > 100 x 100 fields. This suggests that, given certain vulnerable factors (alcohol abuse, aging), there may be a predisposition to greater axonal injury with TBI.

As previously discussed (see Bigler, 1990), there are a number of secondary brain-injury effects related to edema (swelling), brain or meningeal hemorrhages, infection following penetrating injury, the presence of hemorrhages or hematomas, and respiratory complications (hypoxic or anoxic brain injury) because of brainstem or systemic injury. All of these factors appear to be additive to the basic mechanisms of damage as described previously.

In summary, there are several primary mechanisms of cellular injury that either singularly or in combination result in damage to the brain following trauma. As current research has demonstrated, the picture at the microstructural level is much more complicated, intricate, and interwoven than just simple shear/strain injury. Often, the secondary-injury effects (edema, hypoxia, etc.) are then superimposed on the primary injury to compound the damaging effects (see Bigler, 1990).

ADVANCES IN BRAIN IMAGING OF CEREBRAL TRAUMA

The basic clinical findings on computerized tomography (CT) and magnetic resonance imaging have been discussed in detail in previous publications (see Figure 2.5 and Bigler, 1987, 1989, 1990). Since the release of those publications, there has been a shift in focus to quantifying pathological changes via neuroimaging techniques and presenting the data three-dimensionally (3-D; Bigler, 1994a, 1994b; Bigler, Kurth, Blatter, & Abildskov, 1992, 1993).

In the past decade, numerous important advances in computer-assisted methods of analyzing brain imaging data have been made. Examples illustrating several of these advances are presented in Figures 2.6 and 2.7. Based on these methods, a variety of quantitative determinations can be made. These methods are the basis for many of the illustrations that follow.

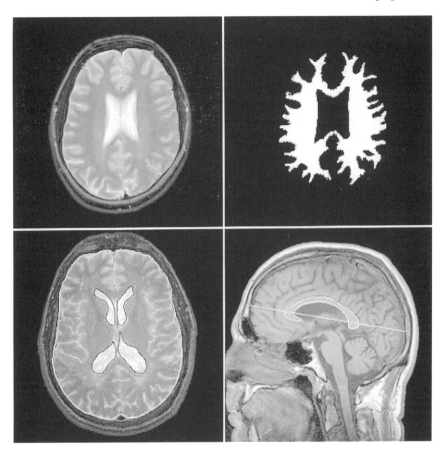

Figure 2.6. Various methods using the threshold technique for image analysis. In the **upper left,** a T-2 weighted image is presented, untouched. A threshold technique **(upper right)** is utilized to separate gray matter and CSF from white matter. Using this threshold principle, the surface area white matter or the ventricular space at this slice level can be calculated and graphically presented. In the **bottom left** figure, outer rim outline of cortical surface area (traced in white) and ventricle outline (traced in black). **(lower right)** Mid-sagittal view depicting a linear (white line) anterior-to-posterior measurement, typically used for head size correction, and a surface area tracing of the corpus callosum (outlined with white line).

Ventricular System Morphometrics

The ventricular system comprises an internal cavitation of the brain embryologically derived from the neural tube (R. A. Fishman, 1992). Figure 2.8 provides several views of the ventricular system in 3-D perspective based on MR imaging taken from a nondisabled individual. In the normal noninjured brain, the ventricles are typically symmetric and, in relationship to the brain, constitute about 1.5% of its total size. However, when the brain is injured, one of the

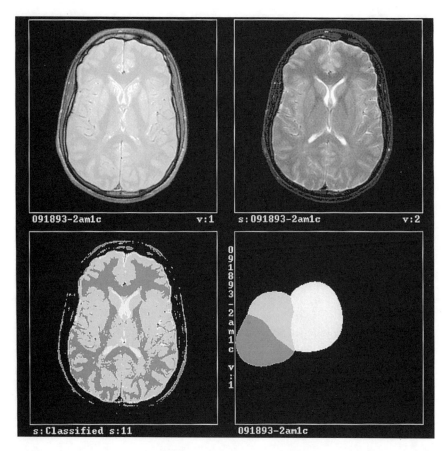

Figure 2.7. Multispectral segmentation of MR images **(upper left)** intermediate and **(upper right)** T-2 weighted spin-echo images at the level of the body of the lateral ventricles. **(lower right)** Plot of two-dimensional feature space where each pixel is plotted with the signal intensity on the T-2 weighted image as the x-axis and the signal intensity on the intermediate weighted image as the y-axis. The location and feature space on the pixels obtained in the user-identified region are shown in their respective shades of gray. **(lower left)** Via application of the segmentation to the entire brain at each registered level, whole brain white matter, gray matter, and CSF values can be obtained. This segmentation was produced using the ANALYZE™ program, which is a registered product of Biomedical Imaging Resources, Mayo Foundation/Clinic (200 First St. SW, Rochester, MN 55905) and is used with their permission.

ventricles increases in size, largely related to the degree of brain tissue atrophy (Bowen et al., in press). There are several reasons for this, as will be explained. The ventricle is filled with cerebrospinal fluid, a watery substance that bathes the internal and outer surface regions of the brain. The continuous production of CSF results in physical support or buoyancy of the brain, but also produces an outward pressure gradient (normally kept in check by the brain tissue and skull).

The outward pressure gradient produces an automatic expansion of the ventricular space as brain tissue wastes away following a serious traumatic brain injury where there is cellular death.

With respect to identifying the pathological changes of cerebral injury, in imaging the ventricular system, the first role—physical support—becomes the most obvious. Because CSF is produced at a constant rate and produces a constant outward pressure, if brain substance degenerates, the ventricles expand. This is demonstrated in Figure 2.9, which compares a preinjury MR scan with one following injury. This was a most fortuitous clinical case in that the individual had an MR brain scan performed prior to a severe traumatic brain injury. (She was having symptoms of dizziness but no abnormalities of the scan were detected.) As can be seen postinjury, there are distinct enlargements throughout the ventricular system in this patient. This ventricular enlargement (hydrocephalus *ex vacuo*) is in response to the loss of brain tissue (referred to as *parenchyma*). Because CSF is under pressure, with parenchymal volume loss there is an outward expansion of the ventricular system to fill this void. Accordingly, ventricular expansion, when not a result of obstructive hydrocephalus or a pathologic overproduction of CSF, is a sign of cerebral tissue loss.

The time frame of degenerative change varies according to individual patient characteristics, severity of injury, and course of treatment (e.g., neurosurgical intervention, treatment for cerebral edema, steroids, etc.), but is usually complete by 3 months postinjury (Bigler et al., 1992). In another clinical case wherein an MR scan was obtained prior to injury, we were able to demonstrate that ventricular changes were about 75% to 90% complete (depending on the target structure measured) by 6 weeks postinjury. This is depicted in Figure 2.10.

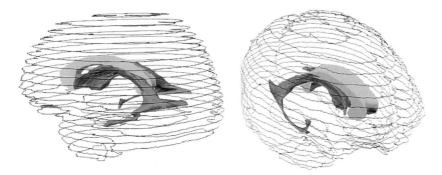

Figure 2.8.   3-D representation of corpus callosum (light gray) to ventricle (dark gray) using MR-based 3-D imaging. **(left)** Lateral view. **(right)** Right superior frontal oblique. Note the intimate anatomic interface between the corpus callosum and ventricular system, in particular the anterior horn (computer graphic work done by Tracy Abildskov).

Pre   Post

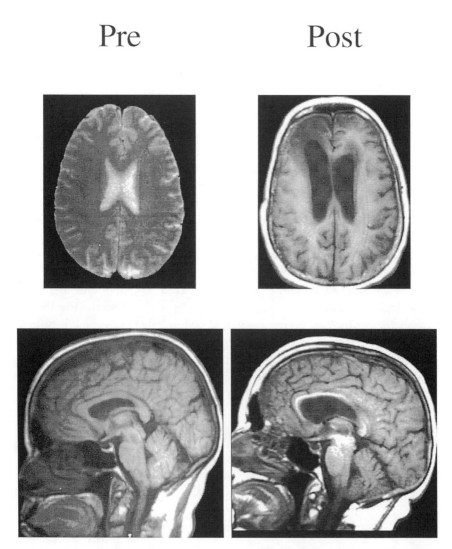

Figure 2.9. **(left)** MR imaging obtained 1 year previous to severe head injury. **(right)** Postinjury anatomic changes several months postinjury. Note the ventricular expansion, wasting of the frontal regions, particularly on the right, and corpus callosum atrophy (based in part on Gale et al., 1994).

Another way to make a ventricular comparison is to utilize the day-of-injury (DOI) scan as an estimate of preinjury brain morphology (see Bigler et al., 1992, 1993; Bigler et al., 1994). In the very acute stages of brain injury, there may be edema, hemorrhages, and formations of hematomas (blood clots). However, these acute effects often take several hours to reach their fullest expression. As most individuals with TBI receive an immediate

CT scan upon hospital admission, the earliest scan (or a scan within a few days of injury), although showing acute pathology, still retains the major ventricular configuration and CSF volume of the brain prior to injury (see Figure 2.5; Bigler et al., 1992; Bigler et al., 1994). Subsequent to the injury, as the brain degenerates over the next several weeks, the ventricular system expands and brain volume recedes. Additionally, this type of study has indicated that the ventricular changes are most likely related to white matter degeneration associated with trauma (Anderson & Bigler, 1994).

This 3-D imaging method of examining the DOI scan with the follow-up MR provides a means of identifying the presence and location of white matter shearing lesions and parenchymal hemorrhages (see Figure 2.11). The case depicted in Figure 2.11 clearly presents the excellent method of lesion identification and comparison over time made possible by this technology. This illus-

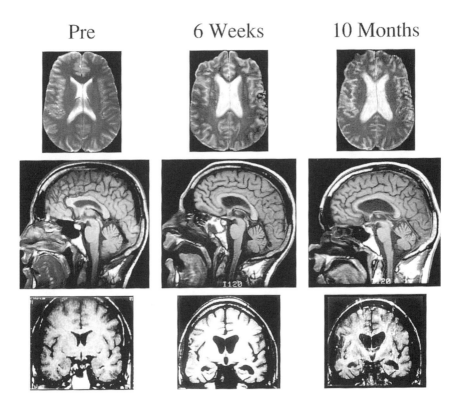

| Pre | 6 Weeks | 10 Months |

Figure 2.10.   MR imaging obtained prior to injury (pre) and then subsequent to injury (6 weeks, and 10 months). Note the considerable expansion of the ventricular system and corpus callosum atrophy. The coronal sections **(bottom)** demonstrate marked ventricular expansion, particularly in the temporal horn region, which is an indirect sign of hippocampal atrophy.

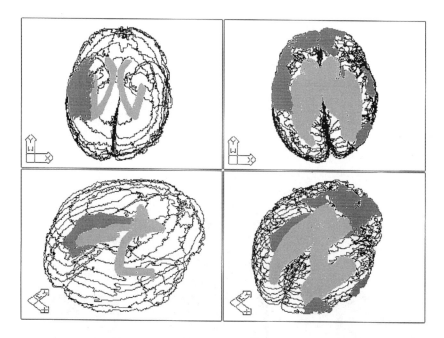

Figure 2.11.   3-D image reconstruction showing DOI on the **left** and follow-up MR on the **right.** The ventricular system is depicted in light gray and areas of cortical encephalomalacia in dark gray. These studies are based on the same patient and images as presented in Figure 2.5. Note the marked expansion of the ventricular system.

tration also demonstrates the greater likelihood of frontal and temporal locus of lesions (Kurth et al., 1994). This observation also relates to the greater likelihood that neurobehavioral deficits will be mediated by pathology within fronto-temporal systems. Often, the greatest degree of ventricular dilation relates to the areas of greater pathology. Because of the frontotemporal locus of pathology, the frontal and temporal horns often exhibit a disproportionate dilation in relation to other aspects of the ventricular system (see Figures 2.2, 2.11, and 2.12).

Normative Database and Morphometric
Analysis of MR Imaging

The key to psychometric principles in behavioral assessment relates to comparison of a given patient with a normative sample. This psychometric principle now has been applied to the normative data that can be obtained from MR imaging. Accordingly, with the data set presented in Figure 2.13,

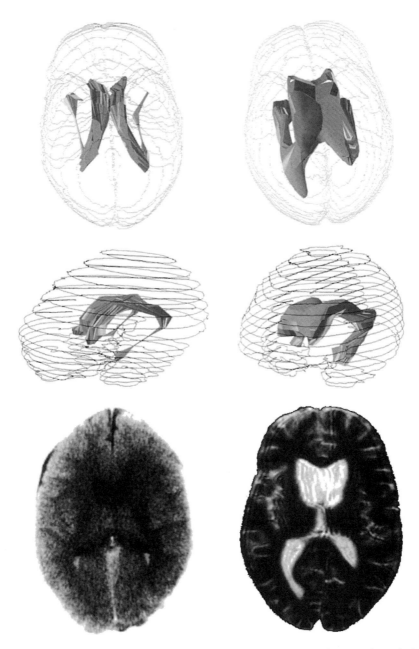

Figure 2.12. 3-D image reconstruction depicting the "classic" frontal-temporal ventricular enlargement typically seen in TBI. DOI is on the **left,** with the 1-year follow-up on the **right.** Note the disproportionate size of the anterior horn of the lateral ventricle in the follow-up MR scan. Such enlargement is an indication of tissue degeneration in the frontal regions of the brain (see Anderson & Bigler, 1994).

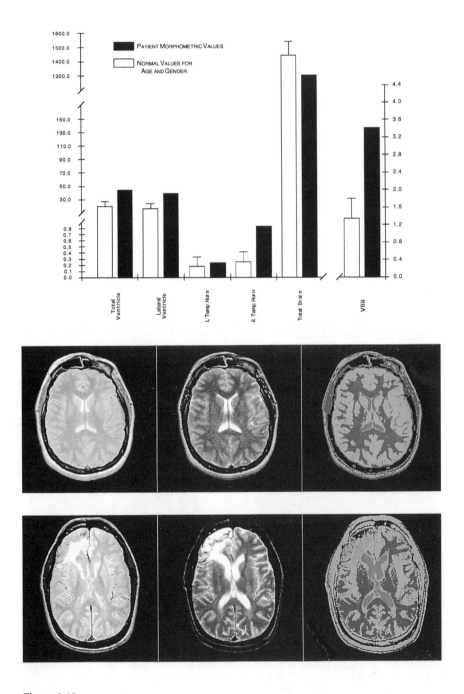

Figure 2.13

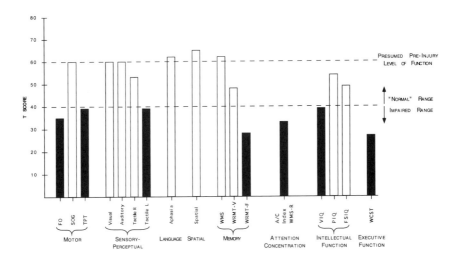

Figure 2.13. **(A)** Bar graph at top left depicts aspects of the patient's quantitative neuroimaging findings of the ventricular system based on volumetric estimates from segmented images. The top row of MR images depicts a medical control subject with proton density weighted MR scan on the left, T-2 weighted scan in the middle, and the "segmented" image differentiating white, gray, and CSF space. The bottom row of images is from the TBI patient with similar-level MR images and a large right frontal lesion (left is on the reader's right). **(B)** Presentation of the patient's neuropsychological data. Neuropsychological performance of the patient depicted in Figure 2.1. The x-axis lists various neuropsychological test findings, with the scores being converted into a *T* score for direct comparison (*M* = 50, *SD* = 10) along the y-axis. Abbreviations: FO = finger oscillation; SOG = strength of grip; TPT = Tactual Performance Test; Aphasia = Aphasia Screening Test; WMS-R = Wechsler Memory Scale–Revised; WRMT-V = Warrington Recognition Memory Test–Verbal; WRMT-F = Warrington Recognition Memory Test–Faces; A/C Index = Attention/Concentration Index; VIQ = Verbal Intellectual Quotient; PIQ = Performance Intellectual Quotient; FSIQ = Full Scale Intellectual Quotient based on the results of the Wechsler Adult Intelligence Scale–Revised; WCST = Wisconsin Card Sorting Test. This neuropsychological profile indicates that the patient has no deficit in basic motor strength as reflected by the intact SOG scores. However, fine motor movement (FO) as well as integrative motor control (TPT) is below what would be expected to be normal. Sensory-perceptual examination reveals intact visual and auditory processing, bilaterally, but the patient has diminished tactile perceptual processing on the left in comparison with the right. No deficits are noted in language, spatial, or General Memory Index score on the WMS-R. However, he clearly has a deficit in facial recognition memory on the Warrington Recognition Memory Test in comparison to a normal WMS-R General Memory Index and a normal performance on the Warrington Recognition Memory Test for Words (Verbal). The patient's Attention/Concentration Index was distinctly impaired on the WMS-R. His intellectual functioning is probably below what would be predicted given his premorbid ability level. He has a distinct deficit in the ability to perform the Wisconsin Card Sorting Test—a task that places demands on flexible thinking and cognitive shifting, typically deficit areas for patients with significant frontal lobe damage. This patient was a very successful contractor and builder who sustained a serious traumatic brain injury in a 70-foot fall while rock climbing. He had graduated from high school and had completed 4 years of college but had not graduated. Both parents were college-educated and his father was a university professor. Accordingly, this patient's preinjury intellectual/cognitive status was felt to be in the above-average range.

a quantitative comparison can be achieved wherein a given patient's MR scan results can be compared with age- and gender-matched controls'. This permits a structure-by-structure comparison using statistical analyses to determine which structures or brain regions are most damaged. Further details of this type of comparison are presented in the figure caption for Figure 2.13. Table 2.1 provides a comparison between selected anatomic structures that have undergone the type of degenerative change that occurs in TBI, and those same structures in age-matched noninjured controls. Two groups were investigated: those whose scans were obtained within 90 days of injury, and those obtained after 90 days. Note the significant reduction in brain volume and the marked increase in ventricular volume, particularly in the group imaged more than 90 days postinjury.

Gale, Johnson, Bigler, and Blatter (1994, 1995b); Johnson, Bigler, Burr, and Blatter (1994); and Johnson, Farnworth, Pinkston, Bigler, and Blatter (1994) utilized this type of morphometric analysis to examine several brain regions in individuals with TBI compared to noninjured controls. Their findings, as does Table 2.1, clearly indicate that CNS trauma results in a variety of nonspecific changes. As presented in Table 2.1, most brain regions exhibit significant degenerative changes in response to injury, particularly with lower Glasgow Coma Scale (GCS) scores. Several of the structures or morphological measures in Table 2.1 that are most significantly associated with trauma also relate to other trauma variables (e.g., GCS, neuropsychological outcome, etc.). Reduction in corpus callosum size (a direct measure of white matter loss; see Figures 2.9 and 2.10) and expansion of the ventricular system (an indirect measure of white matter loss) both relate systematically to GCS as a measure of injury severity, and both correlate with GCS at approximately 0.5 (the GCS correlation positive, the VBR correlation negative; see Anderson & Bigler, 1994; Gale, Burr, Bigler, & Blatter, 1993; Gale et al., 1994). Likewise, morphologic changes in these structures relate to neuropsychological outcome. Because ventricular expansion is an indirect measure of brain mass, particularly white matter loss, it is natural to expect that ventricular measures in the chronic post-TBI state partially predict level of neuropsychological outcome and severity of the original injury. As a general rule, the larger the ventricular system, the greater the amount of tissue loss and the greater the neuropsychological impairment (Anderson & Bigler, 1994; Bigler et al., 1992, 1993; Bigler et al., 1994; Gale et al., 1993; Gale et al., 1994; Johnson et al., 1994).

The other anatomical marker of the severity of injury, from Table 2.1, is the size of the temporal horn. Because of the strategic location of the temporal lobe in the middle fossa, surrounded by bone on the lateral, anterior, and medial surface, the temporal lobe may be most vulnerable to the effects

Table 2.1

Some MRI-Based Anatomic Measures in TBI Patients Compared with Noninjured Controls

Measure	Control		TBI–Early		TBI–Late	
Brain	1343.7	(35.2)	1340.3	(39.3)	1298.22	(55.5)***
Total intracranial vol (C)	1463.1	(150.9)	1446.3	(172.9)	1444.26	(148.9)
Ventrical brain ratio (VBR)	1.3	(0.46)	1.7	(1.0)	2.73	(1.83)***
Total ventricle (C)	17.4	(5.9)	22.7	(13.7)	34.71	(21.6)***
Lateral ventricle (C)	14.6	(5.7)	19.0	(11.3)	29.8	(19.1)***
III ventricle	0.73	(0.26)	1.06	(0.61)	1.72	(0.9)***
IV ventricle	1.66	(0.53)	1.76	(0.79)	1.71	(0.8)
Left temporal horn	0.21	(0.16)	0.37	(0.50)	0.62	(0.9)***
Right temporal horn	0.23	(0.22)	0.44	(0.77)	0.83	(1.9)***
CSF (C)	103.3	(35.2)	106.6	(39.3)	148.7	(55.6)***
Subarachnoid CSF (C)	85.8	(33.2)	83.1	(33.4)	114.1	(41.8)***
Corpus callosum (surface area)	693.9	(91.1)	—	—	598.6	(117.4)
White matter (C)	651.1	(96.2)	648.5	(126.1)	642.1	(92.1)
Gray matter (C)	701.1	(117.1)	691.9	(125.3)	643.2	(66.3)*

Note. Control $n = 128$; TBI–Early $n = 78$; TBI–Late $n = 56$. TBI–Early = Imaging studies done within 90 days of injury; TBI–Late = Imaging studies done $\geq$ 90 days postinjury. C indicates corrected values for head size. Refer to Blatter et al. (1995) for details on head correction procedures.

*$p < .05$. **$p < .01$. ***$p < .001$.

of injury (see Bigler, 1990; Gale, Johnson, Bigler, & Blatter, 1995a). Temporal horn dilation is likely a reflection of nonspecific pathology of the temporal lobe, but it also may reflect degenerative changes of the amygdala-hippocampal-fornix formation because these structures are situated in the floor of the temporal horn (see Figure 2.5). Because the hippocampal structure is critical to memory function, the temporal lobe is critical for language, and both are essential for cognition and human mental function, it is evident

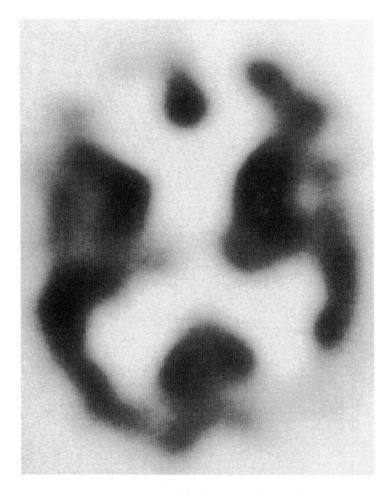

Figure 2.14. SPECT scan in patient discussed in Figures 2.5 and 2.11. The outer rim of the brain should display a rather uniform activation pattern (i.e., black on a gray scale continuum), which is clearly absent anteriorly and posteriorly. This suggests significant metabolic abnormalities that actually extend beyond the boundaries of strict anatomic abnormality, as depicted in Figure 2.5. This case demonstrates how greater clinical yield comes from combining abnormal anatomic findings with physiologic indicators (see Ichise et al., 1994).

that temporal horn dilation may be one of the markers of neurobehavioral and neuropsychological function. Along these lines, we have examined the role of temporal horn dilation and neuropsychological performance (Gale et al., 1993, 1994). The results indicate that, as a general rule, as temporal horn dilation increases, greater neuropsychological impairment results.

Anatomic mapping, as discussed above, is but one aspect of this picture of postinjury pathology. As discussed previously (see Bigler, 1987, 1990), various electrophysiological methods, especially computer-assisted quantitative electroencephalography techniques, provide physiological indices of brain pathology. Neuroimaging techniques based on regional cerebral blood flow or other metabolic measures are now being utilized to a greater degree in the evaluation of the patient with TBI. For example, Figure 2.14 presents the results of such imaging based on single photon emission computed tomography (SPECT) scanning. The importance of SPECT scanning is that it reveals pathologic areas of metabolic functioning or cerebral blood flow that typically extend beyond the actual anatomic boundaries (see Kosslyn et al., 1993). These points are more fully discussed in the caption for Figure 2.14.

SUMMARY

Recent advances at the level of histological and biochemical changes have improved our understanding of the microanatomical changes related to TBI. Coupled with these advancements are improvements in imaging of brain pathology in the TBI victim (see Bigler, 1992, 1994a, 1994b; Levin et al., 1994). Exquisite techniques are now available for imaging, quantification, and presentation of the functional significance of brain pathology in TBI.

PART II

Assessment and Outcome Issues

3. Assessing Children with Traumatic Brain Injury During Rehabilitation: Promoting School and Community Reentry

JANET E. FARMER, DANA S. CLIPPARD,
YVETTE LUEHR-WIEMANN, EDWARD WRIGHT, AND
STEPHANIE OWINGS

Children who sustain moderate to severe traumatic brain injuries (TBI) present unique challenges to rehabilitation and school professionals. Unlike adults with TBI, children are in the midst of rapid developmental changes in physical, cognitive, and behavioral functioning. Childhood brain injury disrupts these developmental processes and sets into action a parallel process—recovery from injury (Lehr, 1990). In the weeks and months that follow an injury, recovery and developmental processes become intertwined and unfold together, each with specific influences on the child.

One of the tasks facing rehabilitation specialists is to identify the initial impact of the injury on the child within the framework of normal developmental expectations. This information allows for appropriate therapeutic interventions during rehabilitation and also provides a baseline to track the course of recovery. A second task is to effectively communicate observations about the child to educators, family members, and others who will support the child's transition back into the home and school community.

The purpose of this chapter is to review a problem-solving, process-oriented approach to child assessment following TBI that can facilitate transition planning (Blosser & DePompei, 1994; Ylvisaker, Hartwick, Ross, & Nussbaum, 1994). This model of assessment is driven not by a specific testing protocol, but by important questions about the individual child's functioning and about available home and school supports. Although the focus of this review is on children with moderate to severe injuries who are treated in rehabilitation, educators may find similar evaluation strategies useful when determining the strengths and needs of other students with TBI who do not participate in rehabilitation. The interested reader is referred to Blosser and DePompei (1994) for an in-depth discussion of problem-solving approaches to assessment and treatment of children with TBI that are applicable in both hospital and community settings.

ASSESSMENT ISSUES DURING REHABILITATION

Traumatic brain injury occurs when an external force causes either transient or permanent impairment in the brain's ability to regulate physical, cognitive, emotional, or behavioral functioning (Savage & Wolcott, 1994). For each child, the actual nature of these changes depends in part on the mechanisms of injury, the specific brain sites affected, and the severity of the injury (see Bigler, chapter 2). In addition, the child's preinjury characteristics, such as age, developmental level, academic achievement, and behavioral adjustment, interact with the brain injury itself to determine the child's initial presentation and long-term outcome (Rivara et al., 1994).

Because the impact of TBI is unique for each child, there is no standard approach to rehabilitation assessment. However, useful guidelines do exist. For example, first, each child's assessment should be individualized and directed toward the goal of recovery from TBI. Individually tailored assessments are conducted for the following purposes:

1. To ensure continued medical stability and physical recovery following injury;
2. To determine the child's baseline pattern of cognitive and behavioral strengths and needs;
3. To document improvements in functioning;
4. To develop a specific plan for rehabilitation interventions;
5. To identify the types of intervention strategies that are most effective (e.g., direct retraining of impaired abilities vs. indirect methods of compensating for weaknesses);

6. To describe environmental, social, and motivational factors that influence performance;
7. To highlight which neurobehavioral changes are likely to have the greatest impact on everyday functioning;
8. To determine needed educational services after hospital discharge; and
9. To contribute to the development of the child's Individualized Education Program (IEP) at the time of discharge (Begali, 1992; Ylvisaker et al., 1990).

Second, because of the broad range and complexity of impairments that can result from TBI, a multidisciplinary team approach is needed. The specialists who assess and treat children in the rehabilitation hospital include physicians, nurses, physical and occupational therapists, psychologists, recreational therapists, and speech/language pathologists. Team communication about child functioning is a fundamental element of rehabilitation, because impairments assessed in one aspect of functioning can greatly influence assessment and treatment in other areas. For example, information that a child is showing language comprehension problems will influence how therapists assess self-care abilities. Furthermore, collaboration among team members allows for a more holistic view of the child across contexts.

Third, family members and educators should be considered integral members of the rehabilitation team and important contributors to the assessment process (Blosser & DePompei, 1994). Interviews with family members can provide rich information about the child's preinjury adjustment at home and school, personal likes and dislikes, and style of coping. These interviews also can inform the rehabilitation team about family factors that may influence the child's outcome, including family coping style; knowledge about brain injury; the presence of stressors such as financial strain or marital discord; social supports; and need for additional resources or assistance. Educators also must become involved early during rehabilitation and actively participate in planning for school reentry. School personnel can provide objective records of preinjury academic functioning, including grades, previous standardized testing, attendance history, and work samples. Teachers can contribute information about preinjury emotional and behavioral adjustment. Observations from family members and educators are valuable throughout rehabilitation as well. For example, they may identify a positive return of functioning during interactions with familiar persons that would otherwise be overlooked, or they may note difficulty with transfer of skills to novel situations outside of the hospital setting.

A final major issue concerning assessment in rehabilitation has to do with strategies for collecting information about cognitive and behavioral changes following TBI. A strong argument can be made for adopting a problem-solving approach to evaluating children following injury (Blosser & DePompei, 1994; Ylvisaker et al., 1994). In this approach, methods of evaluation are determined based on the examiner's knowledge about the common sequelae of TBI. By knowing the appropriate questions to ask at various stages during recovery, therapists can set up hypotheses about expected, age-appropriate behaviors and test each domain of functioning using a range of diagnostic measures. In addition, the team must answer important questions about contextual factors known to influence child outcomes following TBI (Blosser & DePompei, 1994).

Once the important questions are identified, rehabilitation specialists are faced with a decision familiar to educators working with children with special needs: whether to use formal, standardized measures of child functioning or informal, alternative measures (e.g., direct examination of student performance on significant tasks). In educational settings, standardized measures are often used to determine whether a student meets eligibility requirements for special education classification and services. The advantages of norm-referenced testing include the fact that the student is being compared with his or her peers, the uniformity of procedure, and, with careful test selection, the high degree of reliability and validity. The use of standardized instruments also facilitates communication among professionals from varying fields. The disadvantages include that (a) one is sampling isolated bits of student behavior, (b) the focus is on basic skills versus higher order problem solving and reasoning skills, and (c) treatment validity and intervention implications are lacking (Reschly, 1992; Worthen, 1993).

The use of standardized measures with children who have sustained a TBI offers unique considerations. Standardized tests can be used to establish a baseline measure of abilities following injury. A baseline permits documentation of recovery over time, even if the child is assessed by different persons in different settings. These age-normed results provide a frame of reference that can give the child, family, educators, and other team members insight into the extent of change relative to preinjury functioning. Some norm-referenced tests, described in more detail below, have been evaluated specifically for use with children following TBI and can be particularly helpful in documenting changes that might otherwise be missed.

However, great caution is required when considering assessment with standardized tests during rehabilitation (Begali, 1992; Ylvisaker et al., 1994). Children with severe injuries may have such marked cognitive or physical deficits that they are unable to participate adequately in any standardized assessment. The rapid changes experienced by a child during the acute recovery period may limit the usefulness of the results. Further, most standardized measures do not include students with TBI in the normative sample, which compromises validity. Test scores may overestimate classroom performance and create false optimism if there has been a good recovery of previously acquired skills, or if the student benefits from the high structure, short presentations, and one-to-one interactions typical of standardized tests. Finally, because TBI is now a designated special education category under the Individuals with Disabilities Education Act (IDEA; *Federal Register,* 1991), the need for standardized testing to determine eligibility is reduced for children with TBI, particularly those whose injuries require a period of rehabilitation. For these reasons, standardized tests should be used and interpreted judiciously during rehabilitation.

Alternative, informal assessment techniques are crucial for obtaining a full picture of a child's abilities following TBI. This approach requires careful hypothesis formulation about expected competencies at the child's developmental level, followed by the selection of diagnostic tasks to evaluate the child's ability to meet the expectations (Ylvisaker et al., 1990). Such alternative assessment enables clinicians to systematically examine children's cognitive processes (e.g., through learning logs, think-aloud strategies, self-assessment), as well as their product or performance. Using this approach, the examiner can also vary the context and learning environment to determine the impact on performance. Assessment can be continuous, allowing accurate monitoring of progress and response to intervention, which can then be used to make decisions about treatment effectiveness and/or the need for program changes. Informal assessment is particularly important because many of the functional deficits of children with TBI are not demonstrated on formal measures (Crowley & Miles, 1991).

Problems with alternative assessments exist as well. First, this approach to assessment is highly dependent on the therapist's experience and skill, including his or her knowledge of normal development (Ylvisaker et al., 1990). Second, a specialist's experience with the child, either pleasant or unpleasant, may unwittingly bias the results of this type of assessment, which by definition allows for more subjectivity. A multidisciplinary approach to assessment offsets some of these biases, as this practice draws on the strengths of a variety of professionals and minimizes the likelihood of error. Furthermore, videotaping alternative assessment activities provides an opportunity to code or quantify child behavior, track behavioral change, and document the child's progress for family members and educators.

Clearly, neither a single approach to assessment nor a single individual or discipline can address all the issues involved when a child prepares for and returns to school following a TBI. Ideally, the assessment process will involve a strong, collaborative team of family members and professionals who use the best aspects of both formal and informal assessments to achieve benefits for the child.

Tracking the Course of Recovery

In the following sections, the major areas of functioning important to school reentry following TBI—medical/health, intellectual/cognitive, speech/language, academic, sensorimotor, and behavioral domain—will be discussed. These domains parallel the areas that educators must assess prior to developing an IEP for children with special needs. Each section will describe common problems observed in the domain following brain injury, methods of assessment during rehabilitation, and questions to be answered prior to return to school.

Medical/Health Domain

The medical problems associated with traumatic brain injury are numerous. Immediately following brain injury, the unconscious child requires immediate, intensive medical care to prevent complications that can exacerbate the brain damage sustained at the moment of impact. Level of consciousness is typically assessed on admission to the emergency room using the Glasgow Coma Scale (GCS; Teasdale & Jennett, 1974), to determine whether coma is present (GCS = 3–8) or if consciousness is merely altered (GCS = 9–15). This scale measures level of coma by evaluating eye opening, best motor response, and best verbal response (or, in young children, vocalization; Reilly, Simpson, Sprod, & Thomas, 1988). The GCS is important to rehabilitation personnel because it is a useful measure of severity of injury and a predictor of neurobehavioral recovery.

Because most traumatic brain injuries result from motor vehicle accidents, falls, or pedestrian accidents, multiple other injuries must be assessed immediately. The first 48 to 72 hours following injury are most critical to survival following severe injuries. Children with moderate to severe injuries often do not recall this period of time.

After a child is medically stable, transfer to a rehabilitation center is considered if he or she has significant motor, sensory, or cognitive deficits. Recent research has shown that only 42% of children who experienced traumatic head injuries resulting in four or more impairments were discharged from acute medical treatment to rehabilitation (DiScala, Osberg, Gans, Chin, & Grant, 1991). The majority (47%) of the remaining children with similar problems were discharged to home, returning to school without benefit of a transitional period in rehabilitation and presumably placing a substantial strain on the child, educators, and family members.

For children who *are* transferred to a rehabilitation hospital, there is continued medical care and frequent physical, occupational, cognitive, speech, educational, and recreational therapy. Psychological support is provided to the patient and family, and education of peers about TBI is arranged when possible. Initial treatment goals are often determined by the patient's rating on the Rancho Los Amigos Levels of Cognitive Functioning Scale (Hagen, Malkmus, & Durham, 1981), which outlines eight stages of cognitive and behavioral recovery (see Table 3.1). This measure classifies patients based on their level of arousal and attention, responsiveness to stimuli, ability to learn and retain information, and goal-directedness of behaviors. Like adults, children typically follow a fairly predictable pattern of recovery, moving from coma to a period of agitation and disorientation, then to more pur-

Table 3.1
Summary of the Rancho Los Amigos Scale of Cognitive Functioning[a]

Level	Description
I	No response to pain, touch, or sight. Appears asleep.
II	Generalized response to external stimuli. Nonpurposeful inconsistent, and limited responses.
III	Localized response. Blinks to strong light, orients to sound, responds to physical discomfort. May respond inconsistently to simple response commands.
IV	Confused–Agitated. Alert, motorically active, inconsistent and nonpurposeful behaviors that can be aggressive or bizarre, extremely short attention span, and no short-term recall.
V	Confused–Nonagitated. General attention to environment, follows simple commands consistently, but requires frequent redirection due to high distractibility; new information is not retained. May engage in social conversation but with inappropriate verbalizations.
VI	Confused–Appropriate. Inconsistent orientation to time and place, new learning impaired, begins to recall remote memories, follows simple directions, goal-directed behavior with environmental supports and assistance.
VII	Automatic–Appropriate. Performs daily routine in familiar settings in a nonconfused but automatic, robot-like manner. Skills decrease in unfamiliar environment. Judgment impaired.
VIII	Purposeful–Appropriate. Responsive to the environment, but cognitive abilities (e.g., memory, reasoning) may be decreased relative to preinjury levels.

Note. From "Linguistic Competence and Levels of Cognitive Functioning in Adults with Traumatic Closed Head Injury" (p. 189) by E. H. Wiig, E. W. Alexander, and W. Secord in *Neuropsychological Studies of Nonfocal Brain Damage* by H. A. Whitaker (Ed.), 1988, New York: Springer-Verlag. Copyright © 1988 by Springer-Verlag. Adapted with permission.
[a]Hagen, Malkmus, and Durham (1981).

poseful and age-appropriate behaviors. The rate and extent of neurobehavioral recovery depends primarily on the location and severity of injury. Recovery is most rapid in the first 6 to 12 months after injury, though continued gradual improvements can be observed for several years (Fay et al., 1994; Klonoff, Clark, & Klonoff, 1993).

Upon discharge from rehabilitation, residual medical problems likely to be noted at school and to affect participation include seizures, irritability, fatigue, headaches, respiratory problems, hormonal changes, and bowel or bladder incontinence. Posttraumatic seizures occur in a small number of patients after the acute period. Seizures most often occur within the first 6 weeks but can occur in the first 2 years or even later. The seizure types seen include petit mal (staring spells which must be differentiated from inattention), partial–complex (repetitive movements or behaviors with impaired consciousness), and generalized tonic–clonic seizures. Some anticonvulsant medications have sedating side effects that affect attention and learning. Educators and family members must be informed of potential neurological changes and possible side effects of medication, so appropriate treatment can be sought if problems are observed.

Bowel and bladder incontinence occurs less frequently but is problematic socially. The type of abnormality seen is usually urgency incontinence, in which the child has limited warning of an impending bowel movement or bladder emptying. Acceptance and accommodations for this are usually the only necessary treatments. Dysphagia (swallowing abnormality) is common but is frequently resolved or appropriately treated by the time a child reaches school. Frequent wet coughing, gagging, or bouts of asthma/bronchitis/pneumonia should alert the educator to a possible swallowing dysfunction that requires monitoring for safety and referral for medical evaluation. Headaches of many types (migraines, musculoskeletal, visual, or vestibular in origin) can occur. Specific treatment depends upon the headache type, but, in general, rest improves symptoms. Hormonal changes that occur after traumatic brain injury should be considered when there is frequent or infrequent drinking and voiding, poor growth, precocious or delayed puberty, or extreme weight gain. Treatment for these problems is readily available once diagnosed.

Prior to discharge from the hospital, the following medical questions should be answered:

How severe was the injury? What is the prognosis for continued recovery?

What are the major health-related needs of the child? Is an Individual Health Plan needed to establish a protocol for treatment at school?

Are seizures or other neurological problems likely? What changes in behavior would indicate that a physician should be contacted?

Are activity restrictions needed to ensure safety and well-being?

What medications are prescribed? Do they have side effects? Do they need to be administered in the school setting?

Intellectual/Cognitive Domain

Traumatic brain injury places the child at risk for persistent impairments in cognition, which is broadly defined as all mental processes and systems involved in acquiring and using knowledge (Ylvisaker et al., 1990). Under this definition, cognition comprises three areas: (a) basic psychological processes (i.e., orientation, attention, perception, language, memory, and abstract reasoning); (b) component systems (i.e., working memory, long-term memory or knowledge base, response modalities, and executive functions for initiating, planning, and organizing); and (c) integration of these abilities to produce a functional performance (age-appropriate, efficient, and maintained in a variety of settings).

Deficits in each of these areas of cognition are likely to accompany moderate or severe TBI in children (Jaffe et al., 1992, 1993; Klonoff et al., 1993; Levin et al., 1993). Problems are reported most frequently in attention; memory; speed of processing; reasoning and problem solving; and executive functioning (i.e., initiation, planning, organization, persistence, and generalization). These problems tend to persist and interfere with academic progress over time, yet they are not always readily apparent on standardized measures. For example, Jaffe et al. (1992) found that children with moderate or severe injuries improved to the average or near-average range on most formal cognitive tests 1 year after injury, but they displayed continuing deficits on these measures relative to matched controls (Jaffe et al., 1993). Three years after injury, these children demonstrated subtle weaknesses, with uneven performance across multiple areas of cognition and significantly less academic growth relative to their peers (Fay et al., 1994). Children with mild brain injuries typically do not show these types of problems (Polissar et al., 1994). These studies emphasize that extent of brain injury and stage of recovery are important determinants of cognitive functioning. Other research has shown that cognitive outcome is also influenced by such factors as age at injury (younger children typically have worse outcomes) and preinjury functioning (Begali, 1992).

Unfortunately, significant cognitive weaknesses are easily overlooked following TBI, as children often appear intact due to the relatively rapid recovery of mobility, self-care skills, and basic language functioning (Oddy, 1993). In addition, children can display good recovery of preinjury learning, or "remote" memories, even though there may be marked impairments in the abilities required for new learning and successful school performance. Therefore, thorough cognitive assessment is essential following TBI.

In the early stages of recovery, the Children's Orientation and Amnesia Test (COAT; Ewing-Cobbs, Levin, Fletcher, Miner, & Eisenberg, 1990; Iverson, Iverson, Barton, & Farmer, 1994) can be used to measure orientation to person, place, and time, as well as attention/concentration and posttraumatic amnesia (PTA; the length of time until new memories are stored and recalled). The COAT is normed for children ages 3 to 15. The greater the number of days of PTA, the more likely are long-term cognitive deficits and functional impairments. The same information can be obtained for adolescents (>15 years old) using the Galveston Orientation and Amnesia Test (GOAT; Levin, Benton, & Grossman, 1982). The Mini Mental State Examination (Folstein, Folstein, & McHugh, 1975), developed for adults, can also be used with adolescents as a brief screening measure of cognition early in recovery.

When the child is rapidly recovering, cognitive specialists (psychologists, occupational therapists, speech/language therapists, and educators) must rely on informal assessments of cognition. For example, to assess attentional control, length of time on task can be measured under a variety of conditions, ranging from a quiet room with one-to-one assistance to a mock classroom setting with multiple distractors. A pretend-play task, such as having a tea party, can be designed to examine various abilities, including attention, memory for names and faces, word-finding skills, visual discrimination, and problem-solving abilities, as well as ability to integrate skills and generalize learning from other settings. The reader is referred to Ylvisaker et al. (1994) for an extensive review of informal probe tasks to use when assessing cognition at different developmental levels.

Standardized measures of cognition can be used during rehabilitation, once the child is no longer experiencing posttraumatic amnesia and can attend long enough to ensure the validity of testing. For example, the Wechsler Intelligence Scale for Children Third Edition (WISC-III; Wechsler, 1991) provides a baseline measure of global cognitive functioning following injury in school-aged children. A common pattern on the WISC-III among children with TBI is better performance on Verbal subtests, due to the more rapid recovery of previously learned information, but a decline on Performance subtests, due to the demand for novel problem-solving abilities, organization, and speed of processing (Ylvisaker et al., 1994). However, use of intelligence tests alone is never justified. Average scores on this type of measure do not preclude the existence of impairments in functional skills and are not predictive of school success (Fay et al., 1994).

Fortunately, there are several specific cognitive tests that have demonstrated sensitivity to the effects of brain injury in children. For example, more severely injured children have shown changes on measures of attention, such as continuous performance tests (Kaufman, Fletcher, Levin, Miner, & Ewing-Cobbs, 1993; Murphy-Berman & Wright, 1987); memory and new-learning measures, such as the California Verbal Learning Test Children's Version (Delis, Kramer, Kaplan, & Ober, 1989; Fay et al., 1994; Levin et al., 1993); concept formation and problem-solving measures, such as the Wisconsin Card Sorting Test (Heaton, 1981; Levin et al., 1993) and the 20 Questions Test (Denney & Denney, 1973; Levin et al., 1993); planning measures such as the Tower of London (Levin et al., 1994; Shallice, 1982); and measures of cognitive productivity, such as the Controlled Oral Word Association Test (Benton, 1968; Levin et al., 1993) and the Invention of Designs Test (Jones-Gotman & Milner, 1977; Levin et al., 1993).

Neuropsychologists might use these tests in a flexible battery approach designed to clarify a child's cognitive strengths and weaknesses, and then integrate results with formal and informal cognitive evaluations conducted by other team members to develop joint recommendations for the needs of the child upon school reentry. A fixed battery, such as the Halstead-Reitan Neuropsychological Test Battery for Older Children (Reitan & Wolfson, 1992), is not recommended, as this approach is primarily useful in diagnosing brain damage rather than suggesting practical interventions; however, selected subtests, such as the Trail Making Test, the Category Test, and the Tactual Performance Test, can provide additional information about specific cognitive abilities (Fay et al., 1994). These tests can be further supplemented by new measures of children's memory functioning such as the Wide Range Assessment of Memory and Learning (Sheslow & Adams, 1990) or the Test of Memory and Learning (TOMAL; Reynolds & Bigler, 1994).

Prior to transition to school, rehabilitation therapists must answer several key questions regarding the injured child's cognitive abilities, relative to preinjury estimates and to same-age peers:

What is the impact of the brain injury on the child's ability to learn new information in verbal and visual–spatial modalities? Are problems with new learning due primarily to deficits in attention, comprehension, memory, response insufficiency, speed of processing, or reasoning?

Are there differences in immediate versus delayed recall of new material? Does cuing or repetition help? Does the type of material to be recalled make a difference (auditory vs. written; factual information vs. personally relevant material; organized vs. unstructured)? Do incentives improve recall?

What is the child's attentional capacity? Can the child focus and sustain attention, shift attention in a flexible manner, and divide attention when more than one activity must be attended to simultaneously? What contexts promote optimal attention?

Does the child spontaneously plan and organize an approach to tasks? Can the child break large tasks into smaller steps and sequence events temporally? Are there problems with initiating tasks?

Are reasoning and problem-solving abilities intact for everyday activities? For more abstract material?

How efficient is the learner? Will slowed speed of information processing or rate of response impede classroom performance? Will the child need a reduced workload?

Will the child have difficulty organizing, accessing, integrating, or generalizing available cognitive abilities to meet classroom demands?

Speech/Language Functioning

During casual conversation with a student who has sustained a TBI, it may appear that he or she has intact communication skills—the student may understand questions and give sufficient verbal responses. However, with probes to request more specific information, breakdowns in receptive and expressive language skills may be evident.

Linguistic skills that typically return rapidly after TBI include those that are rote, overlearned, and automatic. This includes aspects of phonology, morphology, and syntax. Semantic and pragmatic skills might not be problematic in isolated situations or brief interactions; however, such communication skills are often impaired in more demanding contexts (e.g., with increasing length of material to be understood or expressed, higher levels of language, faster rates of presentation, or more complex dynamics of interaction; Ylvisaker, 1993).

Teachers have reported that language difficulties are significant factors limiting successful school performance in severely brain-injured children (Russell, 1993). The following linguistic deficits are typical in children and adolescents with TBI: impaired language comprehension as a result of decreased attention and speed of processing; problems in higher order language, such as abstraction and making inferences; difficulty with acquisition of age-appropriate receptive expressive linguistic skills, which may be the result of long-term memory deficits; impaired ability to express complex information, state main ideas, or organize verbal and/or written information; problems in word fluency, word retrieval, and confrontational naming; impaired discourse as characterized by confabulations, inappropriate language, tangential speech, and incoherence (irrelevant, lengthy, and fragmented); oral dyspraxia (impaired speech programming); and dysarthria (impaired motor control; Dennis, 1992; Dennis & Barnes, 1990; Jordon, Murdoch, & Buttsworth, 1991; Russell, 1993). Residual cognitive impairments, such as memory and organizational deficits, may make continued language development extremely difficult.

It is important to assess language in different contexts in order to get an accurate understanding of the child's strengths and weaknesses. Several standardized tests are especially useful for examining skills that are typically deficient in children following TBI. For example, the Clinical Evaluation of Language Fundamentals–Revised (CELF-R; Semel, Wiig, & Secord, 1987) assesses phonology, semantics, morphology, syntax, word retrieval, and verbal memory across a variety of receptive and expressive contexts. The Word Test (Jorgenson, Barrett, Huisingh, & Zachman, 1981) and the Test of Language Competence (Wiig & Secord, 1988) evaluate ability to understand and use increasingly complex and abstract language, such as semantic absurdities, inferences, and figurative language.

Informal assessment measures are also necessary for gaining an understanding of language skills in natural, integrative contexts. For example, auditory comprehension can be measured by asking the student questions after he or she has listened to a lecture. In this situation, the student must perform multiple functions. Necessary abilities include adequate attention, comprehension of concrete and figurative language, ability to make inferences, ability to form associations between past and current information, and ability to perform tasks simultaneously (e.g., comprehend and take notes). By manipulating variables such as length of information, visual prompts, and novelty, a reliable impression of receptive language can be formed.

Discourse skills can be examined in a 15- to 20-minute conversation in which abilities related to the introduction, maintenance, and termination of a topic are observed. Successful interaction depends on such skills as the ability to (a) interpret auditory and visual information (facial expressions), (b) rapidly process details, (c) recall and relate past information, and (d) verbalize information fluently with appropriate content. Linguistic strengths and weaknesses, as well as variables that enhance discourse, can be determined by modifying certain factors, such as rate of the speaker's speech; time constraints; familiarity with the topic and communication partner; and demands placed on the student, such as the type of questions asked. A formal measure of language competence in social situations can be obtained using the Pragmatic Protocol (Prutting & Kirchner, 1987), which assesses higher order abilities, such as initiation, maintenance, and appropriate shifting of topic in conversations.

In summary, initial impressions of linguistic skills based on interactions with a student who has sustained a TBI can be deceiving. A representative view of the individual is obtained via examinations of integrative functions. This is achieved through assessment of situations requiring comprehension and expression of information above the sentence level; higher order language; dynamic social interactions; and tasks that demand a significant degree of cognitive and motor skill for success. A variety of communication-related questions should be considered prior to hospital discharge. These may include the following:

What are the child's linguistic strengths and weaknesses? Which have the most effect on academic performance and social interactions?

To what degree is the child's speech production intelligible? What facilitates communication (strategies such as slowing the rate of speech, augmentative communication devices)?

What is the highest level of language (concrete or abstract) that the learner can understand without assistance?

What level of commands does the student follow successfully (two-step, three-step, conditional)?

How do language impairments affect interactions with peers? Adults? One versus several persons? How are these deficits manifested?

Does the student use inappropriate behaviors such as temper tantrums to control or communicate in environments for which she or he has inefficient expressive language skills?

How do such factors as stress; length of material; environmental distractors; interest and motivation levels; presentation style of speakers (teachers, therapists); multimodal presentations (visual, auditory, tactile); and rate of presentation affect receptive and expressive language skills?

What is the relationship among health, motor skills, cognition, and language? For example, do motor demands required for taking notes have a negative impact on comprehension of information presented in lectures?

What strategies facilitate the learner's comprehension and expression (visual cues, repetition, demonstrations, scaffolding, semantic webs, written objectives)?

What are the most and least effective intervention strategies utilized?

Has generalization of newly learned information occurred? If so, how many presentations and what methods were required to achieve this?

Academic Achievement

Academic problems, the need for special education interventions, and school failure are well documented following TBI in children (Hanson & Clippard, 1992). In addition to a loss or reduction of specific skills, deficits in basic cognitive processes, such as attention, organization, and self-regulation, can clearly diminish these children's ability to read, write, or perform mathematical operations (Fay et al., 1994).

Standardized instruments to assess academic achievement may be administered to students with TBI, though there are many limitations and cautions to consider. The Kaufman Test of Educational Achievement (K-TEA; Kaufman & Kaufman, 1985) and the Woodcock-Johnson Psycho-Educational Battery–Revised (Tests of Achievement) (WJ-R; Woodcock & Johnson, 1989) are two widely used achievement measures that are reliable and highly correlated with academic achievement in noninjured children. Among children with TBI, these measures may be helpful in determining the rank order of a student relative to peers, and in quantifying progress over time. However, such achievement tests are likely to overestimate the classroom potential of a child with TBI. They are power tests, administered individually with no time limits; they do not require synthesis of information or decision making, and do not reflect the length of material typically presented in a classroom. Further, they measure previously learned material that the child may recall relatively quickly after TBI, but might not tap what may be significant problems in learning new information. For all these reasons, formal academic tests often have limited utility for students with TBI, especially when the goal of assessment is to define instructional objectives early in recovery.

Performance-based assessment is more likely to identify the effect of TBI on skills necessary for academic progress, and to clarify important areas to target for intervention (Ylvisaker et al., 1990). For example, a miscue analysis (Goodman, Watson, & Burke, 1987) is helpful not only for evaluating recovery of reading skills, but also for examining cognitive and linguistic processes required for academic success. This procedure involves having the student read a text aloud without any help or interference. Deviations (miscues) from the text are marked and analyzed. Immediately after reading, the student retells the story under unaided, aided, and cued conditions.

For students with TBI, the length of the passage may be the first diagnostic challenge, due to reduced attention and memory. Although the passage may need to be shortened, it must still contain a beginning, a middle, and an end. During the oral reading, examiners may note that the reader hesitates and waits for assistance when challenged by unknown vocabulary. Ideally, the examiner would wait and let the student problem solve independently, at which point the child might continue, using strategies he or she had learned previously. In some cases, the student with TBI might become frustrated when adult intervention is not immediately provided. In other instances, the child with TBI might omit complete lines or paragraphs of text, which would indicate that he or she is not attending to, or obtaining sufficient meaning from, the process. When the student retells the passage, the examiner can gain insights into his or her comprehension, narrative language abilities, and memory. Each of these observations, in conjunction with other available data, enables the examiner to gauge the impact of TBI, identify which strategies are working effectively, and determine which conditions facilitate the child's reading performance.

In the area of written expression, many classrooms focus on the product of writing. For students with TBI, assessments should focus on the process of writing. The examiner may first note the effect of acquired physical limitations on the student's willingness and ability to write. Reduced attention and language deficits may impair the writer's ability to generate ideas on a topic during the prewriting stage. Functional activities can be used to examine the effects of writing maps and webs on the student's organization and responsiveness to visual cues during the writing process. Editing and revision processes may determine whether a student recognizes the need for changes and his or her willingness to accept objective feedback from others. The student's strengths and concerns about the mechanics of writing (spelling, capitalization, punctuation) are revealed as well. During a student's hospitalization, clinicians have an opportunity to begin a writing portfolio to document the child's development and recovery, illustrate consistent patterns of strengths and weaknesses, and in general provide pertinent information to the learner, family, and school about instructional needs and necessary accommodations (DeFina, 1991).

The professionals who conduct the mathematics assessment should maintain a holistic view and focus on a broad range of tasks rather than isolated skills. Multiple assessment techniques are recommended, including written, oral, and demonstration formats. The think-aloud method is particularly useful for identifying efficient and inefficient thinking strategies (Crowley & Miles, 1991; Pieper, 1983). With this method, when engaged in a mathematical problem-solving task, the child is asked to say aloud everything she or he thinks or does. Questions and probes can be interjected and are particularly helpful for students who lack awareness of their own performance. Problems can be selected from the learner's school curriculum or from everyday situations that require math reasoning and performance. For example, having a child select a purchase from the gift shop, given a specific occasion and budget, requires a range of functional skills (decision making, math reasoning, social appropriateness) in a real context.

Another strategy for alternative assessment of academic functioning involves incorporating school materials into the evaluation process. This technique can reveal a child's level of skills relative to the general education curriculum and help identify objectives for intervention. Additionally, the use of school texts and assignments can enhance the relevance of cognitive therapies for the child, particularly during the hospital phase of treatment, when insight into changes resulting from TBI is often limited. If rehabilitation personnel lack expertise in some of these areas of performance-based assessment, it may be necessary to invite a skilled teacher from the child's home school district to participate in such assessment activities prior to discharge from rehabilitation.

Assessment of the learning environment is as crucial as assessment of the learner. Numerous studies indicate that environmental factors, such as seating position, room arrangement, spatial density, and classroom organization and management, affect student performance (McKee & Witt, 1990). Ylvisaker et al. (1994) recommended that, during rehabilitation, staff examine situational variables that influence learning and performance by simulating a classroom setting. In this mock classroom, situational variables should be varied to determine (a) the impact of environmental distractions, including the presence of other peers; (b) the optimal length of instructional periods and arrangement of class schedules; (c) effective instructional materials and test formats; (d) appropriate expectations for quality and rate of work production; (e) the need for classroom aids, cuing systems, and/or assistive devices; and (f) factors that influence the child's motivation to learn. The student's responses to situational variables should be documented and incorporated into transition recommendations.

The rehabilitation team needs to be prepared to provide information that considers the following academic issues:

In what content areas (e.g., language arts, mathematics, science) is the child most likely to experience success?

What content areas may prove difficult or overwhelming for the learner? What modifications, if any, would facilitate the child's performance in those areas (reading partners, cooperative learning activities, peer tutoring, metacognitive strategy instruction, calculators)?

Will any classes require a parallel curriculum?

Under what conditions (environmental and/or instructional) can the learner work most independently? For what length of time is it reasonable to expect the child to work independently?

What techniques are recommended for addressing a child's cognitive impairments (e.g., attention, memory, organization) within the context of the curriculum and daily activities within the classroom?

During the initial transition period, what are the instructional priorities for this child (facilitating social relationships, emphasizing task initiation and completion, improving specific academic skills)?

Are there any limitations or considerations that need to be taken into account when assigning homework?

Are special education services required in order to provide an appropriate education? If so, what goals should be considered, what aids and services are necessary to achieve those goals, and what setting constitutes the least restrictive environment?

Sensorimotor Domain

Children with TBI frequently demonstrate a variety of sensory perceptual disturbances that must be assessed and treated in order to facilitate their functional return. Some commonly occurring visual deficits are hemianopsia (blindness to one side of the visual field), diplopia (double vision), blurred vision, and even cortical blindness (loss of the ability to interpret visual information; Baker & Epstein, 1991). Visual perceptual deficits are demonstrated by many children with TBI, including impairments in visual discrimination, visual attention, and visual spatial relations (Trombly, 1989).

Other perceptual deficits following TBI include difficulty with right/left discrimination, diminished body awareness, decreased depth perception, and difficulty with proprioception (knowing where one's body is in space; Trombly, 1989). Hearing loss occurs in about 35% of patients with traumatic brain injury and can be conductive or sensorineural. Auditory perceptual skills, such as the ability to separate target stimuli from background noise and the ability to attend to auditory stimulation, may be impaired. Vestibular disturbances (inner ear problems) are found as much as 6 months posttrauma in 50% of children with TBI (Jaffe & Hays, 1986). Following a TBI, sensitivity to tactile stimulation is often diminished, and the ability to discriminate between sensations (hot from cold, sharp from dull) and infer qualities of objects from touch may be impaired (Cobbs, Fletcher, & Levin, 1986). Even if the child is able to input information from the major senses, the ability to integrate the impulses into meaningful information that can be used in a functional manner may be diminished following trauma to the brain (Pratt & Allen, 1989). Nearly all children require extra time to process sensory information after severe brain injury (Cobbs et al., 1986).

Children often have difficulty acting on sensory information received, due to a number of motor deficits that are common sequelae following more severe injuries. Some examples of motor impairments include quadriparesis (marked loss of function in all four extremities), hemiparesis (loss of function on one side of the body), spasticity (muscle hyperactivity), heterotopic ossification (unusual bone formation in joints or muscles), contractures (inability to move a joint through its entire normal motion), and ataxia (incoordination of fine or gross motor movements). Any of these motor problems can result in decreased mobility, reduced use of an extremity, impaired balance, decreased activity tolerance, high fatigability, or general weakness. Some impairments are painful, which can affect the child's performance in other areas, such as attention to tasks.

The ability to successfully plan and follow through with voluntary movement, or praxis, is often impaired, and some children have difficulty initiating movement following a TBI (Trombly, 1989). Decreased speed of motor output affects a number of children with injury to the brain (Cobbs et al., 1986), and this symptom is often frustrating for parents and teachers. Slowed speed and incoordination may cause difficulty with fine motor tasks, such as handwriting, or gross motor tasks, such as moving efficiently between classes. Sometimes children have problems with bilateral integration and have difficulty coordinating both sides of their body when attempting to participate in functional activities, such as self-care skills (Kovich & Bermann, 1988). When these motor deficits are paired with impulsivity and diminished judgment, which are common neurobehavioral sequelae in children following TBI, safety risks frequently result (Carney & Gerring, 1990).

Standardized assessments are available to establish baseline levels of physical functioning and to measure recovery (Asher, 1989). To assess the child's visual–perceptual and visual–motor skills, tests such as the Motor Free Visual Perception Test (Colarusso & Hammill, 1972) and the Developmental Test of Visual Motor Integration (Beery & Buktenica, 1982) are brief and easy to administer. Gross and fine motor skills can be documented with a measure such as the Bruininks-Oseretsky Test of Motor Proficiency (Bruininks, 1978). Measures of sensory and motor abilities in younger children include the Miller Assessment for Preschoolers (Miller, 1982) and the Peabody Developmental Scales (Folio & Fewell, 1983).

Clinical testing procedures and observations are also used to examine the child's strength and endurance, sensation, postural stability and equilibrium, level of reflex integration, and bilateral integration (DePaepe & Lange,

1994). The child's ability to process sensory information from all systems (including visual, auditory, vestibular, somatosensory, gustatory, and olfactory) can be evaluated by observing the child during multimedia and multisensory play activities (Kovich & Bermann, 1988).

Children with severe motor deficits may need specialized wheelchair and seating systems and must be evaluated in order to determine the positioning that provides the highest level of functional independence (Milner et al., 1990). Information about home and school accessibility for children who will require a wheelchair for mobility must be obtained from parents and school personnel. Many teachers appreciate videotapes, pictures, or diagrams that illustrate the child's sensorimotor abilities and functional skills and depict assistive interventions.

Even with significant recovery, children may return to school with limitations in the physical, sensory, and perceptual domains that will affect their school performance (Coster, Haley, & Baryza, 1994). Questions that need to be answered prior to school reentry include the following:

Is the school accessible to the child? Are there any adaptations that could be made to the school environment to facilitate improved learning for the child?

Can the child tolerate a full day/half day of school?

Will the child be able to safely participate in physical education with peers?

Should adaptations be made to promote safety?

Will the child need assistance with toileting?

Will the child be able to manage the lunch line/lunch tray?

Is special transportation to and from school necessary for the child?

Will the child need special seating to improve school performance? Is it possible to adapt the child's desk to increase function?

Does the child have the fine motor skills necessary for writing and using school supplies appropriately? Would adaptations (built-up handles, computer-assisted word processing) enhance the child's performance?

Will the child be able to attend to his entire visual field? Would positioning the child's desk in a different part of the room assist her in attending to more information?

Will the child be able to copy information from the chalkboard/overhead? Would handouts or verbal instructions make the child more independent?

Behavioral Functioning

Adaptive Behavior. Change in adaptive behavior is common in children with severe brain injury (Papero, Prigatano, Snyder, & Johnson, 1993). Several tools have been developed to examine functional behaviors in young children (Haley, Coster, & Ludlow, 1991). These include the Wee-Functional Independence Measure (Wee-FIM; Braun & Granger, 1991) and the Pediatric Evaluation of Disability Inventory (Haley, Coster, Ludlow, Haltiwanger, & Andrellos, 1992), both designed for children ages 6 months to 7 years. These instruments measure level of performance and extent of caregiver assistance required to complete age-appropriate activities of daily living in areas such as self-care, mobility, and social interactions; thus, they are indicators of severity of disability and can be used to document progress over time.

The Vineland Adaptive Behavior Scales (VABS; Sparrow, Balla, & Cicchetti, 1984) is also a useful measure of behavioral competence after TBI. On the VABS, children with severe TBI have shown significant declines in overall adaptive behavior (composite score of communication, daily living, and socialization skills) relative to premorbid estimates and to the ratings of children with mild or moderate injuries (Asarnow, Satz, Light, Lewis, & Neumann, 1991; Fletcher, Ewing-Cobbs, Miner, Levin, & Eisenberg, 1990; Papero et al., 1993; Perrott, Taylor, & Montes, 1991). Because this measure was designed for children from birth to 19 years, it is especially useful for tracking the impact of TBI on adaptive behavior over the course of development.

Of all the aspects of adaptive behavior, social problems with peers and family members tend to be the most persistent (Deaton & Waaland, 1994). Decreased social competence can be due to declines in awareness of self and others, deficits in processing complex social situations, disorganized social responses, disinhibition, or inflexibility (Papero et al., 1993; Ylvisaker, 1993). These problems in social behavior are often associated with impaired executive functioning and prefrontal brain injury. They are only weakly associated with measures of cognitive functioning, such as IQ, memory, or other neuropsychological tests (Knights et al., 1991; Perrott et al., 1991; Ylvisaker, 1993). Therefore, social integration must be assessed separately from cognitive recovery. Informal observations of the child's social interactions with peers and adults in the rehabilitation setting and during community outings are often quite revealing and should supplement formal assessments of adaptive behavior. Only by watching such everyday interactions can the examiner determine the nature of the social problems and strategies for intervention (Blosser & DePompei, 1994).

Behavioral Adjustment. Although adaptive behavior is often compromised, there is less consensus about whether children with TBI are likely to develop disruptive behaviors or adjustment problems (Asarnow et al., 1991; Fletcher et al., 1990). There have been reports of overactivity, short attention span, immaturity, mood swings, impulsivity, poor judgment, low frustration tolerance, and poor anger control, especially following more severe TBI (Begali, 1992; Knights et al., 1991). In addition, poor self-awareness, decreased initiation, and apathy have commonly been observed. These problems can be especially frustrating because they disrupt the child's motivation to learn and to access needed compensatory strategies.

There are few standardized behavioral measures that have fully captured this type of behavior change. For example, the Child Behavior Checklist (CBCL; Achenbach, 1991) does not typically reflect clinically significant problems on the Internalizing or Externalizing scales following TBI (Fletcher et al., 1990; Rivara et al., 1993). Knights et al. (1991) found decreased attention span and increased disruptive behaviors among severely injured children using the Conners Parent and Teacher Rating Scales (Goyette, Conners, & Ulrich, 1978), compared to preinjury estimates of behavior. Other options for assessment in this domain include nonstandardized checklists designed specifically to assess behavioral problems that are common in children following TBI (e.g., Virginia Department of Education, 1992).

There is a great deal of individual variability in both behavioral adaptation and adjustment following injury. Whether or not a child displays challenging behaviors likely depends on the nature of his or her injury; the child's preinjury behavioral functioning; and environmental factors, such as home and school support (Deaton & Waaland, 1994). Recent empirical studies by Rivara et al. (1992, 1993) have illustrated this multidetermined quality of behavioral outcomes. They found that postinjury problems in school performance and social competence were predicted by preinjury child and family functioning, as well as by injury severity.

These findings suggest that family stress and coping must be examined along with child behavior to identify the potential for poor child outcomes. Family functioning prior to and following TBI has been assessed by Rivara et al. (1993) using the Family Environment Scale (Moos & Moos, 1976). The Family Assessment Device (Epstein, Baldwin, & Bishop, 1983; Kreutzer, Gervasio, & Camplair, 1994) also has demonstrated great promise in studies of adults with TBI and their families. The Parenting Stress Index (Abidin, 1983) has shown sensitivity to changes in parental responses to the injured child (Perrott et al., 1991), and the Family Crisis Oriented Personal Evaluation Scales (F-COPES; McCubbin, Larsen, & Olson, 1985) has been used to identify coping strategies used by families of persons with TBI (Leach, Frank, Bouman, & Farmer, 1994).

Of course, standardized measures of child and family functioning should only supplement clinical interviews and direct behavioral observations (Knights et al., 1991; Rivara et al., 1994). These important contacts allow for assessment of developing (or ongoing) behavioral, emotional, or interpersonal problems in the child. They also permit in-depth assessment of the needs of individual family members and of their knowledge about TBI. Parents and siblings who are knowledgeable about brain functioning and understand the nature of the child's brain injury may cope better than those harboring misconceptions (Deaton & Waaland, 1994). In addition, families that are informed about special education policies and procedures (e.g., requirements for IEP development) are more likely to have appropriate expectations about the role the school can play in their child's recovery, and therefore may be better prepared for the transition (DePompei & Blosser, 1994). Similarly, teachers who are prepared and feel competent to meet the needs of children with TBI are more likely to create a social environment that encourages emotional and behavioral adaptation to injury (DePompei & Blosser, 1993).

The team should evaluate the following child and environmental characteristics to facilitate long-term adjustment:

What are the child's behavioral strengths and weaknesses? Does the child's behavior differ substantially from preinjury, based on parent and teacher reports?

What positive reinforcers or environmental modifications encourage appropriate behaviors (high structure and routine, avoiding difficult activities when the child is especially fatigued)?

What environmental factors decrease inappropriate child behaviors (time-out, redirection)?

Do family members and teachers understand the relationship between brain injury and behavior changes and make accurate attributions about child behavior? For example, is slowed rate of work production related to the brain injury or attributed to laziness and poor motivation?

Do family members have adequate skills for managing the child's behavior? Do teachers?

Are family members coping adequately with changes in the child? What additional supports are needed for the family during rehabilitation and at the time of discharge (training in behavioral management, counseling, support groups, respite care, other interagency support services)?

What is the child's insight into personal changes associated with the injury? Is he or she coping adequately with hospitalization and with disability? Are there effective coping strategies used by the child that parents and teachers should be aware of and support (e.g., allowing the child to try difficult tasks rather than overprotecting)?

How does the child relate to adults and peers? What supports will be needed to facilitate social reintegration (circle of friends, contact with peers after school, peer education)? Is videotaping likely to be a useful strategy to provide feedback regarding social interactions?

Will the child benefit from contact with an adult mentor at school to help organize daily activities and address concerns (social or academic) as they arise? Can the child initiate such contact or should it be planned into the day?

Do parents understand their role as child advocates and active members of the treatment planning team? Is there a need for training in advocacy skills? Is the child allowed to contribute to treatment planning as much as possible?

Are medications needed to help manage attentional or behavioral problems?

SUPPORTING TRANSITION THROUGH COMMUNICATION

For a successful transition from rehabilitation to school and community, assessment information collected about the child with TBI must be effectively communicated to others. This communication process can be complex. The range of problems that can arise following brain injury is large, and every child has a unique set of impairments that must be reviewed. In addition, as indicated in previous sections, standardized assessments alone do not provide sufficient information about the child's performance in functional settings. This requires an increased reliance on alternative assessment procedures, which are time-consuming and must be carefully selected to ensure conceptual clarity. Communication can be hindered by the lack of a common knowledge base and by differing approaches to conceptualizing and remediating the child's problems.

Therefore, families, rehabilitation specialists, and educators must strive to communicate about the child's school and community reentry from the time of hospital admission (DePompei & Blosser, 1994; Janus, 1994). From the onset there should be equal exchanges of information, with the understanding that each individual or agency has expertise important to the transition process. Each participant has the responsibility to facilitate communication and resolve specific problems as they arise (see Appendix for an outline of these roles).

When the communication process starts early, the discharge planning meeting is primarily an opportunity to summarize the child's current capabilities and finalize specific plans for school and community reentry. Rehabilitation specialists should provide updated information on child functioning in the areas required by special educators according to state and federal laws (medical, vision, hearing, intellectual/cognitive, achievement, language, motor, and social/emotional/behavioral areas). This provides a thorough description of the child in a manner that expedites delivery of special education services, if required, and enhances problem solving about the child's needs.

Based on shared knowledge of the child and school/community resources, parents, educators, and therapists can jointly identify educational goals, instructional strategies, classroom placements, possible schedules, and a plan for implementation. The discharge staffing should also be used to specify a plan for future communications among team members, in anticipation of the need to regularly update the child's educational program and monitor social reintegration. A formal IEP may or may not be written at the discharge planning meeting, depending on the school's and family's preferences and needs. At the very least, highlights of the child's strengths, weaknesses, and concerns (e.g., adaptations, motivators, cautions) should be summarized for easy reference by teachers and the IEP team.

For children who are unable to return to school upon discharge from the hospital due to the severity of their injuries, decisions about homebound instruction and therapies must be made. Residential placement may need to be considered in some cases. Although these options should be outlined well before the discharge meeting, this time can be used to finalize plans and to make sure a system of interagency communication is in place to facilitate school reentry as soon as possible.

Parental involvement is key for a student's successful transition from hospital to school, yet some parents may have difficulty participating in their child's educational planning following TBI. Families who are experiencing difficulty adjusting to their child's acquired disabilities, or those who were previously psychologically unavailable, may remain relatively uninvolved in school issues and have difficulty accessing needed community supports (Waaland, Burns, & Cockrell, 1993). DePompei and Blosser (1994) recommended several approaches to intervention for these families, including development of an interagency Individualized Family Intervention Plan, which documents family needs and resources for assistance. It may be necessary to consider such a plan at the time of transition from the hospital to the community. In some cases, a family may be so disengaged that school and rehabilitation professionals are left to provide the best services possible without support from home.

Communication among diverse individuals and agencies poses many challenges. This is especially true following TBI due to the emotional, financial, and time constraints that work against such partnerships (Lash & Scarpino, 1993). However, substantive exchanges of information and proactive problem solving during rehabilitation can help create home and school environments that bridge the transition from hospital to community (Blosser & DePompei, 1994). In addition, the communication networks developed by these efforts can have a more lasting impact if they are also used to foster continued recovery over time. Such support is essential to minimize the negative impact of TBI on development and to enhance the child's opportunities for growth, learning, and acceptance.

Appendix

Tasks and Timeline for the Transition from Rehabilitation to School

Time	Parents	School personnel	Rehabilitation personnel
Upon admission	Sign information releases. Attend therapies to learn child's needs and abilities. Work with staff to learn about TBI.	Send all records. Identify key individual for communication with hospital staff. Indicate school's knowledge of TBI and training needs. Send school materials (books, tapes, etc.) for use in therapy. Share information regarding district special services.	Obtain and send releases to appropriate agencies. Identify key individuals for communication with school staff. Begin sharing information regarding TBI and educational services frequently required. Begin informal and formal assessment and therapy.
Throughout admission	Develop understanding of child and ways to interact that facilitate recovery/performance. Learn about special education services, rights, and procedures. Support child through therapies and social interactions with family and friends.	Maintain contact with rehabilitation staff through visits and/or teleconferences. Visit the student and attend therapies if possible. Begin considering student's needs for return to school (physical, educational, emotional, etc.) and share options available based on knowledge of district resources and schedules. Share information with any personnel that may be working with the student in school.	Educate family and school regarding student's strengths and needs. Identify strategic learning and instructional methods to enhance performance. Begin identifying specific educational considerations needed (length of day, services, environmental accommodations, assistive technology). Prepare videotape demonstrating effective behavioral, physical, or instructional techniques.

(appendix continues)

Time	Parents	School personnel	Rehabilitation personnel
		Request specific written material for educating students with TBI to disseminate to staff.	Inform school of possible services needed and consider dates for a discharge conference.
		Schedule training for staff regarding TBI.	
		Facilitate peer contact by sending audiotapes or videotapes of brief messages or good wishes.	
Near discharge	Develop understanding of child's abilities, emotional status, educational needs, and special; education processes.	Set date for discharge planning meeting and identify personnel who should attend.	Collect work samples or complete portfolio to share with family and school.
	Find support groups/services available in community.	Prepare list of questions remaining for parents and rehabilitation staff.	Compile diagnostic information and program recommendations into a written format consistent with requirements of the Individuals with Disabilities Education Act.
	Identify the family's priorities for the child in light of present status and future goals.	Develop list of possible schedules, instructors, and services to discuss during discharge meeting (including homebound services).	Develop written agenda for discharge planning meeting.
	Meet with rehabilitation personnel to prepare for purpose and format of discharge/IEP meeting.	Identify other agencies that may be necessary to provide services.	If the child cannot return directly to school, collaborate with the school to identify an interim plan.

(appendix continues)

Time	All team members
Discharge planning meeting	Summarize student's strengths and needs.
	Identify a target date for return to school, or finalize interim treatment plans if the student cannot return directly to school.
	Agree upon a prioritized list of educational needs and goals, and what resources are available to address each priority.
	Determine appropriate length of day.
	Identify classes whose content, structure, format, and teaching style are best suited to the student's needs and interests.
	Discuss policies regarding homework and discipline and outline any necessary accommodations.
	Identify a mentor at school who will closely monitor adjustment (educational, emotional, physical).
	Discuss specific plans for facilitating social reintegration and developing a network of peer support.
	Determine systematic methods of communication between home and school, and among home, schools rehabilitation facility, and other pertinent agencies.
	Recommend timeline for IEP review during the initial year.
	Identify key rehabilitation personnel to contact, should an emergency arise.

4. Alcohol and Drug Use Among Young Persons with Traumatic Brain Injury

JEFFREY S. KREUTZER, ADRIENNE D. WITOL, AND
JENNIFER HARRIS MARWITZ

The incidence of traumatic brain injury (TBI) has reached alarming proportions. Researchers estimate that 400,000 people suffer a brain injury each year, 44,000 of whom are in the moderate to severe range (Abrams, Barker, Haffey, & Nelson, 1993). An estimated 1 million to 1.8 million living Americans have sustained moderate to severe brain trauma (Cope & Hall, 1982). Automobile, motorcycle, and bicycle accidents; falls; violence; and recreational injuries are the major causes (Sorenson & Kraus, 1991). Acute medical care and rehabilitation charges are expensive, with estimates ranging from $90,000 to $165,000, depending on cause of injury (Lehmkuhl, Hall, Mann, & Gordon, 1993).

Brain injury is prevalent across all age groups and is the leading cause of death in persons younger than 45 (MacKenzie et al., 1987). Among all age groups, persons between the ages of 15 and 24, followed by individuals ages 5 to 14, are at highest risks for sustaining injury (Sorenson & Kraus, 1991). A recent large-scale, multicenter study revealed that persons ages 16 to 25 constituted more than one third (39%) of persons treated at major trauma centers for brain injury (Ragnarsson, Thomas, & Zasler, 1993). Adolescents with learning disabilities have been identified as being at high risk for incurring traumatic brain injuries (Haas, Cope, & Hall, 1987).

The primary effects of brain injury on neurobehavioral functioning have been well documented. Common physical symptoms include dizziness, balance problems, incoordination, and fatigue. Impairments of attention, memory, learning, motor speed, information processing, and visuoperception have been routinely reported by researchers (e.g., Lezak, 1995; Levin, Benton, & Grossman, 1982). Problems related to self-awareness and executive functioning, lability, irritability, and depression are also common (Thomsen, 1984). On a more global level, high rates of academic failure, unemployment, and family adjustment problems have been reported. To be assured of academic success, many students with traumatic brain injury receive special help from professionals who also serve children with learning disabilities. Estimates of unemployment following severe injury range as high as 70% within the first 7 years (Brooks, Campsie, Symington, Beattie, & McKinlay, 1987). Finally, family adjustment problems are frequently observed, with relatives reporting personal problems relating to frustration, depression, and social isolation (Hall et al., 1994).

Research has identified alcohol use as a common factor among persons with brain injury, relevant to both cause of injury and postinjury adjustment. A review of the literature suggests that between one third and one half of persons with brain injury were intoxicated at the time of injury (Corrigan, 1995). Rimel, Giordani, Barth, and Jane (1982) noted positive blood alcohol findings upon admission for 78% of 199 consecutive patients with moderate brain injury, with 56% meeting the legal criteria for intoxication. Among 538 persons with mild brain injury, the investigators found that 43% met the legal criteria for intoxication. Similarly, Galbraith, Murray, Patel, and Knill-Jones (1976) prospectively studied 918 consecutive admissions of persons with brain injury and found that 62% of the men and 27% of the women with brain injury had positive blood alcohol levels at admission.

The adverse effects of alcohol on early recovery were documented by Sparadeo and Gill (1989). Their investigation revealed that positive blood alcohol levels at admission were associated with higher levels of agitation, lower cognitive status at time of hospital discharge, and longer stays in acute care settings. In addition, Brooks et al. (1989) found that high blood alcohol levels at admission were related to worse performance on postinjury measures of verbal learning and memory. A later study provided evidence that patients with a history of excessive alcohol use have more severe brain abnormalities and a higher mortality rate (Ruff et al., 1990).

Despite concerns about substance abuse, quantitative and prospective studies are rare (Corrigan, 1995). Drubach and colleagues (Drubach, Kelly, Winslow, & Flynn, 1993) found high preinjury abuse rates in a study involving 322 patients averaging 35 years of age. On the basis of family reports and a records review, researchers estimated that 62% had abused alcohol and 37% had abused drugs. Kreutzer, Wehman, Harris, Burns, and Young (1991) examined preinjury drug and alcohol use among 74 adults with traumatic brain injury averaging 24 years of age referred for vocational services. The investigators found that 36% reported preinjury illicit drug use, including marijuana, cocaine, and amphetamines. In addition, 66% were described as moderate or heavy drinkers. Finally, a 37% preinjury alcohol abuse rate and a 9% drug abuse rate were found in a study of 498 adults with brain injury who participated in medical rehabilitation (Wong, Dornan, Schentag, Ip, & Keating, 1993). The investigators obtained data through a medical records review, which may account for relatively low abuse rates.

Fewer studies have focused on postinjury alcohol and drug use rates. Hall et al. (1994) interviewed caregivers 2 years postinjury, on average, to derive information about 51 patients ranging in age from 15 to 77. Using a brief screening instrument, researchers determined that 32% of patients were alcohol dependent and 20% were drug dependent. Kreutzer et al. (1991) reported that, 6 years postinjury, on average, 95% of patients abstained from illicit drugs. For those who used drugs, marijuana was the drug of choice. Fifty percent abstained from alcohol—double the proportion noted preinjury. Twenty-eight percent of the patients remained moderate or heavy drinkers. The high level of continued moderate to heavy use is disconcerting, given persistent reports of increased sensitivity to alcohol after brain injury (Cope & Hall, 1982; Dahmer et al., 1993). Alcohol and illicit drug use is of especially great concern for patients taking prescribed medications (Moore & Polsgrove, 1991; Gold & Gladstein, 1993).

There is little information about substance abuse patterns for adolescents with brain injury, although investigators have reported on alcohol and illicit drug use in the general adolescent population. Focusing on adolescent and adult use patterns, the National Household Survey on Drug Abuse (National Institute on Drug Abuse, 1991) was perhaps the most extensive study of its kind. Interviews were conducted with 1,557 boys and 1,538 girls ages 12 to 17. Asked about usage in the past year, nearly 13% reported marijuana use, 3% reported cocaine use, and 45% used alcohol. Abstinence from alcohol was less common among older persons. For example, only 23% of the 14- and 15-year-olds reported alcohol use in the past month. In contrast, nearly 70% of the 21- to 25-year-olds reported recent use. Mills and Noyes (1984) studied more than 2,000 students, collecting information about substance use within the past year. Among 10th graders, 82% had used alcohol, 42% had used marijuana, and 9% had used cocaine. In the 12th-grade group, 87% had used alcohol, 47% had used marijuana, and 9% had used cocaine. More recently, Robinson et al. (1987) reported that a majority of

10th graders (n = 1,273) had used marijuana but less than 15% had used cocaine during the most recent year. Finally, longitudinal research by Newcomb and Bentler (1987) suggested that illicit drug use declines and alcohol use increases between adolescence and early adulthood.

A number of investigations have focused primarily on patterns of alcohol use (Engs & Hanson, 1988; Hilton, 1987; Robinson et al., 1987). One of the most extensive was a national study conducted by Cahalan and Cisin (1968b). The authors studied drinking frequency and quantity among 2,746 adults ranging from 21 to more than 60 years of age. Within the young adult group (age range = 21 to 29), 30% of females were abstinent and 9% were labeled as heavy drinkers. In contrast, half as many same-age males were abstinent and 28% classified as heavy drinkers. Overall, estimates of abstinence among adolescents have ranged from 13% to 32%, and estimates of moderate and heavy drinkers have ranged from 45% to 76%. In an effort to determine changes in drinking patterns over time, Meilman, Stone, Gaylor, and Turco (1990) assessed alcohol consumption among 17- to 22-year-olds in 1977 and 1987. Based on a cross-sectional methodology, results suggested that the prevalence of heavy use decreased in the late 1980s. In 1977, 16% of the men and 5% of the women could be labeled heavy drinkers. In 1983, approximately 12% of the men and 2% of the women could be classified as heavy drinkers. In 1987, 7% of the men's and 2% of the women's alcohol use fell within the heavy-drinker category.

Research on substance use among youths with neurological disabilities has yielded equivocal findings. For example, Maag, Irvin, Reid, and Vasa (1994) found comparable patterns of substance use among adolescents with and without learning disabilities. Among persons with learning disabilities, 42% used alcohol and 11% used marijuana, whereas half of those without learning disabilities used alcohol and 7% used marijuana. Alternatively, Motet-Grigoras and Schuckit (1986) examined 42 college men with sensory, motor, and metabolic disabilities. In comparison with students without disability, the sample reported drinking at a younger age, along with more drug use, substance-related citations, and symptoms of depression. Some studies have suggested that adolescents with hyperactivity and conduct disorder are at higher risk for substance use (August, Stewart, & Holmes, 1983; Gittleman, Mannuzza, Shenker, & Bonagura, 1985). Others have suggested that rates of alcohol use for persons with neurological disorders are comparable to those of the general population (Alldadi, 1986; Beck, Langford, MacKay, & Sum, 1975; Bruck, 1985; Clampit & Pirkle, 1983).

In summary, adolescents and young adults are at high risk for brain injury and substance use. Substance use following injury contributes to the high incidence of vocational and academic failures. Concerns have repeatedly been expressed about the dangers of alcohol and illicit drug use during recovery. However, little is known about patterns of use among young patients. Knowledge about risk factors, assessment, and intervention can help professionals more effectively overcome obstacles to educational and vocational success.

Overall, there are very few prospective studies on postinjury patterns of substance use. Virtually nothing is known about long-term changes. Investigators have typically combined patients of all ages, and no special attention has been given to the younger patient population. However, this age group faces special problems, given the usual developmental tasks associated with transition from adolescence to adulthood. Brain injury or substance use poses particular problems for persons who wish to become emancipated from their families, establish intimate relationships, complete academic and vocational training, and begin careers.

The purpose of the present study was threefold. First, the pattern of preinjury alcohol and illicit drug use among adolescents and young adults with brain injury was identified. Second, efforts were directed at understanding changes in patterns of usage over time, with special attention given to moderate and heavy users. Preinjury use was twice that of use at 8 and 28 months postinjury (on average). Third, the patterns of substance use of patients taking prescribed medications was examined.

Improved knowledge can enhance future efforts to identify substance use risk factors indigenous to persons with brain injury. Information regarding the nature and incidence of problems will aid allocation of rehabilitation resources and development of substance abuse treatment programs that meet the unique needs of youth with brain trauma.

METHOD

Participants

Outpatients between 16 and 20 years of age at the time of injury were recruited from an outpatient rehabilitation clinic attached to an urban Level I trauma center. The clinic serves persons ages 16 and older. For the present investigation, persons younger than 21 were selected, yielding a sample of 87 participants. Fifty-four percent of the sample were admitted to other hospitals and later referred for outpatient services by physicians. The remaining 46% were directly admitted to the medical center and referred for follow-up after discharge.

The two referral groups were examined to ascertain the comparability of sociodemographic characteristics. Strong similarities were revealed in regard to educational levels, gender composition, and ethnicity. For both groups, the majority of patients were White men, and approximately one third were high school graduates.

Patients receiving follow-up between 2 and 48 months postinjury were included in the current study and grouped on the basis of time postinjury. Fifty-seven patients were seen for follow-up between 2 and 15 months postinjury (M = 8.34 months), and 45 were seen between 16 and 47 months postinjury (M = 28.53 months). A subset of 25 persons was evaluated at both follow-up intervals.

Information about duration of unconsciousness (in days) was used as a primary indicator of injury severity. The full range of brain injury severity was represented in the sample: Thirty-two percent of the patients did not sustain a loss of consciousness. Of the 68% who were unconscious, mean number of days was 19.4 (SD = 30.8, range = 1 to 120). Cause of injury was primarily motor vehicle accidents (90%). Other causes were falls (5%) and gunshot wounds (5%). A history of prior brain injury was reported by 15% of the sample. Admission blood alcohol levels were available for 35 (40%) of the 87 patients. Twenty-one had negative blood alcohol levels, and the remainder had levels ranging from 50 to 195 mg/dl (M = 129.1).

Men constituted 54% of the sample; 77% were White, 21% were Black, and 2% were of other ethnicity. In regard to education, 34% of the sample had not completed a high school education; 30% had completed some college. The remainder were high school graduates without college experience. At the time of injury, 35% were full-time students and 9% were part-time. Overall, 18% had reportedly been held back a grade, and 15% had received special education.

Preinjury, 21% of the sample reported a history of psychological treatment. Of those who had received treatment, 20% related treatment to substance abuse problems. Treatment was also commonly attributed to depression (47%) and anxiety (13%). In regard to arrest history, 18% reported problems with the law.

At follow-up, few participants were living by themselves or with friends. The proportions living with family at first and second follow-up were 88% and 73%, respectively. The proportions living with parents were 86% and 59%, respectively.

Instruments

Information regarding patient and respondent demographics as well as pre- and postinjury psychiatric, employment, academic, and medical histories was obtained. All other data were collected via the General Health and

History Questionnaire (GHHQ; Kreutzer, Leininger, Doherty, & Waaland, 1987). The GHHQ was developed specifically to assess the psychosocial, vocational, and neurobehavioral status of patients with varying ethnic backgrounds and varying levels of injury severity. Several investigations have provided support for the questionnaire's validity and interrater reliability (Kreutzer, Doherty, Harris, & Zasler, 1990; Kreutzer et al., 1991; Sander, Witol & Kreutzer, 1996). Respondents are queried about a patient's pre- and postinjury demographics, substance use, and work and criminal history. Information regarding pre- and postinjury illicit drug use and history of psychiatric or psychological treatment is also obtained.

Contained within the GHHQ is a version of the Quantity–Frequency–Variability Index (QFVI) developed by Cahalan and Cisin (Cahalan & Cisin, 1968a; Cahalan & Cisin, 1968b). On the basis of the quantity and frequency of alcoholic beverages consumed, individuals can be reliably categorized as abstinent or infrequent, light, moderate, or heavy drinkers. The present version was modified to separately examine pre- and postinjury drinking habits. The questionnaire was also adapted for completion by informants as a complement to the original self-report version. The QFVI is especially useful because representative data are available for a large sample of drinkers from the United States population. Moreover, several investigators have used the questionnaire to assess drinking patterns among persons with brain injury (Kreutzer et al., 1990) and other disabilities (Wisconsin Department of Health and Social Services, 1985).

A final section of the GHHQ contains the Neurobehavioral Functioning Inventory (NFI), an extensive behavior and symptom checklist. Items were originally formulated and compiled from interviews with patients with traumatic brain injuries and their families, and from thorough literature reviews. Information is reported pertaining to five categories of information: physical complaints, cognitive function, behavioral status, mood and motivation, and communication skills. Frequency of problem occurrence is rated on a 4-point scale. The present investigation focused only on demographic characteristics, history of psychiatric or psychological treatment, QFVI findings, and information regarding medication and substance use pre- and postinjury.

Procedure

The GHHQ was mailed to participants prior to their scheduled physical and/or neuropsychological examinations. When they arrived for evaluation, their responses to the questionnaire were reviewed for accuracy and completeness. Respondents were asked to clarify or provide additional information when necessary.

Descriptive information pertaining to alcohol and drug use was obtained from the patients. Information regarding educational, neurological, and psychiatric histories was obtained from the patients and from persons the patient identified as a primary caretaker (i.e., had close knowledge of and frequent contact with the patient). Information about duration of unconsciousness, mechanism of injury, and blood alcohol levels was obtained from medical records.

RESULTS

Research on behavioral problems after brain injury has traditionally relied on relatives' reports (Brooks, Campsie, Symington, Beattie, & McKinlay, 1986; Thomsen, 1984). With the recent empowerment movement in brain injury, investigators have increasingly relied on the reports of the injured persons rather than their relatives. Substance abuse investigators have traditionally relied on self-reported drinking information. Research indicates that self-reports and family reports of drinking behavior are generally consistent (Sander, Witol, & Kreutzer, 1996; Maisto, Sobell, & Sobell, 1979).

Self-reported substance use information was the primary focus of the present investigation. In 12% of cases, self-reported information was unavailable. Severe impairment related to injury and unwillingness to provide potentially incriminating information were the primary reasons for incomplete self-report data. To provide a description of the entire sample, we used informants' reports as an alternative and combined them with self-reports for data analysis.

Alcohol Use

Descriptive statistics were computed to describe pre- and postinjury drinking patterns, with QFVI scores used to assign drinking pattern classifications. The percentages of patients in each of the five drinking categories at each time interval are displayed in Table 4.1. Before injury, a large majority (73%) of the sample were drinkers, with more than half (51%) falling within the moderate or heavy classification. During the initial follow-up period, a majority (58%) of patients were abstinent; 25% were labeled as moderate to heavy drinkers. At follow-up, averaging 28 months postinjury, nearly half the sample (49%) was abstinent. Approximately one third were moderate (21%) or heavy (14%) drinkers.

Differences in the proportion of drinkers in each category at each time interval were examined using chi-square analyses. First, comparisons were made between drinking patterns preinjury and those at initial follow-up. A

Table 4.1
Pre- and Postinjury QFVI Classifications

Drinking categories	Preinjury		Initial follow-up		Second follow-up	
	%	n	%	n	%	n
Abstinent	27	23	58	33	49	21
Infrequent	16	14	12	7	9	4
Light	6	5	5	3	7	3
Moderate	37	32	18	10	21	9
Heavy	14	12	7	4	14	6

Note. QFVI = Quantity–Frequency–Variability Index.

substantial decline in drinking frequency and quantity was indicated, $\chi^2(4, N = 86, 57) = 14.87$, $p < .01$. No differences were found when preinjury drinking patterns were compared with second follow-up, or when first follow-up was compared with second ($p > .05$).

To further compare preinjury QFVI classifications with initial follow-up, a second set of descriptive statistics were calculated. Determinations were made as to whether the frequency and quantity of patients' drinking decreased, increased, or remained the same. A majority of patients were assigned to different drinking categories postinjury, with 32% reporting decreased use and 20% reporting increased use. Less than half (48%) of the sample had the same drinking classification before injury and at initial follow-up.

Two subsets of drinkers were examined more closely: persons who were abstinent ($n = 23$) and persons who were moderate or heavy drinkers ($n = 44$) before their injury. For those reporting preinjury abstinence, only one person was a drinker (moderate) at initial follow-up. Three were drinkers at second follow-up, falling within the infrequent or light-drinker classifications. Among the group of moderate or heavy preinjury drinkers, 36% showed no change at initial follow-up and 59% were in the moderate or heavy-drinker category at second follow-up (see Table 4.2). At initial and second follow-up, 43% and 33% were abstinent, respectively.

Illicit Drug Use

Descriptive statistics were calculated to describe pre- and postinjury patterns of illicit drug use, and information was available for 79% of participants ($N = 69/87$). Patients were categorized as either abstinent or users.

Table 4.2
Postinjury Drinking Patterns of Preinjury Moderate/Heavy Drinkers

Drinking categories	Initial follow-up		Second follow-up	
	%	n	%	n
Abstinent	43	19	33	15
Infrequent	14	6	4	2
Light	7	3	4	2
Moderate	25	11	42	18
Heavy	11	5	17	7

Note. N for preinjury moderate/heavy drinkers = 44.

Before injury, 29% reported illicit drug use. Of that group, all used marijuana. Approximately one third (30%) used cocaine and 30% used other illicit drugs (e.g., LSD, amphetamines). Abstinence from illicit drugs was reported by 94% at initial follow-up and 92% at second follow-up. Marijuana remained an overwhelming favorite.

Medications, Drinking, and Illicit Drug Use

Alcohol and illicit drug use can present special risks for persons taking prescribed medications. The subset of patients taking prescribed medications was identified for each follow-up interval. At initial follow-up, 23 persons were reportedly taking medications, and 16 were at second follow-up. Anticonvulsants and antidepressants were the most commonly prescribed medications.

In regard to drinking, the proportions reporting abstinence were 79% at first follow-up and 44% at second follow-up. Among those taking prescribed medications, the proportions of moderate or heavy drinkers at first and second follow-up were 17% and 44%, respectively. In regard to illicit drugs, 96% were abstinent at first follow-up and 87% were abstinent at second follow-up.

DISCUSSION

Research indicates that intoxication increases the risk of accidental injury and death. There is also evidence of high injury and substance use rates among adolescents and young adults. This research has led to questions about whether persons who sustain brain injury have higher preinjury drinking rates than the general population. In the present study, preinjury, 23% of the men and 37% of the women were abstinent. Regardless of gender, the proportion of abstinent persons was 27%. For 16- to 20-year-olds, the National Household Survey on Drug Abuse (National Institute on Drug Abuse, 1991) revealed abstinence rates of 22% to 34%. In a 1987 survey, Meilman et al. (1990) found that less than 4% of university undergraduate men and women were abstinent. In a national survey, Cahalan and Cisin (1968a) found abstinence rates of 16% for men and 30% for women age 21 to 29.

A comparison among studies suggests that abstinence rates for the participants with brain injury in the present study were comparable to those of the general adolescent and young adult population in two ways. First, the gender differences for the general population were also observed for the sample—the proportion of abstinent male patients was substantially lower than that of females. Second, overall abstinence rates for the sample were comparable to those reported in national surveys and large-sample studies.

Many of the patients in the present study were moderate or heavy drinkers preinjury. Comparisons with data provided by other researchers suggest that the proportion of heavy and moderate drinkers in the sample was generally consistent with that reported for the general population. Direct comparisons among studies were difficult because of substantial methodological differences. Investigators have studied different age groups and regions of the country using different assessment methods and labels for consumption levels.

For the present sample, half of the patients were moderate or heavy drinkers preinjury. An examination by gender revealed that 44% of the men were moderate drinkers and 16% heavy drinkers. Among the women, 28% were moderate drinkers and 9% were heavy drinkers. Cahalan and Cisin (1968a) found that 28% of the men and 9% of the women they studied were heavy drinkers. For college students ages 17 to 22, Meilman et al. (1990) found that 69% of the males were moderate drinkers and 7% were heavy drinkers. Among the female college students, 53% fell in the moderate category and 2% fell in the heavy category.

Estimates of illicit drug use among persons ages 15 to 21 have ranged from 17% to 45%. In a study of 10th graders, Robinson et al. (1987) reported that 46% of the boys and 42% of the girls had used marijuana. In regard to cocaine use, 14% of the boys and 15% of the girls reported prior cocaine usage. In the National Household Survey on Drug Use (National Institute on Drug Abuse, 1991), 18% of persons ages 12 to 17 reported use of illicit drugs within the past year. Thirteen percent reported marijuana use and 3% reported cocaine use. Among persons ages 18 to 20, 53% reported prior drug use. Among that group, 30% reported drug use in the past year.

In the present study, 29% of the sample reported drug use within the year prior to injury. As in the general population, marijuana was the most frequently used drug, followed by cocaine. The proportion of persons reporting preinjury illicit drug use was also comparable to that reported in other surveys that have focused on the same age group. Postinjury illicit drug use rates were substantially lower than those for the general population, remaining below 10% at both follow-up intervals.

Researchers have speculated that substance abuse rates increase following traumatic injury. This speculation derives from two sources. First, unusually high alcohol abuse rates have been found among persons with disabilities (Wisconsin Department of Health and Social Services, 1985). Second, clinicians have suggested that alcohol and illicit drugs serve as a means of ameliorating the emotional distress that inevitably follows the onset of acquired disability (Glow, 1989). For the overall sample, the present findings suggested a substantial decrease only at initial follow-up. In comparison with preinjury, more than twice as many persons were abstinent. Nearly 45% of those who were moderate or heavy drinkers preinjury reported abstinence at initial follow-up. A similar pattern was noted for illicit drug usage. Less than 10% of the sample reported illicit drug use at either follow-up interval—a decline compared to 29% preinjury.

Statistical tests did not indicate a difference between drinking patterns at first and second follow-up, or preinjury versus second follow-up. An interesting trend we observed suggested that, over time, postinjury drinking levels return to preinjury rates. Nine percent fewer patients reported abstinence at second follow-up in comparison to first. The proportion of heavy drinkers at second follow-up was double that reported at initial follow-up. Also, identical proportions (14%) of the sample fell within the heavy-drinker category preinjury and at second follow-up.

Data for persons who were abstinent, moderate drinkers, or heavy drinkers were examined separately to develop a better sense of trends over time. That examination revealed that persons who were abstinent preinjury often remained abstinent postinjury. All persons who were abstinent preinjury were also abstinent at initial follow-up. Only 22% of those who were abstinent preinjury were drinkers at the second follow-up, and all of the drinkers fell within the light or infrequent drinking categories.

Preinjury moderate and heavy drinkers were also examined as a separate group. At initial follow-up, 23% fell within the moderate- or heavy-drinker category. More than two thirds fell within the moderate or heavy category at second follow-up, with nearly one third (31%) in the heavy category. The overall pattern of data for abstainers, moderate drinkers, and heavy drinkers strongly suggests that preinjury drinking patterns are important postinjury predictors of consumption.

Commonly prescribed medications for persons with brain injury include antiseizure drugs, antidepressants, anxiolytics, and sleep enhancers (O'Shanick & Zasler, 1990). For the present sample, the most commonly prescribed drugs were antiseizure medications including Tegretol and Phenobarbital. Drinking and ingesting illicit drugs while taking medication is normally contraindicated because of potentially dangerous interactions. Alcohol and illicit drugs can potentiate medications' sedating effects, negate the therapeutic effects of medication, and lower seizure thresholds.

The present findings raise concerns about patients' compliance with physicians' recommendations about alcohol use and prescription medications. Among the patients taking medication at initial follow-up, 4% fell in the moderate- and 13% fell in the heavy-drinker categories. Increasing risk for medical complications over time was evident. At second follow-up, less than 50% of persons taking medication were abstinent. An alarming 44% fell within the moderate- or heavy-drinker categories. On a positive note, nearly 80% of those taking prescribed medication were abstinent at initial follow-up. Additionally, no persons taking medications reported illicit drug use at follow-up.

Study Limitations

Drawing valid inferences from this exploratory investigation requires consideration of the study's limitations. The first set of important issues relates to generalization limitations. The sample containing 87 persons was drawn from a single catchment area, leaving uncertainties about comparability with other regions of the country. Furthermore, follow-up was limited to the first 4 years postinjury, leaving questions about long-term changes. Also, relatively few patients were available for both follow-up evaluations.

Data were derived primarily by self-report, which is subject to bias. Limited self-awareness and memory problems are common sequelae of brain injury. One might argue that patients would be likely to underestimate their own drinking rates, especially in comparison to relatives'. However, a recent study of persons with traumatic brain injury revealed striking similarities between caregiver and patient estimates of postinjury drinking rates (Sander et al., 1996).

The present findings can readily be reexamined in future research. Combining data from several centers to yield a much larger sample will help address generalization issues. Allocation of resources to enhance follow-up rates and extend the follow-up interval will increase the likelihood of a truly longitudinal design reflective of temporal changes. The range of information about substance use can be enhanced in several ways. First, self-report data should be supplemented with historical information about blood alcohol levels, criminal transgressions (e.g., driving under the influence, drunk and disorderly), and medical records pertaining to alcohol-related illnesses (e.g., hospitalization for detoxification). Second, the use of standardized interview procedures can help in assessing whether patients meet established diagnostic criteria for substance abuse disorders. Third, consideration of an individual's injury severity, inpatient status, and partial-day hospitalization status can ensure that drinking estimates at 1 year postinjury were not artificially lowered by lengthy hospitalizations. Finally, the questionnaires used in the present study can be supplemented by others to obtain more extensive, qualitatively different information. The use of scales that yield interval data will enhance the sensitivity of statistical analyses. In all likelihood, a series of studies will be necessary to fully understand the complex relationships among alcohol use, drug use, and brain injury.

Nevertheless, the present study can be considered a relatively unique and important step toward improved understanding of substance use among young persons with brain injury. Quantitative information about alcohol and illicit drug use at three time intervals was obtained. The focus was persons ages 16 to 20 years; the sample was representative of persons at risk for traumatic brain injury, and a full range of injury severity was represented. The sample composition in regard to ethnicity, educational level, and history of previous brain injury was roughly comparable to that reported in other large-sample investigations (Gordon, Mann, & Willer, 1993). Standardized assessment methods and labels for consumption levels developed by other researchers were used, allowing direct comparison with other investigations. Postinjury data were collected using prospective methods. To date, studies of pre- and postinjury substance use among persons with brain injury have been rare.

Clinical Implications

A review of the substance abuse literature and the present findings can serve to guide rehabilitation practice. Men, preinjury moderate and heavy users, and persons taking medications appear to have a higher risk for problems. Carefully monitoring these groups and actively encouraging participation in prevention programs are likely to have important benefits. Also, alcohol usage rates appear to increase over time. Clinicians should consider intensifying monitoring efforts in the long term, especially for those at risk. Additionally, physicians are strongly advised to closely monitor substance use among persons for whom they prescribe medication. Continuing education and family involvement may help prevent potentially dangerous interactions among alcohol, illicit drugs, and prescribed medications.

The present findings suggest that rates of illicit drug use for persons with brain injury decline postinjury and remain lower than those of the general population. Rates of postinjury alcohol use are relatively low within the first year of injury but appear to increase over time. Injury severity, warnings about harmful interactions with prescribed medications, dependence on others, lack of transportation, and limited finances may account for the relatively low alcohol use within the first year postinjury. With long-term improvement, accessibility to alcohol and illicit drugs often increases. Professionals are encouraged to consider increased monitoring with increased independence.

There is evidence that alcohol and illicit drugs pose special dangers for persons with severe injury. Certainly abuse can endanger recovery and reduce the benefits of expensive rehabilitation programs. In addition, persons who continue using drugs and alcohol are increasing their risk for recurrent brain injury (Kreutzer et al., 1990; Nath, Beastal, & Teasdale, 1986).

Even if patients' rates of alcohol use are similar to those of the general population, educating them about their special risks is likely to have myriad benefits. Ultimately, more research is needed to identify use patterns, important risk factors, and elements of successful treatment.

Authors' Note

1. This work was partly supported by Grant Nos. G0087C0219 and H133P2006 form the National Institute on Disability and Rehabilitation Research, U.S. Department of Education.
2. The authors thank Kyle Evans and Grace Sandoz for their assistance in the preparation of this chapter.

5. Long-Term Outcome
After Moderate to Severe Pediatric
Traumatic Brain Injury

GRETA N. WILKENING

Head injuries in children are an unfortunate and common occurrence. Each year, 5 million children in the United States sustain a head injury, with about 200,000 requiring hospitalization (Rossman, 1994). Of these, approximately 20% are described as having an injury of moderate to severe intensity. This chapter discusses the long-term outcome of children with moderate to severe traumatic brain injury (TBI). Although this would appear to be a simple task, a review of the literature quickly reveals methodologic issues that make interpretation difficult; for example, differences between studies in the definition of what constitutes a moderate or a severe head injury make generalization of results problematic.

From an education perspective, the ultimate purpose of reviewing outcome literature is to provide information useful in helping to: (a) anticipate a child's needs as he or she reenters school postinjury, (b) develop plans for monitoring progress, and (c) understand what to expect in terms of probable patterns of strength and weakness. The first portion of this chapter focuses on variables that are predictive of long-term outcome and the second section on the level and pattern of performance that is reported after moderate to severe head injury. Finally, case descriptions illustrating outcome after diffuse or more specific injuries, and after prolonged or more brief periods of recovery, are provided.

HEAD INJURY VARIABLES AS PROGNOSTIC FEATURES

Severity of Injury

The severity of a head injury is most typically characterized by using the Glasgow Coma Scale (GCS; Teasdale & Jennett, 1974). This measure was developed to provide practitioners with a rapid, reliable, and reproducible measure of depth of coma while distinguishing among disturbances in language, consciousness, and motor performance. Clinicians assess these three components of wakefulness independent of one another by judging the type of stimuli required to produce eye opening, the best verbal response, and the best motor response. The composite E + M + V (Eye opening plus Motor response plus Verbal response) has been widely accepted as an indicator of head-injury severity, and GCS score of 8 or less typically indicates that the person has a severe head injury (Levin, Benton, & Grossman, 1982). The criteria for scoring are provided in Table 5.1.

Multiple studies have addressed the relationship between severity of injury—as measured by the GCS—and behavioral/psychological outcome, with compelling evidence of a dose–response relationship (Walker, Storrs, & Mayer, 1983). As in adults, a dose–response relationship appears to exist in children, with those children who evidence the most severe injuries having the most substantial functional deficits. Relationships between GCS score and the following items have been reported:

- Full Scale and Performance IQ (Bawden, Knights, & Winogron, 1985; Levin, Eisenberg, Wigg, & Kobayashi, 1982; McDonald et al., 1994; Winogron, Knights, & Bawden, 1984);
- Performance on the Glasgow Outcome Scale (Esparza et al., 1985);
- Memory (Bassett & Slater, 1990; Levin et al., 1988; McDonald et al., 1994, Levin, Eisenberg, et al., 1982);
- Mortality (Hofer, 1993);
- Academic performance (McDonald et al., 1994);
- Behavior (Mahoney et al., 1983); and
- Speed of response (Bawden et al., 1985).

Levin, Benton, and Grossman (1982) recommended that GCS scores be monitored over time because it is the evolution of coma that appears to be most useful prognostically. McDonald et al. (1994) found that not only did different measures of severity (e.g., initial GCS, GCS eye score, days to

Table 5.1
Glasgow Coma Scale

Activity	Score	Description
Best motor response		
obeys commands	6	follows simple verbal directions
localized pain	5	moves limbs to attempt to escape painful stimuli
withdrawal from pain	4	normal flexor response (abduction)
abnormal flexion	3	"decorticate"—abnormal adduction of shoulder
extensor posturing	2	"decerebrate"—internal rotation of shoulder and pronation of forearm
no response	1	flaccid, without evidence of spinal transection
Best verbal response		
oriented	5	aware of self, environment, time, and situation
confused	4	attention is adequate and patient is responsive, but responses suggest disorientation and confusion
inappropriate	3	understandable articulation, but speech is used in a nonconversational (exclamatory or swearing manner); conversation is not sustained
incomprehensible	2	verbal responses (moaning) but without recognizable words
no response	1	
Eve opening		
spontaneous	4	eyes are open; scored without reference to awareness
to speech	3	eyes are open to speech or shout without implying a response to a direct command
to pain	2	eyes are open with painful stimulus to limbs or chest
none	1	no eye opening, not attributable to swelling

Note. Adapted from "Assessment of Coma and Impaired Consciousness," by G. Teasdale & B. Jennett, 1974, Lancet, 2, pp. 81–84.

reach a GCS of 15) provide varying ability to predict outcome, but the best predictors of outcome at 3 weeks postattainment of orientation were different from those that best predicted outcome at 1 year postattainment of orientation. This study followed 98 children who had sustained traumatic brain injury and 98 controls (matched for age, gender, school grade, and teacher's assessment of academic performance). Injury severity was addressed in 10 ways:

Initial GCS score;

Initial GCS motor score;

Initial GCS eye score;

Initial GCS verbal score;

Duration of loss of consciousness (LOC);

Abbreviated Injury Scale head region score (Committee on Injury Scaling, 1985);

GCS motor score at 3 days postinjury;

Days to reach a GCS of 15;

Days to reach a GCS motor score of 6; and

Days to reach a 75% performance on the Children's Orientation and Amnesia Test (COAT; Ewing-Cobbs, Levin, Fletcher, Miner, & Eisenberg, 1990).

Outcome was assessed via a full neuropsychological exam. The four indices most predictive of early and 1-year outcome were days to an age-adjusted 75% performance on the COAT, days to a GCS score of 15, initial GCS, and LOC duration. These four measures were highly associated with one another. Academic skills and memory performance were most effectively predicted by using multiple variables. Duration of disordered mental status was a stronger predictor of outcome than initial assessment of level of coma (e.g., initial GCS). Not surprisingly, these variables were better able to predict 3-week outcome than long-term outcome. From the point of view of school reentry, it is striking that TBI severity and academic performance at 1 year were highly correlated.

Acute Medical Complications

In addition to consideration of injury severity, knowledge of acute medical variables is significant in the anticipation of functional outcome. Maintenance of normal intracranial pressure in the acute period is considered essential (Levin, Benton, & Grossman, 1982), with elevated intracranial pressure (20mm Hg [mercury] or greater) associated with high mortality and substantial morbidity (Esparza et al., 1985). Increased intracranial pressure also may be associated with the presence of mass lesions (e.g., intracranial hematoma, sub- or epidural hematoma). The presence of intraparenchymal lesions (Choi et al., 1994; Esparza et al. 1985) or intraventricular blood (Ruijis, Gabreëls, & Keyser, 1993) is also predictive of poorer functional outcome. Although extracerebral lesions are associated with relatively good outcome, the presence of such a lesion in association with significant hemispheric swelling suggests a poorer behavioral outcome, presumably secondary to ischemia (Esparza et al., 1985). Diffuse swelling in isolation is thought to be consistent with better outcome, although evidence of diffuse axonal shearing on imaging studies is suggestive of an unfavorable functional outcome.

Although these structural changes, as identified on imaging studies, are useful in anticipating a child's needs postdischarge, professionals responsible for the education of children with such injuries need to be alert to variations that are dependent on the timing of these studies. Changes that are demonstrable on computed tomography (CT) scans vary in direct relationship to the severity of the head injury (Ruijis, Gabreëls, & Thijssen, 1994); however, early CT will fail to detect some lesions, even some clinically severe ones. Repeat imaging via CT may detect lesions in areas that initially were thought to be normal or minimally abnormal (e.g., timing of the CT may alter interpretation of prognosis). Magnetic resonance imaging (MRI) is thought to be more sensitive to the presence of smaller lesions (Ruijis et al., 1994), with focal lesions more evident than would have been predicted on the basis of CT results (Levin et al., 1993; Mendlesohn et al., 1992). As with CT, follow-up MRI scans are more useful in the prediction of quality of recovery than are early studies (Mendelsohn et al., 1992).

Although not predictive of long-term epilepsy, acute posttraumatic seizures can indicate the possibility of poor functional outcome if the metabolic demands of the seizing brain contribute to increased intracranial pressure (Ghajar & Hariri, 1992). Multisystem involvement—particularly the presence of lower limb injuries—is consistent with poorer functional outcome (Greenspan & MacKenzie, 1994). Obviously, children with head injuries may have other problems. Compromised cerebral perfusion secondary to cardiopulmonary disturbances is associated with poorer functional outcome (Ghajar & Hariri, 1992).

Lesion Localization

There is some evidence that the location and size of a focal lesion is predictive of functional outcome. Although multiple studies across many years have demonstrated that the response of the child's physiologically immature brain to injury differs from that of the adult brain, with the congruence between localization and neuropsychologic sequelae less clear and consistent (Wilkening, 1989), there is increasingly compelling evidence that localization of discrete lesions plays a role in functional outcome.

Mendelsohn et al. (1992) and Levin et al. (1993, 1994) demonstrated that focal areas of damage that are measurable on follow-up MRI add to the ability to predict functioning on specific neuropsychological measures, with localization of the lesion contributing to predictive accuracy. Mendelsohn et al. (1992) found that 39 of 55 patients scanned post–head injury (GCS 3–5, $n = 13$; GCS 6–8, $n = 26$; GCS 9–12, $n = 9$; GCS 13–15, $n = 7$) had focal areas of abnormality. More common were anterior lesions involving the frontal lobe. Patients with frontal lesions, or lesions involving the frontal lobes, were more likely to have a speech disturbance. Levin et al. (1993) found that in 40% of their sample MRI revealed lesions confined to or predominantly localized to the frontal region. Knowledge of the size of the frontal lesion enhanced prediction of performance on some measures of "frontal lobe function" when injury severity was known. Lateralization of a frontal lesion was related to the ability to predict performance on some tasks, with left frontal lesion size related to efficiency on the Wisconsin Card Sorting Test (Heaton, Chelune, Talley, Kay, & Curtiss, 1993) and to response inhibition. Right frontal lesion size made an incremental contribution to prediction of verbal fluency and effective use of organizational strategies to assist in memorization. Knowledge of the size of extrafrontal lesions did not contribute to prediction of performance on these specific cognitive measures beyond that made solely on the basis of injury severity. However, greater delineation of the area of abnormality within the frontal lobe (e.g., size of orbital, white matter, or dorsolateral frontal lesions) allowed for prediction of performance on varying aspects of the Tower of London task (a task requiring planning a strategy, identifying subgoals and plans to reach these goals, and holding a plan and the subgoals in working memory; Shallice, 1982) beyond that provided by the severity of injury (Levin et al., 1994).

More recent work in the area of head injury has suggested that, although children do not consistently show the specificity of neuropsychological sequelae following focal lesions that often occurs in adults (Mulhern, Kovnar, Kun, Crisco, & Williams, 1988; Wilkening, 1989), there are patterns that are replicable. The presence of focal lesions mediates performance on sensitive measures, and knowledge of areas of focal disease can contribute to prediction of functional outcome. This may be of special importance in the provision of clinical care to children after moderate to severe head injury. These children do not necessarily show changes on imaging (e.g., CT or MRI), especially early in their course, but it appears that they are likely to have areas of demonstrable focal change later in their course, with predictable functional consequences (Mendelsohn et al., 1992).

Age at Injury

Early experimental animal studies suggested that brain damage acquired early in life was less debilitating than later acquired brain damage. Studies of young children, however, indicated that there is no general sparing of cognition after early brain disease (Levin et al., 1994). Children with leukemia who received cranial radiation as part of their prophylactic central nervous system (CNS) treatment (Fletcher & Copeland, 1988; Silber, et al., 1992), children with liver disease (Stewart, Campbell, McCallon, Waller, & Andrews, 1992), and children with brain tumors (Ellenberg, McComb, Siegel, & Stone, 1987; Ris & Noll, 1994) all appear to have poorer cognitive outcomes if they are younger at the time of diagnosis or treatment than children with similar diagnoses or treatment who receive a CNS injury at a later age. The results from studies of children with head injuries are consistent with this pattern.

Children who sustain moderate to severe head injuries when they are younger have not been found to have a sparing of cognition (Levin, Eisenberg, et al., 1982, 1994). Indeed, more severe cognitive impairment is seen in children who are injured when they are less than 13 years of age. These children exhibit long-term deficits in recognition memory that are not seen in adolescents with injuries of a similar magnitude (Levin, Eisenberg, et al., 1982). Brink, Garrett, Hale, Woo-Sam, and Nickel (1970) reported that younger children with injuries equivalent to those of older children (based on length of coma) demonstrated a greater decrement in intellectual function post–severe head injury.

Additional studies by Levin, Eisenberg, et al. (1982) and Levin et al. (1988, 1993) demonstrated that the recovery pattern may vary as a function of age at injury. For example, memory difficulties were found to be more specific in adolescent patients (Levin, Eisenberg, et al., 1982, 1988). (It should be noted that this may reflect in part the normally late emergence of better articulated memory strategies. Young children thus would not demonstrate failure compared with same-age controls because they could not yet be expected to have skills in this area.) Frontal lobe skills may be discriminatively disturbed in children with severe injuries who were less than 10 years old at the time of injury (Levin et al., 1993). These children were found to produce more perseverative responses and to have greater difficulty on tests requiring the use of alternative strategies. They demonstrated decreased verbal fluency and poorer use of semantic strategies compared to same-age peers.

An associated, significant factor in understanding and predicting outcome in children of different ages at the time of injury is the epidemiology of head injury. Younger children are more likely to be injured in falls, whereas adolescents are more likely to be injured in high-acceleration motor vehicle accidents (Levin, Eisenberg, et al., 1982). It may be that the resulting injuries are different.

PATTERN AND TEMPO OF RECOVERY

Long-term, chronic deficits are an anticipated sequelae of moderate to severe head injury in children, but these children do demonstrate improvement and recovery over time. The level of deficit and the school needs of a child once he or she has left the acute care setting reflect the point in the recovery process when he or she is evaluated. Many studies have suggested that the vast majority of the recovery that will be seen is evident in the first 3 to 6 months postinjury (Chadwick, Rutter, Thompson, & Shaffer, 1981). There is subsequent ongoing recovery, but the pace is slower (Choi et al., 1994). It should be noted that teachers often describe increased difficulty over time (Rivara et al., 1993), which perhaps is secondary to delayed recognition of deficits or appears as expectations for the child become more stringent with increasing age or time since injury.

NONTRAUMA PROGNOSTIC VARIABLES

Premorbid Level of Function

Recent studies have used controls so as to not confound new versus long-term difficulties experienced by children or adolescents post–head injury. There is some reason to think that children who sustain head injuries are not a "typical" population. In a study of children with head injuries that were retrospectively identified, Greenspan and MacKenzie (1994) found that, 1 year prior to injury, these children were enrolled in special education classes at more than twice the national average. Brown, Chadwick, Shaffer, Rutter, and Traub (1981) found that children with mild to moderate head injury were more likely to show evidence of behavioral difficulties prior to their injury. These children can be expected to have increased disturbances subsequent to a moderate to severe head injury, and the debilitating effects (both cognitive and behavioral) may be potentiated by the underlying premorbid disturbance (Rivara et al., 1994).

Psychosocial Factors

As stated previously, a dose–response relationship between injury severity and outcome has been documented, but only a portion of the variation in functioning can be explained on this basis (Rivara et al., 1994). Child-related premorbid factors (intellectual ability, previously developed skills, psychological adjustment) likely play an important role. Another potential mediator of outcome is psychosocial functioning of the family (Brown et al., 1981; Fletcher, Ewing-Cobbs, Miner, Levin, & Eisenberg, 1990; Rivara et al., 1994).

Greenspan and MacKenzie (1994) found an association between poverty and poorer functional status 1 year postinjury, regardless of injury severity. Children from homes with fewer economic resources were more likely to demonstrate behavioral difficulties, to have ongoing health concerns, and to be enrolled in special education classes. Family functioning (e.g., the stability and strength of relationships), the level of stress, and the resources for coping with stress, in combination with the child's pre-injury status as well as severity of injury, appear to be potent predictors of a child's adaptive functioning post–severe head injury. Family functioning is most useful in the prediction of behavioral adjustment, particularly in children with moderate head injury (Rivara et al., 1993). Brown et al. (1981) found that the adjustment of children with severe brain injury seemed to reflect underlying neuropathology and was less contingent upon family functioning than that of children with moderate brain injury. Families described as less "rigid" appeared to adapt best to the demands of parenting a child with a brain injury and were most able to respond to the needs such children impose (Rivara et al., 1994).

MODERATE TO SEVERE HEAD INJURIES: LEVEL AND PATTERN OF FUNCTION

A description of the variables that contribute to outcome provides a basis for understanding brain injury recovery, but many questions still need to be asked:

What, in a general way, does one expect to see in children who sustain a moderate to severe head injury?

How do they function cognitively?

Do they progress academically?

Assuming the recovery of constant awareness and responsiveness, would such
children be expected to function autonomously?

How different are they likely to be from their same-age peers?

Motor impairment as a consequence of moderate to severe head injury is
generally one of the earlier and better resolving complications (Brink et al., 1970;
Rossman, 1994). Despite this, children with childhood brain injury have ongoing motor deficits that affect both gross- and fine-motor skills (Chaplin, Deitz,
& Jaffe, 1993). Although some children will have obvious disturbances (e.g., a
hemiparesis, spasticity, or significant ataxia), even those with less apparent difficulties tend to be different from their matched controls on tasks that emphasize
speed of movement or hand–eye coordination. The level of motor disturbance is
related to injury severity as manifested by length of coma (Brink et al., 1970).

Many studies of children with a head injury have reported the intellectual status of these children. Although average IQs were frequently reported,
the distribution was atypical, with more children performing at below-average
levels than anticipated, based on the normal distribution. This was true when
no controls were employed, leading to the question, Were the group of children in the study representative? However, this also occurred when matched
controls were used, suggesting that children who have sustained moderate to
severe head injury do sustain some loss of intellectual function.

In one of the earlier studies of IQ post–severe head injury (mean duration of
coma, 7 weeks), Brink et al. (1970) reported that 66% of this population was
functioning in the normal to borderline range of intellectual functioning 1 year
later. Wingron et al. (1984) reported mean Full Scale IQs of 94 and 82 in children with moderate and severe head injuries, respectively. Performance IQ (PIQ)
demonstrated a dose–response relationship, with PIQ poorer in the group with
severe injuries than in the group with moderate injuries. This pattern of greater
PIQ sensitivity to the debilitating effects of head injury has been reported by others (Chadwick et al., 1981). Levin, Eisenberg, et al. (1982) found age differences
in terms of intellectual performance post–head injury. Children with GCS scores
≤ 8 had mean Verbal IQs (VIQs) and PIQs of 90 and 87, respectively. Adolescents
had mean VIQs and PIQs of 98 and 105, respectively, when assessed subsequent
to injuries also producing GCS scores of ≤ 8. Although these average scores are
encouraging, it must be remembered that 33% of the children with severe head
injuries had VIQs below 80, and 40% had PIQs below 80, clearly an abnormal
and negatively skewed distribution. Fay et al. (1994) reported on children 3 years
post–head injury. They found VIQs, PIQs, and mean Full Scale IQs of 95, 94,
and 97, respectively, in children with a severe head injury. These scores were significantly different from the average scores of matched controls.

The degree of deficit evident in children who sustained a moderate to severe head injury was also apparent in studies that assessed subtle but clearly potent aspects of functioning. Speed of processing, particularly on tasks requiring greater cognitive analysis, was slower in these children than in matched controls (Fay et al., 1994) or less severely injured children (Bawden et al., 1985). Performance on tasks such as Coding was often overtly abnormal.

Basset and Slater (1990), Fay et al. (1994), Jaffe et al. (1993), and Levin, Eisenberg, et al. (1982, 1993) all reported memory problems in children with moderate to severe TBI. Levin et al. (1988) noted a dose–response relationship between injury severity and the level of memory disorder. Children with mild to moderate head injuries appeared to show relatively good recovery of memory skill (Levin et al., 1988) although this was not a consistent finding among researchers (Basset & Slater, 1990). Fay et al. (1994) found that, at 3 years postinjury, children who had suffered moderate head injury had impaired verbal memory as compared with matched controls.

The literature strongly suggests ongoing difficulties with new problem solving and adaptive capacity. Levin et al. (1993, 1994) identified specific difficulties with rule-based learning and decreased verbal fluency in youngsters with head injury, particularly those involving frontal lesions. Fay et al. (1994) found impoverished performance on the Trail Making and Category tests (Reitan & Davison, 1974), again suggestive of a disturbance in the ability to readily complete rule-based tasks, learn from experience, and adapt to new and variable situations.

Academic deficits have also been reported (Fay et al., 1994; Greenspan & MacKenzie, 1994). Fay et al. reported mean levels of performance to be within normal limits, but Greenspan and MacKenzie described an unusually high frequency of special education involvement: At 1 year postinjury, 30% of a group of children with head injuries required special education intervention. There was a dose–response relationship, with 78% of the children with the most severe injuries enrolled in special education.

Unfortunately, the degree of difference in academic performance between children with a head injury and their matched controls appears to increase over time (Fay et al., 1994). This is not interpreted as representing deterioration, but rather as reflecting the difficulty these youngsters have in adequately accommodating to the demand for increased facility or complexity.

Most of the just described findings have been identified only when comparing children with varying degrees of injury to one another or by comparing children with a head injury with matched, uninjured controls. Often, absolute performance of the "injured" group (or groups) was normal when compared with population means.

The quantitative extent of the deficits seen in children with moderate or severe TBI is often unremarkable and impressive in its suggestion of a good recovery. Unfortunately, the pervasiveness and consistency of the identified deficits is equally impressive, emphasizing the frequently debilitating effects of such injury on day-to-day performance. Although children with these injuries often perform adequately on standardized tests, comparisons with adequately composed control groups strongly suggest that, post-injury, children with moderate or severe TBI are different from their pre-morbid selves and from other children.

Although most children with a severe head injury will gain some level of responsiveness—and it is these children that are described in the previous paragraphs—there are children who remain in a persistent vegetative state. Such children do not evidence purposeful awareness of, nor psychological interaction with, their environment. They may have primitive, nonpurposeful reactions, including spontaneous eye opening, sleep–wake cycles, crying, chewing, or swallowing. In a follow-up study of such children, Fields, Coble, Pollack, Cuerdon, and Kaufman (1993) found that, after the first year at home, 10 of the 13 children followed were receiving special education services, occupational therapy, physical therapy, or speech therapy. Eight of the 10 children were receiving these services at school. This is a fairly rare occurrence, but schools do need to anticipate the possibility that they will be required to provide services to children who are entirely dependent, and are anticipated to remain dependent, as a consequence of severe head injuries.

From an education perspective, the behavioral problems reported to occur in youngsters who have sustained moderate to severe head injury are of great importance. Brown et al. (1981) found new psychiatric disorders to be two to three times more common in children with a severe head injury when compared with children with orthopedic difficulties or youngsters with mild head injury. Posttraumatic behavioral concerns commonly include increased aggressiveness, poor control of anger, increased activity, difficulties with sustained attention and concentration, and social isolation and inappropriate behaviors (Michaud, Rivara, Jaffe, Falte, & Dailey, 1993). Fletcher et al. (1990) found a weak association between cognitive and behavioral change in the long term, but Brown et al. (1981) reported that significant changes in cognitive function during the acute phases (suggestive of a more significant neurologic insult) were associated with long-term behavioral difficulties (e.g., there appeared to be a dose–response relationship between injury severity and behavioral changes; see Michaud et al., 1993).

Although a variety of behavioral problems have been reported in children with histories of moderate to severe head injury, these children are best typified as evidencing a disturbance in "executive functions," or those skills that in adults are thought to be mediated by the frontal lobes. As a group, youngsters with moderate to severe TBI experience greater difficulty in self-observation and modulating affect (Filley, Cranberg, Alexander, & Hart, 1987), focusing on pertinent and relevant information while ignoring equally compelling but less salient stimuli, evaluating the adequacy of their own responses, and learning from experience. They tend to be impulsive and have poor judgment.

The generally consistent evidence of a dose–response relationship between moderate to severe head injury and behavioral outcome emphasizes the "organic" nature of these behavioral disturbances. Poorer behavioral outcome is associated with more significant structural change as evidenced on a CT scan (Filley et al., 1987). It is also true, however, that the premorbid adjustment of the child, and of the family, exerts a moderating influence and should be considered in assessing etiology and in treatment planning (Brown et al., 1981; Rivara et al., 1994). Brown et al. (1981) did not find the persistence of behavioral symptoms to discriminate behavioral dysfunction related to a head injury from psychiatric symptoms thought to be unrelated to the injury.

Group data are useful in helping us to anticipate and understand specific pathologies, but they are limited in the ability to help us plan for individual children (Fay et al., 1994). Assessing a child subsequent to a head injury requires evaluating him or her as a unique individual. Knowing what is "expectable" should assist us in: (a) not attributing deficits to a head injury that are unlikely to have been caused by that injury, and (b) establishing rational goals. Because the varying consequences of moderate to severe injury can be best understood in the context of specific children, I have included several case studies here.

Case Example 1: S. W.

S.W. was a 9-year-old male who was injured in an automobile–pedestrian accident. At the scene he was unresponsive, with decerebrate posturing. Evaluation in the emergency room revealed multisystem involvement, and S.W.'s family was given a very guarded prognosis. An MRI scan of the brain revealed cerebral swelling and bilateral frontal, right parieteal, and cerebellar hemorrhages. He was taken to the intensive care unit, pharmacologically paralyzed, and placed on a respirator to control intracranial pressure. His initial pressure was between 50mm and 60mm Hg, which is high. His stay in the intensive care unit was notable for ongoing difficulty in managing his intracranial pressure, with frequent spikes to between 30mm and 40mm Hg. By Day 10 postinjury, S.W. had been successfully taken off the respirator and transferred to the pediatric ward. He was ambulating without difficulty, although the physical therapist noted poor judgment regarding attention to danger. S.W. was independent for activities of daily life, and he was talking and responsive. During an interview on Day 13 postinjury, S.W. was noted to be oriented to person but not to place or time. Total score on the Children's Orientation and Amnesia Test was 88 (the average for his age group = 115, standard deviation = 6). He knew he was in the hospital, but not which hospital, and he did not know the year, month, season, or time of day. He had apparent ongoing posttraumatic amnesia, being unable to remember who had come to visit.

Pre-accident history was significant for S.W.—his mother's pregnancy had only lasted 32 weeks—and he had required 2 months in the newborn intensive care unit. Early development was described as unremarkable. S.W. had recently completed the third grade. He had not been placed in special education, but he had been in a special tutoring program in math and reading. As early as first grade there had been concerns regarding S.W.'s attention. No social difficulties were reported. S.W.'s family denied specific behavioral concerns, although they did note that he had been in trouble at school for fighting. In addition, there had been substantial family stress, as S.W.'s father had moved in and out of the home.

S.W. was discharged from the hospital 14 days postinjury. He continued to be disorganized, confused, and mildly amnesiac. Occupational and physical therapies were discontinued prior to discharge, as he had no identified needs in these areas. On testing completed just prior to discharge, S.W. had a Verbal IQ of 70, a Performance IQ of 70, and a Full-Scale IQ of 68. His academic testing revealed better functioning, with reading skills at a solid third-grade level.

S.W.'s injury was clearly quite serious. Initial GCS was 2 (1 eye opening and 1 best motor response; best verbal response could not be assessed because S.W. was on a respirator and could not speak around the tube). His GCS remained below 8 until 6 days postaccident. Strikingly, by Day 13 postaccident, S.W. remained disoriented, as assessed by the COAT. He displayed a number of symptoms that were disconcerting and suggestive of poorer outcome. Specifically, medical staff had difficulty in maintaining normal intracranial pressure, and there was accompanying compromised cerebral blood flow. He sustained bleeding into brain tissue and had focal damage to both frontal lobes, which is consistent with long-term difficulties in response inhibition, planning, and flexibility in thinking. In addition, his premorbid history was significant for the suggestion of both behavioral and learning needs, and he had a newborn history often associated with learning difficulties. The family also had chronic social problems. Thus, S.W.'s prognosis for good school adjustment is poor.

Follow-Up. S.W. was seen for repeat evaluation at 1 year postaccident. He had recently had an MRI scan that revealed bifrontal changes in the brain with evidence that cortex had been damaged and replaced by scar tissue. When S.W. returned to school 10 months prior to evaluation, he was initially placed in a general education classroom without additional supports. Both social and academic difficulties occurred, and he was placed in a multi-age classroom with learning disability resource support. S.W. was described by his mother as "goofy," with a tendency to engage in inappropriate discussions. Children who had been friends began avoiding him. Memory problems were described, specifically, difficulty remembering what he had been told to do. S.W. was scheduled to enter fifth grade shortly after this follow-up exam.

At the time of this assessment, S.W. appeared to be a small, attractive young boy without external evidence of his significant injury. He appeared agitated, moving constantly, touching things, and standing up without any apparent reason. He was not oppositional and could be redirected. His thinking was disorganized and confused; for example, he thought that a "surprise box" from which he wished to take home a large stuffed bear dressed as a football player might be hidden behind a wall clock. He often would begin a task and then lost track of what he was doing. For example, he began copying a figure as directed but halfway through started coloring his copy.

S.W.'s evaluation demonstrated significant, ongoing difficulties. He had a Verbal IQ of 74 and a Performance IQ of 81 on the Wechsler Intelligence Scale for Children–Third Edition (WISC-III; Wechsler, 1991) evidencing improvement in problem solving, which was consistent with a resolving head injury. The lack of change in verbal skill suggested that S.W. might have had premorbid deficits that contributed to his lack of improvement in this area, a finding corroborated by school personnel, who described pre-accident language difficulties. Academically, S.W. had made minimal growth over the preceding year—failing to add reading or math skills and showing only limited improvement in spelling skills.

Although S.W. had no overt hemiparesis, specific motor assessment revealed left-sided slowing, a functional concern in this left-handed child. No specific sensory deficits were identified.

S.W. had intact understanding of language, but he displayed expressive difficulties consistent with the frontal damage seen on the MRI scan, and qualitative frontal disinhibition. S.W. could recognize objects without difficulty and showed no specific spatial confusion. However, he displayed substantial confusion when copying a complex figure and was unable to arrange details in an organized fashion.

S.W. required specific, ongoing instruction and reminders to follow rules. He was slow to learn a new, unique response mode. He was able to complete only four categories (out of six) on the Wisconsin Card Sorting Test, making numerous perseverations (repeating the same error despite being told he was wrong). On a continuous performance measure, S.W. demonstrated normal accuracy, but this was accomplished by slowing his response time, and the variability of his speed of responses was unusually high.

S.W. slowly acquired new verbal information on the California Verbal Learning Test (Delis, Kramer, Kaplan, & Ober, 1994). His learning curve was inconsistent and flat, but he did not forget at an unusually rapid rate. S.W.'s disturbance represents poor ability to encode (e.g., put memories into storage). Not only could he not spontaneously recall information, he also could not recognize it. S.W.'s lack of self-monitoring and his disorganization were striking. He "recalled" words that were never presented to him and seemed unaware and unperturbed that he was recalling items that were semantically discrepant from what he actually had been told.

S.W.'s mother completed the Child Behavior Checklist (Achenbach, 1991). She described S.W. as a child with substantial difficulties attending to important stimuli, as well as a tendency to engage in odd behaviors. She endorsed items seen in other children with aggressive, acting-out behavior.

Although S.W. has had a "good" recovery (e.g., he is ambulatory, independent for self-care, and able to engage in age-appropriate activities), he clearly has substantial and debilitating deficits that will have an impact on his school functioning. He does not meet standard definitions for a learning disability (his intellectual performance and achievement are consistent), but he is having, and will continue to have, problems in acquiring basic academic skills. He demonstrates behavioral and thinking problems related to his frontal lobe damage. Given that he is 1 year postinjury, and that there is evidence of changes in brain structure, little spontaneous recovery is anticipated. Rehabilitation strategies emphasizing careful structuring of the environment to assist S.W. in organization and self-monitoring will be useful, and compensatory strategies should be emphasized. Both the family and the school should be given information regarding S.W.'s cognitive and perceptual needs, as well as support for behavior management techniques.

Case Example 2: D.X.

D.X., a boy 6 years 11 months in age, was seen for assessment approximately 10 days post–head injury. He was hit in the head by a foul ball at a baseball game. D.X. sustained an immediate, brief loss of consciousness but then began crying. He remained responsive for the next 20 minutes but began vomiting and became less responsive. He was brought to the hospital via ambulance, sedated, intubated, and hyperventilated to control intracranial pressure. His GCS score upon admission was 10. Imaging studies demonstrated a left temporal contusion. He was rapidly extubated and showed good resolution of his depressed level of consciousness. D.X. was discharged 5 days postinjury; at that time, he had word-finding problems and difficulty remembering verbal information over a 5-minute interval. He had no demonstrable motor abnormalities.

D.X.'s premorbid history was unremarkable. His mother had a normal, full-term pregnancy, labor, and delivery. He had had no prior significant illnesses or any hospitalizations. His early development was reported to have been normal. At the time of his injury, D.X. had just begun attending first grade. He had attended an academically oriented kindergarten and entered first grade reading and writing at a level that his first grade teacher considered to have been above average. D.X. lives with his mother and father. They indicated that there had not been any premorbid social or behavioral concerns.

In assessment, D.X. presented as a vivacious, engaging youngster who expressed a sense of confidence about his skills. At times, he was overly intrusive in his questions—not rude, but inappropriately familiar in a new environment with strangers. He had frequent difficulty in recalling specific words, which was consistent with the focality of his injury. D.X. had a hard time attending to tasks, tending to change the subject or ask irrelevant questions.

D.X.'s evaluation, which was done during an early stage of his recovery, indicated some abnormalities. Generally, the level of his performance was normal (i.e., he successfully completed as many items as most other children his age); however, the pattern of his performance was unusual. It suggested that his skills at the point of his assessment were adequate, but his current performance represented a decrement from his premorbid status.

Specifically, D.X. had academic skills that were well above grade level, consistently 2 standard deviations above the mean. In contrast, his Performance IQ, although normal, was slightly below average (WISC-III Performance IQ was 95). As is often seen post–head injury, the ability to solve new and unique problems, as measured by Performance IQ, was poorer than his Verbal IQ score (WISC-III Verbal IQ was 107). That this was true despite D.X.'s clear, specific acquired language difficulties (e.g., aphasia) emphasized that this current performance represented a decremental change in skill.

D.X.'s receptive language was unremarkable. Expressively he had a mild repetition disturbance and a clear dysnomia (word-finding difficulty). He could not think of the words "fireman" ("the water guys") or "volcano" ("a hot lava"). He was able to learn new information without difficulty but could not retrieve that information when he was not focusing on it (e.g., he lost information unusually fast). He remembered only what was within his span of attention. D.X. also had difficulties with recognizing previously presented information.

D.X. had clear difficulties following a recent head injury of moderate severity. He had deficits that were specifically associated with an area of damage to the left temporal lobe, a language disturbance (aphasia), and a memory disorder. He had difficulties that may be related to the more diffuse effects of his injury (e.g., greater difficulty with new problem solving and increased implusiveness). He was followed up very shortly after the injury, and it is anticipated that D.X. will show ongoing recovery, although long-term sequelae are anticipated due to the specificity of his deficits and the degree of measurable injury.

Case Example 3: A.B.

A.B. was 14 years 2 months of age at the time of his evaluation, which occurred approximately 7 1/2 years after a severe head injury sustained during a motor vehicle accident. A.B. was in a coma for 4 weeks immediately after his injury. His records indicated that an initial CT scan revealed a fracture on the left side of his skull, with a deep right-temporal intracerebral hemorrhage. He had also sustained a posterior fossa hemorrhage. An MRI scan done 10 days later revealed bilateral posterior hemorrhages. A.B. had had left-sided seizures that began approximately 10 days after the accident and continued. They did not respond to treatment. He also had a left hemiparesis and a left homonymous hemianopsia (he could not see in the left visual field). Initially, he was discharged from the acute-care hospital to a rehabilitation hospital. At that time he was independent for most activities of daily living and was talking but not walking (secondary to a broken hip). He remained at the rehabilitation hospital for 3 months. He quickly regained reading and spelling skills during this period and returned to school upon his discharge.

A.B.'s mother had had a normal, full-term pregnancy, labor, and delivery. A.B. had had no significant illness, and no hospitalizations prior to his injury. He was taking Neurontin® and Depakote® at the time of his evaluation, but he had ongoing, although infrequent, seizures.

A.B.'s early development was reported to have been within normal limits. Early school records revealed that he had been performing exceptionally well prior to the accident, with achievement on standardized tests at the 95th to 98th percentiles in all domains.

At the time of his evaluation, A.B. lived with his father, stepmother, sister, and two stepsisters. (His mother had died in the accident in which A.B. was injured.) He was enrolled in the eighth grade and received resource room assistance about half time.

Current concerns included A.B.'s difficulty in remembering new information, his lack of initiation of activities, apathy, slow speech, and decreased social interaction. He tended to repeat the same comment perseveratively.

A.B. presented as a polite, attentive young man who, after a brief break in the assessment procedure, did not recognize the examiner, confusing her with another woman with short hair. He tended to discount his problems, explaining his visual-field defect by noting that his eyes were blurry. He expected the examiner to be familiar with situations and settings that she clearly could not be expected to know, for example, the house around the corner from his family's. He was fully cooperative and he interacted well with the examiners.

A.B.'s performance demonstrated the devastating nature of his head injury. Although his IQs just after the accident were in the low-normal range, demonstrating his ability when he could rely on old, overlearned skills, his performance on this evaluation was in the clearly impaired range, with a striking disturbance in visual–spatial skills related to his right hemisphere hemorrhage. A.B. had a VIQ of 74 and a PIQ of 48.

Although language was an area of strength for A.B., he had readily apparent difficulties in this area. For example, he had difficulty retrieving the names of objects, with skills at the 6- to 7-year-old level. He had no receptive language disturbance.

A.B. appeared to have a mild visual agnosia (i.e., he could perceive and describe what he was seeing but could not always ascertain the meaning of what he was viewing). He had problems in organizing details within space and could not get the parts of a complicated figure in appropriate relationship to one another, although he did relatively well recognizing the individual parts. A.B. was performing well academically. His reading recognition skills, which were good, were at the sixth-grade level. His reading comprehension skills were at the late third-grade level. Not surprisingly, given A.B.'s relatively stronger language skills, his spelling was at the late eighth-grade level. In contrast, A.B.'s arithmetic skills were more consistently limited, being at the third-grade level.

A.B. had profound verbal and visual memory disorders. He not only could not retrieve information, but also had difficulty recognizing information to which he had been previously exposed. He learned new verbal information slowly and forgot what he had acquired unusually quickly. During learning trials, he seemed to learn only what was within his span of attention—what he was exposed to most recently. His memory disorder was disproportionately large and suggested a specific amnesia.

A.B. had trouble solving new problems. It was difficult for him to change his strategy for solving a problem even when it was made clear to him that he was being unsuccessful. He tended to perseverate on a response set that was not allowing him to reach a stated goal.

A.B. had consistent left-sided manual motor difficulties. He also was slow on his right side, although the deficit was less. He thus had bilateral motor difficulties, with the left greater than the right. In addition to his left visual-field defect, A.B. also had left-sided auditory and tactile suppressions: He tended to neglect and ignore stimuli on the left.

A.B.'s assessment results, as well as his parents' description of his behavior, indicated that he had sustained a significant derangement of skills as a consequence of his injury. Now at 7 years postinjury, A.B. is unlikely to show significant functional improvement in those identified deficits. His verbal overlearned skills are basically intact, although his impoverished memory has not allowed him to learn new age-appropriate verbal information. He has both diffuse difficulties and a disturbance attributable to his right hemisphere hemorrhage. Specifically, he has difficulties in left-sided motor and sensory functioning, a lack of awareness of his own deficits, and a problem in making sense of visual information, contributing to an arithmetic disturbance. A.B.'s social isolation is not surprising, given his difficulties in understanding and responding to unique situations, in changing his responses if they are inadequate, and in maintaining a continuous memory of ongoing events.

A.B. will be limited in terms of living situations and employment. Safety issues secondary to his left-sided neglect need to be considered. A functionally based school and vocational curriculum, as well as a program aimed at learning specific, functionally important verbal information was recommended. Development of recreational activities in which A.B. can be successful was suggested.

SUMMARY

The three children just described in the case examples, none of whom is atypical of those with moderate to severe head injuries, will clearly require long-term monitoring and school intervention. Like others who sustain damage to the brain, these children—one acutely injured with the expectation of resolution of some symptoms; one demonstrating some, but not complete, recovery and resolution; and one evidencing stable deficits—have dramatically changed functioning with alterations in perception, cognition, and behavior. School intervention, as well as environmental changes, will be required for optimum independence and adjustment.

Schools must be prepared for the return and ongoing education of children with moderate to severe brain injury. Current literature suggests these children will probably have difficult-to-measure, but substantial, changes in functioning and will require the coordinated, concerted efforts of numerous school personnel—including special educators, psychologists, physical and occupational therapists, speech–language therapists, and social workers—as well as their families. School programming should address the specific needs of each child, with attention to premorbid factors, injury severity and focality, ongoing medical issues (e.g., seizures), time since injury, and family resources. Current evaluation results, combined with consideration of peri-injury variables predictive of future problems, should be considered in order to establish achievable, realistic goals.

6. Neuropsychological Consequences of Traumatic Brain Injury in Children and Adolescents

JANIECE LORD-MAES AND JOHN E. OBRZUT

Injury to the head is one of the leading causes of disability in the industrialized nations (Johnson, 1992) and a significant cause of death and disability among children and adolescents in the United States (Goldstein & Levin, 1991). Martin (1988) estimated that each year 1 million children experience sustained closed-head injuries. A plethora of research on TBI has escalated in an attempt to understand the full ramifications of cerebral insult. Depth and duration of consciousness and age at the time of injury are factors in neurodiagnostic and neuroprognostic decisions regarding recovery and ultimate outcomes of head injury. Age of onset, for example, can significantly alter the course of growth, and qualitative differences can be found not only between children and adults but between adolescent and preadolescent youth with TBI.

Parents, relatives, or teachers may not fully appreciate the impact of head injury on cognition or on the student's performance in the academic setting. Frequently, a child's physical recovery from closed-head injury creates expectations for adequate cognitive and behavioral functioning in parents, and teachers. However, a normal physical appearance can mask underlying cognitive deficits (Johnson, 1992). Various neuropsychological measures are increasingly identifying more specific cognitive dysfunction following brain injury (see Bigler, 1988, 1992; Obrzut & Hynd, 1987; and Farmer &

Peterson, 1995, for reviews). Katz, Goldstein, Rudisin, and Bailey (1993) stated that "neuropsychological assessment has proved to be a way of examining the cognitive structure" and has "the capability of identifying the strengths and weaknesses in cognitive function" (p. 65). Insight regarding injury to the cortical and subcortical structures is being obtained from a wide variety of scientific disciplines, such as neurology, behavioral medicine, psychiatry, psychology, and neuropsychology. From such multivaried databases, clearer patterns have emerged in the identification of brain–process relationships. Recent findings related to hemisphere specialization (i.e., laterality), behavioral correlates of focal damage, and behavioral sequelae of cognitive dysfunction resulting from TBI have added much to our knowledge base.

The intent of this chapter is to address the advances derived from the study of neuropsychology and the associated neuroscientific information related to cognitive function and dysfunction in school-age children and adolescents (6 to 18 years of age) who have experienced some form of TBI. Developments in assessment for individuals with acquired cerebral trauma as well as implications for learning and the cognitive sequelae will be included.

BEHAVIORAL AND COGNITIVE OUTCOMES WITH TBI

Recent advancements in noninvasive imaging techniques such as X-ray computed tomography (CT) scans, position emission tomography (PET) scans, and magnetic resonance imaging (MRI; Jaffee, 1982; Martin & Brust, 1985) have provided a quantitative electrodiagnostic picture of the brain (John, 1986; John, Princhep, Eastman, Friedman, & Kaye, 1983). Bigler (1988) contended that this advancement in technology relative to brain imaging (anatomy and function) has allowed some delineation of structural effects following TBI. Consequently, steady improvements in the medical management of brain-injured children have occurred.

Correlational studies using MRIs of individuals with TBI have demonstrated an association with cognitive performance. For example, MRIs have documented localization of lesion (Levin et al., 1993; Wilson, Teasdale, Hadley, Wiedmann, & Lang, 1994), and associations with specific language impairments (Chapman et al., 1992) and depth and location of lesion in relation to hemispheric disconnection effects (Levin et al., 1989).

Although technological advancements have provided new information about brain structure and function with adult samples, the absence of demonstrable changes is common on CT scans of children with head injury (Johnson, 1992). However, the lack of such evidence should not lead to the assumption that there is no brain damage, because behavioral differences and cognitive changes in postmorbid functioning have been documented in cognitive and neuropsychological assessments of children with TBI (see Dalby & Obrzut, 1991).

From a less structural point of view, TBI has been found to be associated with a variety of neuropsychological outcomes in children, including poor performance on speeded tasks, memory impairment, decreased recall, and difficulties in processing novel or complex visual–spatial stimuli (Dalby & Obrzut, 1991; Ewing-Cobbs, Fletcher, & Levin, 1986; Lehr, 1990; Reeder & Logue, 1994). More recently, 5- to 16-year-old patients have been found to display inadequate perceptual processing (Mattson, Levin, & Breitmeyer, 1994), with specific impairment of visual memory (Levin et al., 1994a). A strong relationship was found among declines in adaptive functioning, measures of intelligence, motor and language abilities, and the extent of severity of head injury (impaired consciousness for a 24-hour minimum). In addition, motor and expressive language functions were compromised the most from head injury in 4-month-old to 5-year-old children, regardless of the severity of injury (Ewing-Cobbs, Miner, Fletcher, & Levin, 1989). Other studies with children who have sustained TBI have also indicated such outcomes as speech and language deficits that result in communication disorders (Szekeres & Meserve, 1994; Ylvisaker & Feeney, 1994).

AGE DIFFERENCES WITH TBI

Age differences have been recognized as an important variable in studies investigating the behavioral sequelae that follow TBI. The measurable cognitive outcomes of TBI are often different for a child when compared with those of adolescents or adults. The brain injury sustained by a child occurs concurrently with development and thus may create an incomplete collection of abilities (Brazzelli, Colombo, Della Sala, & Spinnier, 1994; Johnson, 1992; Levin, 1991; Segalowitz & Brown, 1991).

Segalowitz and Brown (1991) reviewed cognitive differences among high school youth with TBI and pointed out the significance of age at time of injury. Over 60% of the student body responding to the survey had experienced a head injury at an early age (average age = 9 years). The age at injury and the length of unconsciousness as a result of the injury correlated inversely; more boys than girls experienced both head injury and unconsciousness. More specifically, the "age of injury and years since injury both correlated with the ranking of mathematics" (p. 554); the earlier the injury, the lower the preference for mathematics. Interestingly, Segalowitz and

Brown used only cases in which injury occurred after the age of 1. Their decision was based on earlier reported findings (Huttenlocher, 1990) indicating that there was a radical difference in the processes of recovery after this age. Segalowitz and Brown also found a significant relationship between the incidence of head injury and several developmental factors, such as hyperactivity, stuttering, and mixed-handedness. A greater likelihood of mixed-handedness, as opposed to consistent left- or right-handedness, especially for boys, was found to correlate with closed-head injury, $p < .01$, and with duration of unconsciousness, $p < .002$. Evidence also supported the relationship of hyperactivity and stuttering to the occurrence of head injury (but not with each other). Thus, Segalowitz and Brown concluded that the head injury incidence found in their study was "high enough to be considered as a factor in developmental disabilities, especially those related to hyperactivity and stuttering" (p. 556).

A significant difference in receptive language function was demonstrated between infants (less than 3 months old) and toddlers (Ewing-Cobbs et al., 1989). Those who sustained TBI during infancy had greater difficulty developing receptive and expressive language, whereas those who sustained TBI as toddlers showed a better improvement rate in receptive language. Age differences also were shown in the recovery of writing skills between preadolescents and adolescents, all with TBI: The preadolescents did not recover as quickly as the adolescents (Ewing-Cobbs, Levin, Eisenberg, & Fletcher, 1987).

Slower recovery on specific cognitive tasks (motor and visual–spatial) has recently been found with younger adolescents than with older adolescents who experienced a similar degree of severe head injury (Thompson, Francis, Steubing, & Fletcher, 1994). Furthermore, Thompson et al. investigated the change in factors affecting recovery following head injury in children through adolescence. An analysis of repeated neuropsychological assessments of motor, visual–spatial, and somatosensory skills revealed that younger children with severe injuries recovered slower than not only older children with similar injuries, but also than children of the same age with milder head injuries. Thus support was given to the belief that there is increased vulnerability of rapidly emerging skills in young children. From this research, it seems that neurological development continues until at least 12 years of age, and that the frontal lobes are the last neurological structures to mature, around the 12- to 14-year age period.

In other work, the severity of pediatric closed-head injury and age of the affected child were found to be strongly associated with cognitive performance as measured on the Tower of London task (Levin et al., 1994b). Likewise, performance on a visual–motor task significantly improved with age in children with closed-head injury (Levin et al., 1994a), and a marked deficit in performance on a test for attentional functioning was found in younger children when compared with adolescents, 6 months postinjury (Kaufman, Fletcher, Levin, Miner, & Ewing-Cobbs, 1993).

Johnson's (1992) research concerning children with head injury who later return to school suggested that head injuries may have long-term effects, (e.g., memory and language deficits) not readily apparent in the acute stage. Children may present severe learning difficulties years later, when the injury has been forgotten or discounted. The simple act of returning to school is not an acceptable index for recovery.

Verduyn, Hilt, Roberts, and Roberts (1992) described 17 subjects who had experienced cerebral damage. The subjects developed multiple partial seizure (MPS)–like symptoms subsequent to a closed-head injury. Neurobehavioral disorders were described in the context of dysphoric mood, aggressive outbursts, and affective lability. The most frequently endorsed symptoms were brief memory gaps, subjective mental decline, word-finding lapses, episodic complaints, severe headaches, confusional spells, the illusion of involvement in peripheral vision, temper outburst, pain, and dysphoria. It became exceedingly difficult for families to cope with the individuals' unpredictable affective episodes.

As with many studies of individuals who have sustained head injury, the behavioral outcomes described in Verduyn et al.'s (1992) study failed to show a consistent pattern of depressed overall intellectual capacity, yet evidence of perceptual/cognitive dysfunction was revealed on neuropsychological testing. Individuals in their study displayed an average intellectual range with severe attentional dysfunction, memory impairment, and some degree of impairment on tests presumably measuring frontal-lobe function (Controlled One Word Association and Design Fluency). Deficits in attention (Goodyear & Hynd, 1992; Kaufman et al., 1993; Murray, Shum, & McFarland, 1992; Wood, 1989), memory (Meyers & Levin, 1992) and language impairments (Brazzelli et al., 1994; Chapman et al., 1992), and evidence of frontal lobe dysfunction (Hebb, 1949; Kelly, Best, & Kirk, 1989; Levin, 1991; Mattson & Levin, 1990; Shue & Douglas, 1992; Vikki & Holst, 1989; Villa, Gainotti, DeBonis, & Marra, 1990) have been reported frequently in subjects who have suffered a minor closed-head injury (e.g., due to motor vehicle accidents, school fights, physical abuse, pedestrian car accidents). Comparatively speaking, these cognitive dysfunctions also have been reported by individuals diagnosed with attention-deficit/hyperactivity disorder (ADHD; Goodyear & Hynd, 1992; Kaufman et al., 1993) and learning disabilities (LD; Arffa, Fitzhugh-Bell, & Black, 1989; Gaddes & Edgell, 1994; Kupfermann, 1985; Obrzut & Hynd, 1983; Selz & Reitan, 1979; Williams, Gridley, & Fitzhugh-Bell, 1992).

LEARNING DISORDERS AND BRAIN DYSFUNCTION

Cognitive dysfunctions identified among individuals who experience LD are closely aligned with the cognitive outcomes found in many individuals with brain damage. Earlier reviews describe evidence supporting the relationship between brain dysfunction and LD (see Obrzut & Hynd, 1987; Rourke, 1987). Such evidence originated from research on subtypes of children who experience specific LD. However, because there has been a continued lack of consensus on the etiological issues of learning problems, some researchers have continued to further investigate specific subtypes of LD in relation to brain dysfunction.

Arffa et al. (1989) recently utilized cluster analyses to identify subtypes of LD in children who had sustained brain injury. Of the five clusters, no single one identified subjects who experienced LD or brain damage exclusively, although quantitative and qualitative differences were found between clusters. For example, in contrast to Cluster I (identifying half of the subjects with LD and two thirds of those with brain trauma), Cluster II (consisting mainly of subjects with brain trauma) displayed considerably depressed scores in visual processing, conceptual reasoning, and spatial skills; these appeared as relative strengths in Cluster I. Cluster III (comprising a greater portion of subjects with LD) demonstrated a measured outcome of advanced strength for motor skills, with deficits in auditory sequencing, tactile perception, and visual–conceptual skills. These results indicated that subjects who experienced LD and brain trauma demonstrated many functional similarities across clusters, and, by inference, suggest similarities in functional neuropsychological organization.

More recently, a cluster analysis was conducted with children and adolescents who had sustained injury to the brain (Williams et al., 1992). Four interpretable clusters emerged. The first contained those individuals who performed within normal limits on all measures and demonstrated strong nonverbal and spatial skills relative to the other clusters. The second cluster was composed of those who demonstrated higher verbal skills relative to nonverbal skills, relatively poor arithmetic scores, marked motor and sensory deficits, and behavior within normal limits. The third cluster consisted of those individuals who had a higher percentage of documented brain damage; in addition, their inattentiveness scores were clinically elevated. The fourth cluster contained individuals who had the poorest Full Scale IQs, Verbal IQs, and achievement scores, along with clinically significant behavior problems on three of the four factors of the Conners Behavior Rating Scale (CBRS; Conners, 1973). The emerging four clusters did not identify either subject group exclusively, although outcomes from intellectual, neuropsychological, and behavioral testing displayed patterns of similarity between the groups. Williams et al. found similar patterns of performance between subjects with LD and subjects with hard neurological signs. They interpreted this as a parallel between cognitive functions and possible underlying cerebral structure. Results from the study provided support for the idea of a parallel existence of cerebral function and/or structure between subjects who experience LD and those who have sustained brain injury.

Regarding the addition in the Williams et al. (1992) study of the CBRS as a measure of socioemotional functioning, the findings showed that 51% of the subjects scored within normal limits when the CBRS was included in the first analysis. In the second analysis, which did not include a socioemotional variable, 65% of the subjects scored within normal limits. These findings suggest that the addition of behavioral information contributes to a further delineation of subgroups within TBI and LD populations. Such information could, in turn, significantly influence behavioral management of subgroups of children with TBI. These results are comparable to those of previous work using cluster analysis, and they support empirical studies that have evidenced an elevated frequency of emotional disorders in subjects who have neuropsychological deficits (Fuerst, Fisk, & Rourke, 1989; Spreen, 1989).

Furthermore, two clusters found in the analysis with no socioemotional component provided differentiating characteristics between Verbal IQ and Performance IQ scores, as measured on the Wechsler Intelligence Scale for Children–Revised (WISC-R; Wechsler, 1974) and neuropsychological differences between clusters. Higher verbal skills and language abilities in one cluster were contrasted with higher performance skills and nonverbal abilities in a second cluster. These cognitive differences support earlier studies and may be related to functional hemispheric specialization.

HEMISPHERIC SPECIALIZATION WITH TBI

Functional asymmetries have been widely associated with hemispheric specialization in a normally developed cerebrum (Bradshaw & Nettleton, 1981; Geschwind, 1979; Obrzut, Hynd, Obrzut, & Pirozzolo, 1981). Although Obrzut (1987) contended that evidence has not proved an association between cognitive ability and laterality performance, he also believed it would be premature to entertain the notion that no such relationship exists. Recent studies continue to investigate the associations between functional asymmetries derived from cognitive deficits identified in subjects with left- or right-hemisphere lesions.

From a developmental perspective, Thal et al. (1991) studied lexical development in children younger than 3 years old. Results showed a heavy reliance on well-practiced but underanalyzed speech formulae in children with right-hemisphere damage (RHD). Greater delays in expressive language, and more protracted delays, were found in children with left-hemisphere damage (LHD), although the latter showed better comprehension than children with RHD.

Stiles and Nass (1991) examined spatial grouping ability in slightly older children, 3- to 5-year-olds with congenital focal brain injury. No difference was found in degree of active play among the subjects, although a systematic difference was found in the final construction. Subjects with RHD demonstrated a difference in ability to organize objects into coherent spatial groupings, whereas subjects with LHD demonstrated a significantly poorer performance in their ability with local relations within the spatial arrays. These results were interpreted as showing the occurrence of spatial integrative deficits in subjects with RHD and spatial encoding deficits in subjects with LHD. Another investigation found phonological aspects of language-processing deficits in 8- to 18-year-old children with left-hemisphere lesions, while visuospatial operations were unaffected. This suggests that phonological aspects of language continue to be predominantly mediated by the left hemisphere (Papanicolaou, DiScenna, Gillespie, & Aram, 1990).

Right-hemisphere injury is associated with a greater risk to overall intellectual development, especially if the injury occurs early in a child's development. Aram and Eisele (1994) tested 26 children (6 to 12 years old) with unilateral brain lesions and found that the right-lesioned subjects scored lower on an intelligence test than the left-lesioned subjects. Additionally, Eisele and Aram (1993) investigated the differential effects of early hemisphere damage on expressive and lexical comprehension measures in children with unilateral brain injury. The researchers found that subjects with left-hemisphere lesions performed comparably to control subjects on the lexical comprehension measure. Right-lesioned subjects, however, scored lower than either of the other two groups on both measures—expressive and lexical comprehension. The authors interpreted these results as support for a specialized role of the right hemisphere in acquisition of word meaning. However, when spontaneous conversational speech was compared in children with either left or right unilateral brain lesions, results showed the left-lesioned subjects to have a slower rate of speech.

Hom and Reitan (1982) studied lateralized cerebral lesions and concluded that there is right-hemispheric specialization for tactile–perceptual skills. However, in 1992, Reitan, Wolfson, and Hom presented new data supporting an equivalent dominance status for sensorimotor deficits. In essence, whereas the right hemisphere seems dominant for tactile–perceptual abilities, the left hemisphere functions more efficiently than the right when it is required to resist bilateral simultaneous stimulation. Reitan et al.'s data described for the first time a behavioral dimension, sensory–perceptual in nature as opposed to language, in which the left hemisphere seems to maintain dominance.

Hemispheric specialization of emotion and temperament also has been quantitatively studied in young preschool- and school-age children with brain damage, as well as in adolescents and adults, with parallel findings. From a developmental perspective, Nass and Koch (1987) explored right-hemisphere specialization for attention and emotion in 1- to 3-year-old toddlers. These authors demonstrated that cerebral asymmetries are discernible as early as the toddler years, and that the children with right-hemisphere damage demonstrated significantly more negative temperaments with respect to mood and rhythmicity.

RECENT DEVELOPMENTS IN TBI ASSESSMENT

A current popular approach to measuring the outcome status of TBI is the neuropsychological approach (Gaddes & Edgell, 1994; Johnson, 1992; Obrzut & Hynd, 1987; Williams et al., 1992). According to Obrzut and Hynd, assessment from a neuropsychological perspective is beneficial in the diagnosis of strengths and weaknesses, giving a broader knowledge base from which to interpret psychoeducational data and thereby elucidating more precisely the complexities of a brain–process relationship. Johnson (1992) further suggested that many cognitive functions from posttraumatic disturbances are not detected by routine clinical neurological examination and are more likely to be identified by neuropsychological assessment.

The challenge facing neuropsychologists working with individuals with TBI is to accurately predict the recovery of cognitive functioning. Empirical research has confirmed that neuropsychological tests and/or measures are valid predictors of cognitive outcome (Ewing-Cobbs & Fletcher, 1990; Obrzut & Hynd, 1987; Ylvisaker, Kolpan, & Rosenthal, 1994). For example, Karzmark (1992) reviewed a number of studies that examined the relationship of injury-related variables to long-term cognitive outcome as measured by neuropsychological tests. Results from these studies indicated that injury-related variables (e.g., posttraumatic amnesia [PTA]) may be robust predictors of outcome. However, Karzmark also found that cognitive variables had the same predictive strength as injury-related variables. Participants' performance on a brief cognitive evaluation conducted soon after they suffered a cerebral trauma was significantly predictive of global cognitive outcomes 6 to 7 months postinjury (Karzmark, 1992). In addition, the results confirmed the predictive validity of early cognitive tests for later memory performance.

Sherer, Parsons, Nixon, and Adams (1991) reviewed the clinical validity of the Speech Sounds Perception Test (SSPT) and Seashore Rhythm Test (SRT) of the Halstead Reitan Neuropsychological Test Battery (HRNB; Reitan & Wolfson, 1985). Although the SSPT is consistently endorsed as a measure of hemispheric laterality, Sherer et al.'s review found that the clinical validity of the SSPT is inconsistently supported by empirical studies. In addition, Sherer et al. indicated that their literature review failed to reveal a single empirical study supporting an association of SSPT and SRT with "alertness and concentration." They therefore conducted their own study to investigate SSPT's ability to discriminate between left- and right-sided brain damage, and whether the SSPT and SRT are related to, or are measures of, alertness and concentration. The findings supported the use of SSPT and SRT as general indicators of brain damage rather than as measures of lateralized functioning. Similarly, Sherer, Scott, Parsons, and Adams (1994) studied selected tests from HRNB and tested the relative sensitivity of the Wechsler Adult Intelligence Scale–Revised (WAIS-R; Wechsler, 1981) subtests in discriminating the effects of brain damage from no brain damage. Results indicated that both measures were equivalent in the subtests' ability to discriminate the groups; therefore, no support was given to the proposal that the WAIS-R had poorer sensitivity.

Neuropsychological assessment is often the approach employed to show long-term cognitive difficulties in children who have sustained a brain injury. Children/adolescents might appear to be physically unaffected but neuropsychological measures will display deficits in cognitive outcomes. The neuropsychological assessment of cognitive skills and performance abilities does not always take the form of a battery of combined tests with standardized norms, such as the HRNB. Often the assessments include an evaluation of deficits in intelligence, academic performance, adaptive problem solving, memory, speed or information processing, language, and perceptual–motor skills (Dalby & Obrzut, 1991; Farmer & Peterson, 1995).

The intellectual measures used are often one of the Wechsler scales (i.e., Wechsler, 1974, 1987). Wechsler's tests of intelligence are considered to be of great practical benefit relative to guiding the management of children with TBI if the results are utilized to generate hypotheses and are based on a broad factorial structure (Johnson, 1992). IQ scores can obscure a child's neuropsychological status or misrepresent the cognitive functions of the brain following TBI (Lezak, 1988). Several researchers suggest that children with TBI demonstrate lowered Wechsler Performance scores (Banich, Levine, Kim, & Huttenlocher, 1990; Farmer & Peterson, 1995; Johnson, 1992) without consideration of the multifactorial nature of the performance subtests. Johnson suggested that the Performance IQ score decrement could be due to a variety of other problems, such as speed of response, sequencing, perceptual planning, or abstract or meaningful analysis difficulties. Conversely, many children with TBI could perform adequately on standard IQ tests despite residual weaknesses in cognitive domains, such as attention, memory, and executive functions (Ewing-Cobbs & Fletcher, 1990). Thus, the head injury may be subtle but significant for the affected child. Intellectual measures can be sensitive to TBI and show a decline in cognitive abilities. Children with a head injury may show an average IQ profile, which masks other specific cognitive weaknesses (Ewing-Cobbs & Fletcher, 1990).

Banich et al. (1990) provided preliminary longitudinal data to suggest a "fall off" in IQ directly related to the degree of neurological problems in children with acquired or congenital unilateral brain lesions. The effects of unilateral lesions on subsequent intellectual functioning was shown to have differential effects depending on the age at time of injury: Subjects with pre- or perinatal unilateral brain lesions had lower IQs, associated with elapsed time since injury. Infants who sustained brain damage after birth had lowered IQs more closely associated with lesion size. Aram and Eisele (1994) also reported on the intellectual stability of 26 children and adolescents following unilateral hemispheric damage. Subjects were administered the Wechsler intelligence scales at two points in time. These authors found that left-lesioned subjects exhibited no difference across time among the three IQ scores (Verbal, Performance, and Full Scale), whereas right-lesioned subjects exhibited noticeable decreases in each of the three IQ measures across Time 1 and Time 2 testing. Overall, there was tentative support for "verbal sparing" (p. 93), poorer development of certain intellectual functions following right-hemisphere damage, and a documented stable pattern of intellectual performance over time in children with acquired (or congenital) unilateral lesions.

The disturbance of memory is a common cognitive outcome of closed-head injury. Lewin (1968) asserted that memory impairment is the most significant area of difficulty for remediation in closed-head injury. Therefore, accurate identification of specific memory impairments becomes essential. Preliminary studies with the Wechsler Memory Scale–Revised (WMS-R; Wechsler, 1987) have shown encouraging results with adolescents with head injury.

Along this line, Reid and Kelly (1993) assessed the validity of the WMS-R with a sample that included control participants and older adolescents who had recently sustained a head injury. The relationship between the participants' performance on the WMS-R and severity of injury and day-to-day memory performance was evaluated. Results showed that the subjects with closed-head injury performed consistently in the impaired range on all five WMS-R indices. Given the changes in the WMS revised edition, memory can now be examined from a multifactorial perspective. Thus, close scrutiny of the data revealed specific deficits in memory processes. For example, particular difficulty in the *delayed memory* component was found, as were significant discrepancies among specific component scores, suggesting that the WMS-R is potentially useful for treatment planning with older adolescents who have sustained a head injury (Reid & Kelly, 1993).

WECHSLER SCALE CLASSIFICATION WITH TBI

In terms of diagnostic classification of brain injury, a unique subtest pattern formulated from scores on the WAIS was found to be related to left temporal lobe damage (Dobbins & Russell, 1990). However, in an attempt to improve the predictive power of this established index, Russell and Russell (1993) added Digit Span (DS) to the subtest pattern. The subtest pattern was then placed into the following formula:

$$(V + I)/2 - (D+S)/2 < 0 = LTD,$$

where V = Vocabulary, I = Information, D = Digit Span, S = Similarities, and LTD = left temporal lobe damage. As predicted, the results supported the validity of the index for LTD; and the addition of DS increased the predictive validity of the previously formulated index. Furthermore, the positive results confirmed that Vocabulary and Information are functions likely controlled by the left temporal lobe, whereas the DS subtest functions seem to be under the control of the left parietal lobe (Russell & Russell, 1993). Furthermore, the study established that adolescents and adults with LD also display this pattern.

Donders (1993) explored the factor structure of the WISC-R with 108 participants diagnosed with TBI, ranging from 6 to 16 years in age. A principal components factor analysis of the 11 subtests yielded three factors that subsequently were subjected to varimax rotation. Whereas the first (verbal comprehension; .66 to .81) and second (perceptual organization; .64 to .81) factors were identified by high loadings, the third and final factor (freedom from distractibility) revealed only moderate loadings (.45 to .58).

Investigating the potential validity of the third factor was considered important for a population of children with TBI because of the frequently reported attention and concentration problems in children with head injury. Cognitive deficits such as these are often considered among the most serious problems following injury to the head (Fletcher & Levin, 1988). Donders' results provided preliminary support for Kaufman's three-factor model on the WISC-R (Factor 1, verbal comprehension; Factor 2, perceptual organization; Factor 3, freedom from distractibility) as applied to children who have acquired brain injury. The subtest loading for Factor 3 was further qualified. Similar to previous studies, Donders points out that arithmetic and coding had a modest loading on one or two other factors). Thus, it would seem premature to assume that a specific freedom from distractibility factor exists for children who experience TBI.

An abbreviated form of the WISC-R, the Hobby Split-Half Short Form, has also been investigated in relation to its utility with children and adolescents with severe brain injury (Hooper & Roof, 1993). The overall agreement rate between the standard administration and the Hobby Short Form was 76.7%. All correlations between the two forms ranged from .83 to .99, and all t tests between subtests were nonsignificant, with the exception of Object Assembly, where the Split-Half Form was found to be slightly higher. The findings suggest that scores from the Hobby Short Form are statistically and clinically consistent with the scores from the complete WISC-R battery, and examiners can use the form with individuals with brain injury in a reliable manner.

SUMMARY AND CONCLUSIONS

In summary, TBI in the United States is one of the leading causes of disability in children. The disability resulting from a traumatic impact to the head may be more complex than can be judged by physical appearances, conventional educational assessment techniques, or even general neurological evaluations. Subtle cognitive dysfunction can result from a closed-head injury that can drastically change an individual's learning ability. The behavioral outcome in children following such an acquired head injury has been found to be associated with a variety of neuropsychological deficits, including poor performance on speeded tasks, memory impairment, and difficulties in processing novel or complex visual–spatial stimuli. These deficits may not reveal themselves in the acute stage; however, children may present severe learning difficulties years later.

The resulting cognitive dysfunction following TBI may fail to show up on routine intellectual assessments. The attentional dysfunction, memory impairment, language impairment, auditory processing deficits, and evidence of frontal lobe dysfunction commonly reported in individuals with TBI may only be revealed through the use of neuropsychological evaluations. Such evaluative procedures are also of benefit when diagnosing and prescribing treatment plans for children and adolescents who experience ADHD and LD. Comparatively speaking, the cognitive dysfunction associated with TBI also has been reported by individuals diagnosed with ADHD and LD. Documents in the literature continue to show support for a direct relationship between brain deficits and learning problems. Recent evidence has utilized cluster analysis to identify subtypes of LD in children diagnosed with acquired brain damage. Various clusters have been identified, and the findings suggest that the addition of behavioral information contributes to a further delineation of these subgroups.

Empirical investigations of deficits in brain function have increased the amount of useful information concerning individual differences in cognitive function. For example, cognitive outcomes from studies using participants with brain injury have added considerable information to individual differences in hemispheric specialization. Specifically, empirical studies of subjects with left-hemisphere lesions have demonstrated that these individuals experience greater delays in expressive language when compared to subjects with right-hemisphere lesions. Subjects with left-hemisphere lesions show better language comprehension, slower rates of speech, greater encoding deficits, and deficits in phonological aspects of language processing; however, intellectual development is at greater risk with early right-hemisphere damage, and empirical support can be found for a specialized role of the right hemisphere relative to acquisition of word meaning.

The literature on cognitive functioning following TBI is ever increasing. More research is required in order for us to understand the outcomes of acquired brain injury in all individuals, and specifically in children whose cognitive structure has not yet fully developed. The primary challenge facing educators working with individuals who have suffered TBI is to accurately assess the nature and extent of injury and to predict rates of recovery.

7. Childhood Traumatic Brain Injury: Initial Impact on the Family

SHARI L. WADE, H. GERRY TAYLOR, DENNIS DROTAR,
TERRY STANCIN, AND KEITH OWEN YEATES

Traumatic brain injury (TBI) is a major source of morbidity and mortality among children (Goldstein & Levin, 1987). Although most of the more than 100,000 children hospitalized for TBI each year enjoy substantial recovery, those with moderate to severe injuries are at marked risk for ongoing neuropsychological, behavioral, and academic problems. However, injury severity accounts for only a modest portion of the variance in child outcomes, and a wide range of functioning is observed even among the most severely injured children (Fletcher & Levin, 1988; Levin, Benton, & Grossman, 1982). Moreover, many children manifest long-term behavioral problems despite apparent cognitive recovery.

A number of investigators have speculated that initial cognitive impairments and behavior changes in the child disrupt family life and adversely affect parent adjustment and parent–child interactions (Boll, 1983; Brooks, 1991; Brown, Chadwick, Schaffer, Rutter, & Traub, 1981; Fletcher, Ewing-Cobbs, Miner, Levin, & Eisenberg, 1990; Perrott, Taylor, & Montes, 1991; Rutter, 1981). These changes, in turn, may negatively affect the child's subsequent psychological adjustment in spite of cognitive recovery. Despite the important role the family plays in the child's recovery, few investigators have assessed the effects of TBI on the family (see Wade, Drotar, Taylor, & Stancin, 1995, for a complete review).

With a single exception, existing studies of the effects of pediatric TBI on families have been limited by retrospective designs or a reliance on clinical observations to the exclusion of empirically validated measures (Perrott et al., 1991; Rutter, Chadwick, & Shaffer, 1983). In the only study to date to incorporate both a prospective design and standardized assessments of family functioning, Rivara and co-investigators (Rivara et al., 1992) followed children and their families for a year, beginning at the time of the TBI. Initial assessments were conducted shortly after the injury to obtain measures of preinjury family functioning. These assessments were repeated at 3 and 12 months following the injury. Family measures included standardized self-report measures of family environment, and interviewer ratings of family functioning. The effects of the child's injury on family functioning were evaluated by examining changes in the family measures over time. A comparison of children with severe TBI with children with mild or moderate TBI revealed a deterioration in family functioning (as determined by interviewer ratings) among the more severely injured children. Changes in family functioning were not observed on parent self-report measures. Rivara and colleagues also noted that preinjury family functioning and coping, along with ratings of the child's premorbid behavior, predicted which families would be the most adversely affected, above and beyond injury severity. These data indicate that TBI has a decided impact on families, and point to the potential moderating role of family resources and coping on TBI outcomes.

Clinical reports of family functioning following pediatric TBI, investigations of TBI in adults, and descriptive studies of the impact of pediatric trauma on the family also provide direction for future empirical studies of the effects of pediatric TBI on families (Livingston & Brooks, 1988; Oddy, Humphrey, & Uttley, 1978; Rivara, 1994; Waaland & Kreutzer, 1988). Taken together, the results from these divergent literatures suggest that TBI, and traumatic injuries more broadly, are associated with psychological distress in the primary caregiver and concomitant marital tensions and strain. Evidence also indicates that family roles, responsibilities, and interactions may be altered, with adverse consequences for healthy siblings (Harris, Schwaitzberg, Seman, & Herman, 1989). However, across studies, many families exhibit considerable resiliency in the face of trauma, manifesting no long-term negative effects. Thus, it is incumbent upon researchers to identify factors that distinguish families who cope well from those who experience ongoing difficulties. The identification of predictors of long-term adjustment is crucial for the design and implementation of family-focused interventions following TBI. Toward this end, a comprehensive model of family adaptation to TBI would consider stressors and resources likely to influence outcome, such as preinjury family functioning, injury-related burden, chronic life stresses confronting the family, social supports, community resources, and therapeutic and rehabilitative services (see Wade et al., 1995, for one framework).

The effects of TBI on the family are also likely to vary as a function of the amount of time that has elapsed since the injury. The tasks and stresses associated with an acute hospitalization are quite different from those arising from chronic neuropsychological and behavioral deficits (Rolland, 1987). Findings from the literature on TBI in adults indicate that family distress and dysfunction may intensify rather than diminish over time (Brooks, 1991). Furthermore, a family's ability to successfully cope with the initial demands of the injury may have important implications for its long-term adaptation (Rivara et al., 1992). Thus, future research must distinguish initial effects of pediatric TBI on families from ongoing and chronic concerns.

The current report has three primary goals:

1. To detail the effects of TBI on families during the initial phase of the child's recovery;
2. To identify factors associated with initial family adaptation; and
3. To consider the implications of these findings for interventions with families.

These results represent the initial findings from a prospective, longitudinal study of the effects of severe and moderate TBI on the family, compared with traumatic orthopedic injuries not involving the central nervous system (CNS). The findings from this project extend the work of previous investigators in several important respects. An orthopedically injured sample was recruited to enable us to disentangle the consequences for the family of a neurological injury from those arising from other non-CNS injuries requiring acute hospitalization and disruptions in family routine. Further, care was taken to assess a wide range of injury-specific and global family outcomes, including injury-related burden and stress, family functioning, and parental mental health. Finally the relationship between preinjury family resources and stresses and the impact of TBI on families was examined, facilitating identification of those at high risk.

One of our hypotheses was that severe TBI would adversely affect the family social environment and would result in greater parental burden and psychological distress than either moderate TBI or orthopedic injuries not involving CNS insult. A second hypothesis was that family resources and coping, chronic stresses, and family supports would influence family adjustment following TBI.

METHOD

Participants

The current findings are based on the information gathered from the families of 96 children with moderate to severe TBI and 69 children with orthopedic injuries who served as a comparison group. Eligibility criteria for both the TBI and orthopedic injury (ORTHO) groups included (a) age between 6 and 12 years of at the time of injury, (b) no evidence of child abuse or a previous history of neurological disease or neurosensory impairment, and (c) English as the primary language spoken at home. Recruitment into the TBI group also required documentation of moderate-to-severe TBI. Consistent with previous investigations, severe injuries were defined as those in which the initial Glasgow Coma Scale (GCS; Jennett & Bond, 1975) score was 8 or less (Fletcher et al., 1990; Fletcher & Levin, 1988). Moderate injuries were defined as those in which the initial GCS score ranged from 9 to 12 or in which a higher GCS rating was accompanied by seizures or other signs of neurological dysfunction, skull fracture, intracranial mass lesion, diffuse cerebral swelling, or documented loss of consciousness for more than 15 minutes. Children with types of TBI other than closed-head injuries were excluded. Inclusion in the ORTHO group additionally required a documented bone fracture requiring an overnight hospital stay and the absence of any evidence of loss of consciousness or other findings suggestive of brain injury.

Table 7.1 presents demographic and injury characteristics for the TBI and ORTHO groups. As Table 7.1 indicates, the groups were comparable with respect to most key demographic factors. The only exception to this was the fact that there was a significantly higher proportion of Black children in the ORTHO group compared with the TBI group. Because of this difference between the groups, a composite measure of sociodemographic status that incorporates race was used as a covariate in all analyses. As anticipated, the groups differed significantly with respect to indices of injury severity and length of hospitalization. The Injury Severity Score (ISS; Mayer, Matlack, Johnson, & Walker, 1980) reported in Table 7.1 was calculated based on non-TBI-related injuries only, to permit comparison of the TBI and ORTHO groups in terms of other multisystem injuries, including the severity of any orthopedic injuries accompanying TBI. As evident in group comparisons on this measure, the group with severe TBI was comparable to the ORTHO group with respect to other traumatic injuries, but the group with moderate TBI had less severe other injuries than either of the other two groups.

Table 7.1
Background Characteristics of Children with Moderate TBI, Severe TBI,
and Orthopedic Injuries

Characteristic	Severe TBI	Moderate TBI	Orthopedic
Mean age at injury ($\pm$ SD)	9.4 years (2.2)	9.9 years (1.9)	9.2 years (1.9)
Mean injury severity score ($\pm$ SD)*	9.0 (10.6)	2.1 (3.7)	7.6 (3.2)
Mean days in hospital ($\pm$ SD)*	13.4 (9.3)	6.6 (7.1)	12.9 (12.5)
Gender of child	71% male	73% male	61% male
Ethnicity	76% White	82% White	59% White
Proportion of two-parent families	55%	71%	62%
Hollinghead Four Factor SES	33.3	34.1	33.5
Percentage receiving public assistance	38%	20%	29%

Note. TBI = traumatic brain injury.
*Group differences significant, $p < .05$.

Procedure

All age-appropriate admissions at two regional children's hospitals and a large county hospital were monitored for potential eligibility. Once children meeting study criteria were medically stable, informed consent was obtained and the following procedures were carried out: (a) Parents were interviewed regarding the perceived burden of the injury; (b) parents completed questionnaires pertaining to the child's preinjury behavior, preinjury family functioning, parental psychological distress, and sociodemographic status; (c) forms were mailed to schools to obtain teacher ratings of preinjury behavior and school performance; and (d) the child's medical chart was reviewed.

Baseline assessments of the child's cognitive and neuropsychological functioning and academic achievement were conducted as soon as possible (in the case of the TBI group, once posttraumatic amnesia had resolved). Mean time between injury and baseline assessment was .7 months for the total sample ($SD = .4$). The two injury groups did not differ in this regard. Other aspects of the preinjury family environment, including preinjury family stressors and resources, social networks, and parenting styles, were also assessed at baseline. Additional information obtained from parents at this time included parent perceptions of the child's postinjury health status, information regarding concurrent parental psychological distress and coping mechanisms, and parent perceptions of the impact of the injury on the family since the child's discharge from the hospital.

Although parent measures collected at the hospitalization and baseline assessments were readministered at 6 and 12 months, only a portion of these follow-up assessments are as yet complete; hence, the current article focuses on only the initial impact of TBI on families. The child's biological mother served as the primary informant in 90% of the TBI cases and 93% of the orthopedic cases.

Measures of Preinjury Status

The McMaster Family Assessment Device (FAD; Byles, Byrne, Boyle, & Oxford, 1988; Miller, Bishop, Epstein, & Keitner, 1985) was used to assess family functioning across a variety of domains. The FAD is a 53-item self-report measure composed of seven subscales related to family interactions and environment. The subscales of the FAD have been shown to have good internal consistency and stability over time. Moreover, responses are only weakly correlated with measures of social desirability. Construct validity is suggested by the relationship of the FAD with other measures of family environment, as well as measures of individual functioning. Parents were asked to complete the FAD at baseline to establish the family's functioning prior to the injury. The 12-item General Functioning subscale was used to summarize preinjury family health.

The Life Stressors and Social Resources Inventory (LISRES; Moos, Fenn, Billings, & Moos, 1989) was administered as an interview to assess life events and social supports. The LISRES is an extensive interview measure that generates subscores for stressors and resources across the following domains: (a) personal health, (b) home and neighborhood, (c) work, (d) finances, (e) spouse or partner, (f) children, (g) relatives, and (h) friends and social activities. The LISRES, which has satisfactory internal consistency and moderate to high temporal stability, has been shown to predict changes over time in the functioning of adults with alcoholism and depression. Averages of the stressor and resource subscales were constructed to serve as summary indices of chronic stressors and social resources, respectively.

Sociodemographic status (SDS) was assessed by means of a summary index used in previous studies of children at biological risk for cognitive and academic difficulties (Hack et al., 1994) and was calculated on the basis of maternal education, race, and marital status.

Measures of Injury Impact and Coping

The Family Burden of Injury Interview (FBII; Taylor et al., in press) was developed to assess the unique burdens and challenges of pediatric TBI for families (see Drotar et al., 1996, for a complete description of FBII development). Slightly different sets of questions were administered during hospitalization and postdischarge assessments, reflecting changes in the concerns confronting parents after the child returns home. At both assessments, parents were also asked a series of open-ended questions about concerns, types of help needed, and the aspects of the injury found to be most difficult. The hospitalization FBII generates six subscale scores corresponding to the following sources of injury-related stress: (a) changes in school and work schedules, (b) the child's recovery and adjustment, (c) siblings' reactions and behavior, (d) the reactions of extended family and friends, (e) changes in daily routine, and (f) the spouse's reactions. The post-discharge FBH generates five subscores corresponding to injury-related stress in the following areas: (1) changes in routine and work and school schedules, (2) concerns with the child's recovery and adjustment, (3) the reactions of extended family and friends, (4) the spouse's reactions, and (5) siblings' reactions and behavior.

The Impact on Family Scale, Version G (IOF-G; Stein & Jessop, 1985) provided a previously validated measure of the impact of pediatric disability on the family. The scale generates a Total Impact score and subscale scores on the following four dimensions: Caretaker Burden, Familial Burden, Financial Impact, and Disruption of Planning. For each item, parents indicate the extent to which they agree with a statement regarding the child who was injured and then report whether they believe that their rating is related to the child's injury. The subscales were derived from factor analyses and demonstrate good internal consistency. The Total Impact score served as a summary measure of family impact in the current analyses.

The Brief Symptom Inventory (BSI; Derogatis & Melisaratos, 1983) was selected to assess parent psychological adjustment. The BSI is a widely used 53-item, self-report questionnaire designed to tap a range of psychiatric symptoms. It yields three global indices and nine subscale scores. Established cutoffs are available to identify individuals with symptoms likely to warrant clinical attention. Cronbach's alpha for global and individual scales ranges from .71 to .83, and test–retest reliability ranges from .68 to .91. Validity has been demonstrated through its correlation with content scales and cluster scores of the MMPI. The BSI was chosen for the current study because of its brevity and sensitivity to change. Based on the recommendations of Derogatis and Spencer (1982), clinical "caseness," that is, symptom levels likely to warrant clinical attention, was defined as Global Severity Index $T \geq 63$ or T scores on two or more subscales ≥ 63.

The COPE (Carver, Scheier, & Weintraub, 1989) was used to assess the caregiver's coping style in response to the injury and its sequelae. The COPE is a 52-item, self-report inventory measuring 13 distinct aspects of coping behavior within the broader dimensions of problem-focused (or active) coping, emotion-focused coping, and maladaptive coping. The subscales have been shown to have good internal consistency and moderate to high stability over time (Carver et al., 1989).

Analyses

Differences in family stress and burden among the moderate TBI, severe TBI, and ORTHO groups were assessed using an ANCOVA. SDS served as the covariate in these analyses. The Tukey test was used for post hoc comparisons. To control for Type I error, Bonferroni adjusted alpha levels were employed in analyzing multiple measure domains. Thus, the alpha level for comparisons of the six FBII subscales at hospitalization was set at $p < .008$, whereas the alpha level for the five FBII subscales from baseline was set at $p < .01$. The alpha level for comparisons of outcomes in domains represented by a single summary score (e.g., BSI and lOF) remained at $p < .05$. Chi-square analyses were used to make comparisons among the groups on the frequencies of specific open-ended responses on the FBII. Hierarchical multiple regression analyses were used to identify social–environmental predictors of family burden and distress, after controlling for injury factors and sociodemographic status.

RESULTS

Injury-Related Burden and Stress During Hospitalization

Table 7.2 depicts the average stress levels in each of the six domains of the hospitalization FBII for families of children with severe TBI, moderate TBI, and orthopedic injuries. Comparisons of stress levels among the three groups were made using an ANCOVA, controlling for the effects of SDS. As predicted, the families of children with severe TBI experienced significantly more stress overall than the families of children in the other two groups. After adjusting the alpha level to account for multiple comparisons, no differences were found among the groups in stress levels on subscales of the FBII.

Table 7.2
Injury-Related Burden and Stress from the FBII at the Time of Hospitalization

	Severe TBI		Moderate TBI		Orthopedic	
Source of stress	M	(SD)	M	(SD)	M	(SD)
Work and school	1.1	(1.3)	1.1	(1.3)	.97	(1.4)
Concern for child	1.9	(1.3)	1.4	(1.1)	1.3	(.97)
Siblings' reactions	.88	(.78)	.67	(.79)	.48	(.57)
Others' reactions	1.4	(1.1)	1.0	(1.2)	.88	(.88)
Routine and chores	1.5	(1.1)	1.4	(1.0)	1.5	(1.2)
Spouse's reactions	1.3	(1.2)	.82	(.89)	.73	(.79)
Total stress*	1.3	(.67)	1.0	(.58)	.94	(.56)

Note. FBII = Family Burden of Injury Interview; TBI = traumatic brain injury. *FBII* Subscale Ratings of Stress: 0 = *not at all stressful;* 1 = *a bit stressful;* 2 = *fairly stressful;* 3 = *quite stressful;* 4 = *extremely stressful.* *Indicates group difference *p* < .008. According to post hoc analyses, stress was greater with severe TBI than with moderate TBI or orthopedic injury.

However, there was a trend for parents in the severe TBI group to endorse higher levels of stress in the domains of (a) concern for the injured child, $F = 5.00$, $df = 164$, $p = .008$, and (b) reactions of siblings, $F = 3.8$, $df = 146$, $p = .02$; spouse, $F = 3.0$, $df = 110$, $p = .05$; and other family members, $F = 3.6$, $df = 164$, $p = .03$, to the injury. Parents in all three groups experienced comparable levels of stress associated with disruptions in work and school schedules and alterations in the daily routine.

Interestingly, even among the caregivers of children with severe TBI, average ratings of stress arising from injury-related burden tended to fall into the low to moderate range (.88 to 1.9). However, there was considerable variability in parents' perceptions of stress. For example, despite a mean rating of only 1.9, 25% of the parents of children with severe TBI rated concern for the injured child as quite or extremely stressful, as compared to 8% of the parents of children with moderate TBI and less than 2% of the parents of children with orthopedic injuries.

Injury-Related Burden and Stress at Baseline

At the time of the baseline assessment, the families of children with severe TBI continued to report higher overall levels of stress than the families of children in the other two groups (see Table 7.3). The families of children with severe TBI also acknowledged higher levels of stress in two specific domains: concerns regarding the injured child's recovery and adjustment, and the reactions of extended family and friends to the injury.

Specific Parental Concerns

The vast majority (95%) of parents reported persistent concerns in response to open-ended questions on the baseline FBII (see Table 7.4). Their concerns were largely consistent with the pattern of stresses revealed in the structured portion of the FBII. The most common area of concern for

Table 7.3
Injury-Related Burden and Stress from the FBII at the Baseline Interview

Source of stress	Severe TBI		Moderate TBI		Orthopedic	
	M	(SD)	M	(SD)	M	(SD)
Routine/schedules	1.5	(1.1)	.89	(.81)	1.2	(1.1)
Concern for child**	1.7	(1.1)	1.2	(.73)	1.1	(.84)
Others' reactions	.75	(.86)	.38	(.49)	.26	(.46)
Spouse's reactions	1.4	(1.1)	.90	(.59)	1.0	(.96)
Siblings' reactions	1.0	(1.0)	.69	(.82)	.71	(.77)
Total stress**	1.3	(.78)	.83	(.49)	.91	(.68)

Note. FBII = Family Burden of Injury Interview; TBI = traumatic brain injury. *FBII* Subscale Ratings of Stress: 0 = *not at all stressful;* 1 = *a bit stressful;* 2 = *fairly stressful;* 3 = *quite stressful;* 4 = *extremely stressful.* **Indicates group difference $p < .01$. According to post hoc analyses, stress was greater with severe TBI than with moderate TBI or orthopedic injuries.

Table 7.4
Reported Frequency of Families' Concern Following Injury[a]

Area of concern	Severe TBI		Moderate TBI		Orthopedic	
	n	%	n	%	n	%
Full recovery	11	27	18	36	15	22
Specific deficits	5	12	6	12	13	19
School reentry	7	17	5	10	7	10
Child's adjustment	4	10	7	14	8	12
Fears of reinjury	4	10	4	8	4	6
Physical restrictions	1	2	3	6	2	3
Returning to normal	3	7	3	6	7	10
Sibling/family	3	7	2	4	7	10
Finance/bills	3	7	2	4	4	6
No concerns	2	5	2	4	4	6

Note. No group difference was significant at the $p < .05$ level. TBI = traumatic brain injury.
[a]Based on responses to open-ended questions.

parents of children in all three groups was whether the child would fully re-cover, noted by 27% of the severe TBI group, 36% of the moderate TBI group, and 22% of the ORTHO group. Further, 22% of parents of children with severe TBI, 26% of parents of children with moderate TBI, and 31% of parents of children with orthopedic injuries voiced medical or developmental concerns, anxiety about behavior changes, or concern about how the child was coping with the injury. Some areas not queried in the structured part of the FBII were also noted, such as fears of reinjury and concerns about school reen-try and academic success. Chi-square analyses failed to reveal any significant differences among the groups in terms of the nature of concerns reported.

Types of Help Requested by Families

A significantly higher proportion (63%) of the parents of children with severe TBI, compared with the parents of children in the moderate TBI or ORTHO groups (46% and 40%, respectively), expressed a desire, in response to the open-ended questions of the FBII at baseline, for some type of help or assistance, $\chi^2 df$ (1) = 6.54; $p < .05$ (see Table 7.5). Concrete ser-vices, such as childcare and housekeeping, and financial assistance repre-sented the most commonly cited needs. These needs were noted by 29% of the group with severe TBI, 16% of the group with moderate TBI, and 19% of the ORTHO group. An additional 15% of the severe TBI group, 16% of the moderate TBI group, and 4% of the ORTHO group indicated a desire for additional medical information, ongoing monitoring of the child's con-dition, or assistance in setting up rehabilitation services. The need for coun-seling or emotional support was expressed by only six families in the severe TBI group (15%), three families in the moderate TBI group (6%), and four families in the ORTHO group (6%). The groups differed significantly only with respect to the need for medical information and monitoring, which was noted more frequently among the families of children with moderate TBI.

Impact on the Family

An ANCOVA revealed differences on the IOF-G Total Impact score that were consistent with the differences found on the FBII, $F = 5.3$, $df = 166$, $p < .01$. Mean Total Impact scores for the severe TBI, moderate TBI, and ORTHO groups were 2.4 ($SD = .45$), 2.1 ($SD = .30$), and 2.3 ($SD = .47$), respectively. According to post hoc comparisons, the families of chil-dren with severe TBI reported significantly more injury-related effects than families of children with less severe TBI.

Table 7.5
Rates of Types of Help Requested by Families Following Injury

Type of help	Severe TBI		Moderate TBI		Orthopedic	
	n	%	*n*	%	*n*	%
Financial	5	12	6	12	7	10
Information/monitoring*	2	5	6	12	0	0
Rehabilitation	4	10	2	4	3	4
Support/therapy	6	15	3	6	4	6
Academic	3	7	0	0	1	1
Childcare	4	10	1	2	6	9
Housekeeping	3	7	1	2	0	0
No help needed	15	37	27	54	41	60

*Indicates group differences significant at $p < .05$.

Parent Psychological Distress

Group differences on the BSI Global Severity Index approached significance, $F = 3.1$, $df = 163$, $p = .052$. Means for the severe TBI, moderate TBI, and ORTHO groups, respectively, were 56.7 ($SD = 9.4$), 56.5 ($SD = 10.0$), and 53.3 ($SD = 12.7$). Follow-up analyses comparing the moderate and severe TBI groups with the ORTHO group indicated significantly higher global severity scores among the parents of children with TBI, after controlling for SDS (ANCOVA: $F = 6.0$, $df = 163$, $p = .01$).

As hypothesized, group differences on the Anxiety subscale of the BSI were marginally significant, $F = 3.0$, $df = 163$, $p = .051$. Means for this measure for the severe TBI, moderate TBI, and ORTHO groups, respectively, were 56.7 ($SD = 9.8$), 56.6 ($SD = 10.0$), and 53.2 ($SD = 11.7$). Follow-up analyses comparing the moderate and severe TBI groups with the ORTHO group revealed significantly higher scores on the anxiety subscale among parents following TBI (ANCOVA: $F = 6.1$, $df = 163$, $p = .01$). The groups did not differ with respect to depressive symptomatology.

In a proportion of cases, scores on the BSI satisfied the criteria for clinical caseness as defined earlier. Specifically, 45% of parents in the severe TBI group met these criteria, compared with 45% of the moderate TBI group and 33% of the ORTHO group. Differences among the groups in the proportion of parents exceeding the criteria for clinical caseness, although they were in the predicted direction, did not reach statistical significance when tested via logistical regression controlling for SDS.

Predictors of Family Sequelae Following TBI

Based on previous literature, it was hypothesized that the impact of TBI on the family would be determined by the injury's severity as well as characteristics of the social environment, including the presence of other family stresses and the availability of resources with which to respond to the demands of the injury and other stressors. Effective premorbid family functioning, family and community supports, and family coping strengths in response to the injury were identified as resources that could serve to mitigate the impact of the injury on the family.

As indicated in Table 7.6, the BSI, IOF, and FBII subscales were only modestly correlated with one another, suggesting that they measured distinct aspects of the family sequelae of TBI. Therefore, separate regression analyses were performed for each of the major family outcomes: (a) the total stress arising from injury-related burdens as assessed by the baseline FBII, (b) the Total Impact score from the IOF-G, and (c) parental psychological distress as measured by the BSI Global Severity Index. In each analysis, SDS was entered first to control for the effects of race and social class. On the second step, the lowest Glasgow Coma Scale score (LGCS) was entered as a measure of the severity of the TBI. Next, severity of other injuries, as measured by the non-head-injury ISS, was entered into the regression equation. Other family stressors and resources, including social and community supports as assessed by the LISRES, preinjury family functioning as assessed by the FAD General

Table 7.6
Bivariate Relationships of the Primary Outcome Measures

Measure	Total impact	BSI GSI	FBII Routines	Child	Others	Siblings	Spouse
Total impact	1.00	.32	.62	.34	.28	.39	.38
BSI GSI		1.00	.26	.38	.18	.22	.37
FBII routines			1.00	.48	.47	.56	.56
FBII child				1.00	.62	.53	.58
FBII others					1.00	.52	.46
FBII sibling						1.00	.50
FBII spouse							1.00

Note. All correlations are significant, $p < .05$, two-tailed. FBII = Family Burden of Injury Interview; Total impact = summary score from the IOF-G; BSI GSI = Brief Symptom Inventory Global Severity Index; FBII Routines = stress with changes in daily routines; Child = stress regarding the child's recovery and adjustment; Others = stress regarding the reactions of extended family and friends; Siblings = stress regarding the reactions and behavior of siblings; Spouse = stress regarding spouse's reaction.

Functioning Index, and injury-related coping style as measured by the COPE, were then entered in stepwise fashion.

As shown in Table 7.7, SDS was not a significant predictor of any of the family outcomes following TBI. Controlling for SDS, the severity of TBI accounted for 9% of the variance in the Overall injury-related stress score from the FBII and 11% of the variance in the Total Impact of the injury as assessed by the IOF-G. Severity of TBI was unrelated to the Global Severity Index of the BSI. The severity of other traumatic injuries accounted for additional variance in the Total Impact score and Global Severity Index, but not in Overall injury-related stress on the FBII. Most important, even after taking social factors and injury factors into account, all three family outcomes were associated with some aspect of the family's preinjury social environment or injury-related coping. Specifically chronic life stress accounted for 8% of additional variance in total burden from the baseline FBII and for 14% of variance in the IOF-G Total Impact score. Maladaptive coping accounted for 18% of additional variance in the BSI Global Severity Index. Specifically, higher levels of injury-related stress on a family were associated with more chronic

Table 7.7
Hierarchical Regression Analyses Predicting Family Outcomes

Family outcome	Predictor	R^2	R^2 change
FBII total stress			
	SDS	.001	.001
	LGCS*	.09	.09
	ISS	.12	.03
	Chronic stressors**	.21	.08
IOF total negative impact			
	SDS	.03	.03
	LGCS**	.14	.11
	ISS*	.18	.04
	Chronic stressors***	.32	.14
BSI Global Severity Index			
	SDS	.04	.04
	LGCS	.04	.00
	ISS	.11	.07
	Maladaptive coping***	.28	.18

Note. FBII = Family Burden of Injury Interview; SDS = Index of Sociodemographic Status; LGCS = lowest Glasgow Coma Scale; ISS = the modified Injury Severity Scale score with injuries to the head/neck region removed; Chronic stressors = an average of the stressors subscales from the LISRES; Maladaptive coping = the sum of the behavioral disengagement, emotional disengagement, and venting of emotions subscales from the COPE.
*$p < .05$. **$p < .01$. ***$p < .001$.

environmental stress. Finally, greater parental psychological distress was associated with coping characterized by mental or behavioral disengagement or venting of emotions. Although preinjury family functioning and support from family and friends were correlated with the negative impact of TBI on the family and parental psychological symptoms, they did not account for unique variance in the regressions after controlling for SDS and injury severity. Together, SDS, injury severity, and family status measures accounted for 21%, 32%, and 28% of the variance in injury-related burden, negative family impact of injury, and parent psychological symptoms, respectively.

DISCUSSION

The results of the current study support and extend the existing literature regarding the effects of pediatric TBI on families. Consistent with previous findings, the current data indicate that severe TBI is a significant family burden and source of stress during the acute hospitalization, as well as several weeks following discharge. Further initial family burdens and stress arising from severe TBI are quantitatively and qualitatively different from those associated with non-neurological trauma. In addition to generating marked concern regarding the child's recovery, severe TBI was more likely to become a source of stress in interactions with other family members, such as siblings and grandparents. However, severe TBI and orthopedic injuries resulted in comparable alterations in family schedules and routines, underscoring that stress is common to any acute trauma. The unique stresses associated with severe TBI appear to be psychological (e.g., anxiety about the future) and interpersonal in nature.

The findings from this study also underscore the multidimensional nature of stress arising from TBI. A factor analysis of the FBII interviews at hospitalization and baseline indicated that family burden and stress arising from TBI fell into a variety of distinct domains, including worries about the injured child, interpersonal stresses with other family members, and disruptions in family routines and school and work schedules. Moreover, the low intercorrelations of the FBII subscale scores with measures of parental distress and global impact on the family (shown in Table 7.6) suggest that the family outcome measures are tapping different aspects of distress/impact. This pattern of findings strongly argues for a comprehensive approach to the measurement of family adaptation, rather than relying on a unitary measure.

The parents of children with either severe or moderate TBI reported significantly elevated levels of psychological distress on the BSI compared with parents of children with orthopedic injuries. Moreover, 45% of the parents in the TBI group exceeded the clinical cutoff on this measure. Despite this high level of parent distress, very few parents or children received any type of counseling in the time period immediately following the accident. Parents' self-reports regarding the type of assistance that was needed following hospital discharge underscored the discrepancy between the level of emotional distress in the family and the type of help sought. These findings suggest that the psychological impact of TBI on the family cannot be understood by merely asking families what type of help is needed. It may be that parents have difficulty articulating psychological needs. Conversely, they may perceive emotional distress as normal for individuals in their situation, thereby making it something that needs to be endured rather than addressed via professional intervention. Despite the fact that the parents' concerns and distress were often of an emotional nature, they were much more able to express concrete, nonpsychological needs. These findings suggest that a comprehensive-care approach is required, in which parents are given anticipatory guidance about the stresses and emotional sequelae that are likely to arise following TBI. This approach, together with opportunities to express their fears, may reduce the psychological morbidity seen in parents. Anecdotally, parents reported benefiting from the opportunity to discuss their anxiety and concerns with the study interviewers, suggesting the potential utility of supportive counseling.

The results of the regression analysis suggest that risks for adverse family consequences may vary to some extent, depending on the type of family outcome considered. Injury-related burden, as measured by the FBII, and overall negative impact of the injury were predicted by chronic life stress, whereas parental psychological symptoms following the child's injury were associated with maladaptive coping styles. It is perhaps not surprising that the burdens arising from the injury are perceived as more stressful by individuals who already have stressful lives. Moreover, chronic stresses with spouses or in-laws may be exacerbated by the demands placed on the family by the child's injury. The association between maladaptive coping strategies and parental psychological distress raises intriguing questions about the role of coping style in individual and family adaptation. However, in interpreting the relationship of coping to parental adjustment, it is important to note that these measures were collected at the same point in time, thereby precluding causal interpretations. Further, without preinjury data regarding parental functioning, it is not possible to determine to what extent parental psychological difficulties were present prior to the injury. Although the importance of preinjury family functioning has been noted by previous investigators (Rivara et al., 1992), premorbid family functioning did not independently contribute to the outcomes investigated in the current study. However, family functioning was correlated with parental psychological distress and over-all impact of the injury in univariate correlations, and may be a more impor-tant determinant of long-term adaptation.

The findings from this study, although preliminary, have important implications for intervention with families following TBI, and traumatic injuries generally. Many more families have unmet psychological needs than are currently receiving services. Families of children with severe injuries or multiple other stressors appear to be at particular risk and therefore warrant closer attention. Health care providers cannot rely on families to directly express their emotional needs and therefore must probe emotional concerns and distress more directly. As this project continues to collect prospective data on family adaptation to traumatic injury, pathways and timing for successful family interventions should become clearer. Future analyses will also enable us to determine if the distress seen in parents diminishes over time, and to eval-uate the impact of such parental morbidity on the child's recovery.

AUTHORS' NOTES

1. Work on this chapter was supported by Grant No. MCJ-390611, Maternal and Child Health Bureau (Title V, Social Security Act), Health Resources and Services Administration, Department of Health and Human Services.
2. The authors wish to acknowledge the contributions of Nori Mercuri-Minich, Elizabeth Shaver, Madeline Polonia, and Christopher Schatschneider.

PART III

Intervention

8. Interventions for Students with Traumatic Brain Injury: Managing Behavioral Disturbances

THOMAS J. KEHLE, ELAINE CLARK, AND
WILLIAM R. JENSON

Traumatic brain injury (TBI) is the most common cause of acquired disability in childhood and adolescence (Michaud, Duhaime, & Batshaw, 1993). Although the nature and severity of the disability is largely a function of the neuropathological features of the injury itself, cognitive and behavioral problems are fairly common (Di Scala, Osberg, Gans, Chin, & Grant, 1991). Cognitive problems, although considered by many to be the most disabling sequelae of injury (Capruso & Levin, 1992), are not the only problems that cause concern. According to Levin (1987), family members are more distressed by the behavioral disturbances. This is not surprising, given the fact that research has shown that parents of children and adolescents who sustain a TBI report the same behaviors in their children as parents who have children in behavior disorders (BD) classrooms (Michaud, Rivara, Jaffe, Fay, & Dailey, 1993). Both groups of parents describe their children as having poor attention and concentration, distractibility, hyperactivity, irritability, low frustration tolerance, poor motivation, apathy, poor anger control, aggression, and anxiety, and as experiencing social isolation and resorting to substance abuse (McAllister, 1992; Michaud, Duhaime, & Batshaw, 1993; Rosenthal & Bond, 1990).

In addition to the externalizing behaviors that children with TBI are reported to show, many have internalizing problems as well. McKinlay, Brooks, Bond, Martinage, and Marshall (1981) found that approximately 70% of their sample displayed irritability. Silver and Yudofsky (1987) found about the same rate of aggression in their sample. Although irritability is not targeted for intervention as often as aggressiveness is, it is commonly found to be a precursor to more disruptive and assaultive behaviors (McKinlay et al., 1981). Behavioral problems, whether externalizing or internalizing, do not resolve as quickly or spontaneously as some other problems (e.g., motor control; Di Scala et al., 1991). If cognitive deficits underlie or contribute in some way to the behavioral disturbances, then recovery is going to take even longer—at least as long as resolving the cognitive impairments. Cognitive deficits often take the longest time to recover from the impact of injury (Di Scala et al., 1991). Perhaps, this is due in part to the fact that so many variables determine the outcome from cognitive disabilities. Besides the injury itself, researchers have shown that variables as diverse as the number of parents living in a household can affect the outcome; for example, younger children from single-parent homes experience less complete cognitive recovery than older children from two-parent households (Tompkins, Holland, Ratcliff, & Costello, 1990).

Although behavior problems in TBI populations have been the topic of discussion in many articles and the subject of numerous scientific investigations, studies that specifically address the validity of interventions with this population are almost nonexistent. Because behavior problems can seriously limit these students' academic and social success (Rosenthal & Bond, 1990), it is critical that educators use the most effective management strategies available. Given the fact that scant empirical data exist to support the use of one strategy over another, educators will have to rely on strategies that have been empirically supported with other populations of children and adolescents who have behavior problems (i.e., behavior disorders). Although there are no data to even suggest a "preferred," let alone best, practice with children and adolescents who suffer the consequences of TBI, what is known about the impact of TBI on behavior and cognition may be helpful in adapting interventions that are accepted practice for reducing maladaptive behaviors and increasing desired behaviors. This chapter emphasizes the need to adapt behavioral strategies in accordance with the cognitive deficits that these students commonly have. These deficits not only have the potential to affect behaviors, including emotional expression, but also can interfere with planned treatments. Mapou (1992), however, noted that treating behavior problems associated with cognitive deficits may actually be easier than trying to treat long-standing personality traits or well-established behavior patterns.

Behavioral Sequelae

Defining the Problem

Researchers have found an excessive rate of behavior disturbance in children who sustain a severe TBI even if they have had no prior history of behavior problems, developmental problems, or central nervous system damage, including head injury (Asarnow, Satz, Light, & Lewis, 1991). Certain populations, however, have been shown to be at substantially greater risk for developing behavior problems following injury. Young males from impoverished and dysfunctional families are an example of this higher risk category (Michaud, Rivara, et al., 1993). Although some have argued that preexisting problems, such as poor judgment or impulsivity, predispose children and adolescents to injury (Rosenthal & Bond, 1990), a causal relationship has not been established. According to Donders (1992), relatively few individuals with TBI have prior histories of behavioral disorders. This conclusion was drawn from a study showing that less than 11% of the participants were described by parents and teachers as having behavior problems before their injuries. Regardless of the exact nature of the relationship between prior behaviors and sequelae following TBI, research has shown that when prior problems did exist, or a person had a predisposition for disturbance (e.g., lack of environmental support and deprivation), the outcome tends to be worse than in cases where there is no such prior history (McAllister, 1992).

Worse outcome is not associated only with premorbid characteristics; it is also strongly associated with the severity of the injury. Research has documented that the more severe the injury, the more likely it is that a child or an adolescent will have behavioral sequelae (Asarnow et al., 1991; Fay et al., 1994; Fletcher, Ewing-Cobbs, Miner, Levin, & Eisenberg, 1993). Researchers have also shown that once present, these behavior problems tend to persist, and may even get worse over time. According to a study by Brown, Chadwick, Shaffer, Rutter, and Traub (1981), over a 2-year period, children with severe TBI showed about a 300% increase in behavior problems. Fay et al. (1994) at the University of Washington also showed that some children with moderate or severe TBI continued to have behavioral problems 3 years after injury. In the Washington study, the participants with moderate or severe TBI performed worse than matched controls on 40 of 53 variables. The data demonstrated that, in addition to behavioral problems, intelligence, adaptive problem solving, memory, achievement, motor performance, and independent living skills were impaired.

Although some researchers have indicated that regardless of injury severity, children who sustain a TBI are more likely than their uninjured peers to be left with functional limitations, including behavioral problems (Greenspan & MacKenzie, 1994), those studies are relatively few in number. The studies that do exist often rely on questionable methodology, such as telephone interviews with parents. Prospective studies of mildly injured children that include face-to-face assessments tend to show that mild injuries have negligible effects on behavior (Jaffe et al., 1993; Knights et al., 1991). Further, these studies demonstrate that children and adolescents with mild TBI are indistinguishable from peers without TBI histories (Bijur, Haslum, & Golding, 1990). In a study comparing mild TBI with other hospitalized populations, after controlling for hyperactivity before the age of 5, Bijur et al. found that children treated for burns and lacerations did as poorly as or worse than children with TBI on measures of behavior and cognition.

It is unclear what explains the report of behavioral disturbances and cognitive problems in children and adolescents who sustain mild TBI. Some are of the opinion that the measures used are not sensitive enough to assess subtle problems, while others believe that parents tend to overreport problems as a result of the emotionally charged nature of the injury (Casey, Ludwig, & McCormick, 1986). According to Casey et al., TBI is often associated with abrupt behavioral changes, including loss of intellect and serious behavior problems, thereby causing parents to overreport, and over-attribute to injury, problem behaviors. This, however, is not always the case. In fact, at times, parents or school personnel do not believe the TBI to be the cause of a child's disruptive behavior (Michaud, Rivara, et al., 1993). This may be due to the fact that dysfunctional behaviors are not immediately apparent. According to Michaud, Rivara, et al., the longer the interval between the age of a TBI and the onset of behavioral and academic problems, the less likely it is that problems will be attributed to the brain injury. The researchers found, however, that the likelihood of having had a prior TBI among special education students in BD classes is three times higher than the rate of TBI in general classrooms.

NEUROPATHOLOGICAL CONSIDERATIONS

Research has shown that as damage increases (e.g., affecting diffuse areas of the brain), so does the probability that behavior problems will occur (Wood, 1987). Although the relationship between behavioral sequelae and damage to frontal and temporal regions has been well established, relationships between other areas of the brain and behavior are not as clear (Mapou,

1992). Mapou contended that, whereas some areas do not have much impact on behavior, other areas account for most of behavior. He argued that damage to the frontal region alone could account for the majority of behavior problems seen in populations with TBI.

Given the fact that damage almost always occurs in the frontal region, and very frequently occurs in the temporal area, regardless of the location of impact to the skull (Mapou, 1992), certain sequelae can be expected. Although no particular behavioral patterns have been found following injury, researchers have found patterns of cognitive impairments (Dalby & Obrzut, 1991). When frontal regions of the brain are damaged, impairments in attention, executive functioning, reasoning, and problem solving can be expected (Levin, 1987). Similarly, when damage takes place in the temporal regions, problems with new learning and memory consolidation can occur (Levin, 1987). Although such damage can have a direct impact on behavior (e.g., poor emotional control), it is difficult to predict the exact nature of these behaviors unless cognitive factors are taken into account. Consideration of cognitive deficits, in fact, may prove critical for designing effective behavioral interventions.

Cognitive Deficits That Affect Behavioral Sequelae

A number of cognitive problems need to be considered in terms of potential for affecting behavior. Poor attention is a particularly important factor to consider. Problems with attention are commonly seen following TBI (Jaffe et al., 1993) and can be one of the greatest barriers to treatment. Inattention reduces individuals' ability to comprehend what is taking place in their environment and reduces their chances of benefiting from learning experiences. When inattention is left untreated, learning can be seriously disrupted, which, in turn, can disrupt behavior. It is not surprising to find that irritability and aggression are common among TBI populations who have impaired attention (Mapou, 1992).

Other cognitive deficits that have the potential to interfere with appropriate behavioral responses pertain to executive functions. These functions are important for behavioral control, as they involve planning, initiating, and executing goal-directed behaviors. These problems, which are rather common in individuals who sustain a TBI (Levin, 1987), can impair a person's ability to mentally solve problems and to act on those solutions. For some, there is not even the motivation to engage in purposeful behaviors. As with poor executive functioning, it is fairly obvious to see how poor insight and judgment can interfere with appropriate behavioral responding. As

Mapou (1992) noted, these problems can lead to circular arguments and escalating behaviors.

Problems with learning new information, or even remembering old, can be devastating to a person's progress and can lead to problems with self-esteem and depression. Even certain therapies may be less effective as a result of the person's inability to retain information. Problems with learning and memory not only are frustrating but also reduce the chance that a person will be able to learn from his or her own experiences.

INTERVENTION STRATEGIES

Examples of Common Behavioral Sequelae

Although the behavioral sequelae following injury are diverse, some behaviors are particularly relevant to a discussion of intervention strategies; aggression and noncompliance are two of these. These behaviors are highly interrelated and appear to be a combination of neurophysiological, constitutional, and environmental factors. Neither behavior, however, appears to be linked to any specific cause of brain injury. Aggression and noncompliance have been found in children who suffer head injuries, but also in children who have central nervous system infections, hemorrhages, and hypoxia (Wood, 1987). They also occur in populations with no known history of central nervous system involvement (Kehle, Clark, Jenson, & Wampold, 1986). It can therefore be assumed that any focal or diffuse brain damage that affects the systems involved in the regulation of emotion and behavior can cause behavioral disturbances such as these (McAllister, 1992).

According to Wood (1987), aggression in children and adolescents with TBI often takes one of two forms. The first is impulsive, unprovoked aggression, or what he called "episodic dyscontrol" (p. 141). The second is an overreaction to situations due to poor emotional control. The first type tends to involve more random acts of violence and destructiveness, whereas the second seems to be more provoked. Often, the second type is also initially manifested as irritability, which tends to escalate into an angrier emotional response. Although both types of aggression are seen in a variety of injuries, the former is often associated with temporal lobe damage, whereas the latter has been associated with damage to the frontal lobes (Mapou, 1992).

Noncompliance is a more pervasive childhood behavior that is learned and reinforced when escalating noncompliance and disruptiveness terminates behavioral commands (Rhode, Jenson, & Reavis, 1993). Noncompliance can, however, be secondary to brain injuries that affect cognitive skills involved in the assessment of social situations (e.g., processing information, reading social cues, understanding cause and effect, remembering and generalizing from one situation to the next; Begali, 1992).

Antecedent Classroom-Based Strategies

With regard to the treatment of behavioral sequelae in TBI populations, Franzen and Lovell (1987) outlined two general principles. The first involves reducing the antecedents that elicit inappropriate behavior, such as noncompliance. The second principle involves reducing the probability that an inappropriate behavior, such as aggression, will be reinforced in the first place. Installing effective classroom-based antecedent strategies is an example of the first principle. These preplanned classroom strategies are fundamental, and their effectiveness is largely related to the degree that they correctly anticipate problem behaviors. Examples of these proactive intervention strategies include the public posting of classroom rules, classroom scheduling, structuring classroom space, and teacher movement about the room (Rhode et al., 1993). For students who have problems with reasoning and problem solving, or have difficulty remembering, these strategies may be helpful.

Publicly Posted Rules. Publicly posted classroom rules function to define expected student behaviors. Posting rules in the classroom also serves to remind students who might otherwise forget them. Although the reasons for the rules should be clearly explained, for students with reasoning problems this may not be relevant. Such students should not, however, have a problem understanding the consequences for compliance or noncompliance if they are concrete and presented clearly. Several characteristics of good proactive rules are important for the student with TBI. These include being specific, tying rules to consequences, making sure rule breakage is measurable, and, if possible, stating the rules in a positive manner (Rhode et al., 1993). For students who have problems controlling their emotions, especially anger, positive statements are likely to be important. Students with problems comprehending will probably find the specific and concrete nature of the rules to be quite beneficial. Keeping the number of rules short can also help the student who has difficulty learning and remembering.

Scheduling. The time devoted to instructional activities should typically constitute no less than 70% of the school day (Rhode et al., 1993). However, students with TBI may not have the attentional capacity to tolerate this amount, and thus adaptations will have to be made. The amount and degree of student engagement in instructional activities can be improved by augmenting the curriculum with peer tutoring and cooperative learning approaches. This may also help to increase a student's awareness of behavioral expectations of the class and improve his or her compliance. For students who can attend well, using interactive software may be of some benefit for improving class performance by addressing underlying cognitive processing problems.

Structuring Class Space and Teacher Movement Around the Room. When assigning student seating, teachers should place students who have disruptive behaviors near them and away from other students with behavior problems. According to Rhode et al. (1993), seating students near teachers allows for better anticipation of problem behaviors and more opportunity for reinforcing appropriate behaviors. For the student who has problems initiating behaviors, this will be particularly important. Reducing distractions will also benefit those students who have attentional and memory problems. In addition, there is considerable evidence in support of the relationship between teacher movement around the room and appropriate social behavior (Rhode et al., 1993). For these students, opportunities for repetition and frequent reinforcement will be a benefit. Positive antecedent strategies are employed to communicate to the student that appropriate and functional behavior will be expected, appreciated, and rewarded. The knowledge of such reward promotes student motivation and improves compliance. Recognition of appropriate behavior should, therefore, be continuous and embedded in the teacher–student dialogue.

Consequential Classroom-Based Interventions

Effective Use of Teacher Reprimands. The most common and preferred method that teachers employ to deal with student noncompliance and aggressiveness is a reprimand. Typically, embedded within the reprimand is the threat of punishment if student compliance is not forthcoming (Reavis, Jenson, Kukic, & Morgan, 1993). Incredibly, elementary and junior high school teachers deliver a reprimand every 2 minutes, on average. In senior high, the rate falls to one every 4 minutes (Reavis et al., 1993; White, 1975). The frequency of reprimands is, to a degree, correlated with the student's ability level (Heller & White, 1975). It has been shown that students who have cognitive disabilities or significant social skill deficits are more likely to receive substantially higher rates of teacher reprimands. This is a particular concern for some students with TBI. Malec (1984) warned that punishers can have a negative effect on these students' mood, initiative, and self-esteem. Deaton (1994) stressed the importance of using positive reinforcements to change the behavior of children with TBI.

Because the appropriate use of reprimands, however, has been shown to temporarily improve student compliance and has also improved academic competence (Reavis et al., 1993; Van Houten, Nau, MacKenzie-Keating, Sameoto, & Calavecchie, 1982), this strategy should not be neglected. The use of reprimands, though, should be infrequent and should be used when other, more positive interventions have failed. To ensure that reprimands have a positive, enduring effect, they should (a) be employed sparingly and in combination with other strategies (Van Houten & Doley, 1983), (b) include the use of preplanned and reasonable consequences if indicated, (c) be monitored so that the rate of reprimands relative to reinforcing statements is at a substantially lower rate, and (d) be presented correctly (Reavis et al., 1993).

The correct presentation of a reprimand involves several variables, including the distance the teacher stands from the student who is to be reprimanded, the amount of time given to the student to comply, how the teacher faces the student, and the tone of the reprimand (Reavis et al., 1993). Student compliance rates increase when reprimands are embedded in a precision request that is in the form of a statement rather than a question. Rather than asking the student if he or she wants to do something, it is more effective to tell the student it is now time to do something. This may be critical for individuals who have difficulty organizing their thoughts and problem solving. After the request is made, the teacher should wait approximately 3 to 5 seconds in order to give the student sufficient time to respond. The reprimand or request should be made after establishing eye contact with the student. It is also important to make the command within a distance of approximately 3 feet. The request typically should not be made more than two times; however, if attentional problems are interfering with a student's compliance, then further repetitions may be necessary. If judged appropriate, touching a student's shoulder immediately prior to the request or reprimand also enhances the student's compliance. The tone of the teacher's voice should be firm, relatively quiet, and lacking emotionality.

In addition to the above, initially requesting compliance from normally tractable students who are seated near the noncompliant student will increase the probability that that student will acquiesce to the teacher's request. In addition, the teacher can build a momentum of compliance by having the noncompliant student respond to positive and enjoyable requests immediately prior to a less preferred or aversive request (Reavis et al., 1993).

Incorporating specificity into reprimands and requests for compliance increases the probability that a student will respond in a positive manner. It is more effective to describe the exact behavior desired than to give general or vague reprimands. The teacher should also socially reinforce student compliance with a request or reprimand. A preplanned negative consequence, such as time-out, however, can help to ensure compliance if the student is not responsive to reprimands or requests for compliance after being given ample direction and opportunity to respond. Time-out for students with TBI, as for all students, must be used in a manner that ensures student safety.

Precision Requests and "Sure I Will." Precision requests can be employed to increase appropriate classroom behaviors and decrease inappropriate behaviors. In combination with the previous suggestions regarding the use of reprimands, precision requests incorporate the following sequence (Reavis et al., 1993):

(1) If a second request is needed, use the key word,"need."
(2) If the request is followed, use a social reinforcer (e.g., praise).
(3) If the request is not followed, use a mild pre-planned negative consequence.
(4) After the negative consequence has been delivered, repeat the request cycle again until the student follows the request. (p. 5)

One difficulty with noncompliant and aggressive students is teaching them to substitute appropriate and adaptive behaviors for the inappropriate and maladaptive behaviors. Use of the "Sure I Will" program along with precision requests facilitates this substitution (Rhode et al., 1993). "Sure I Will" is the process of teaching the student to respond to teacher requests for compliance with the response, "Sure I will," or a similar statement (e.g., "No problem," "Okey dokey," etc.) implying a timely and willing acquiescence. If the student is randomly reinforced for stating, "Sure I will," and the whole procedure is combined with a precision request, compliance rates should be expected to improve (Rhode et al., 1993). According to Rhode et al. (1993), simply uttering the phrase "Sure I will" assists the student in starting the requested behavior and is incompatible with noncompliant and argumentative behaviors. For students who have problems with attention, this element will likely be important. The teacher should reward only genuine "Sure I will"–type responses. After implementation, the criteria for reinforcement should be gradually increased until rewards are given for only exceptional performance. The program can be combined with the use of "mystery motivators" and/or a response–cost procedure to further increase its effectiveness in reducing the student's noncompliance. Using mystery motivators, as described by Rhode et al., entails writing the name of a desirable reinforcer on a piece of paper and sealing this inside an envelope. The envelope is then displayed in a prominent location in the classroom or home (e.g., on the chalkboard or refrigerator). The teacher then takes a monthly calendar and randomly places an *X* on the days when reinforcers will be given. All days are then covered up by using something like a self-sticking dot. The student is given the mystery motivator envelope only on days that he or she has earned a reward and the *X* appears for that day. If no *X* appears, then the student waits for the next day to peel off a dot.

This system creates high anticipation and a visual reminder of what has to be done to earn a chance at the mystery motivator. In cases where reinforcements are difficult to select, or novelty is required (e.g., students with impaired executive functions), mystery motivators may prove to be an effective strategy.

Effective Use of Teacher Praise. One of the most basic and common strategies employed in educational settings for children with behavior disorders is the use of praise. Praise is defined as any behavior, verbal or nonverbal, that communicates approval. Its effectiveness has been well documented (e.g., Shutte & Hopkins, 1970), despite the fact that teachers use praise relatively infrequently (Thomas, Becker, & Armstrong, 1968). At each successive grade level, praise is used with decreasing frequency (White, 1975). Reavis et al. (1993) outlined an I-FEED-V procedure for the effective implementation of praise. Praise should be delivered *i*mmediately, *f*requently, with *e*nthusiasm, and after establishing *e*ye-contact with the student. Further, the teacher should *d*escribe in detail the appropriate behavior and should use a *v*ariety of statements when communicating praise.

Reavis et al. (1993) suggested that praise statements should exceed reprimand statements by a 4 to 1 margin. If this does not work for the student who requires more consistent reinforcement, alter the ratio (e.g., to 8 to 1). Also, the teacher should be sensitive to the individual student in regard to when praise is appropriate: For some students, public praise would not be rewarding but, rather, would be embarrassing. For example, students who are sensitive about their loss in functioning may not find this attention rewarding. In these cases, praise should be delivered in an unobtrusive manner (Reavis et al., 1993).

Augmented Self-Modeling. Observational learning is the behavioral or cognitive change that occurs as a result of observing and copying a model's behavior. The model can be live, filmed, or even imagined. The relatively efficient learning that occurs as a result of observing and copying other students' behaviors is related to the degree the student (a) identifies with the model, (b) has an incentive to imitate the model, (c) attends to the model, and (d) has an opportunity to practice and match the model's behavior (Bandura, 1986). These variables can be maximized by employing the student as his or her own model. Self-modeling is accomplished by constructing edited videotapes depicting the student exhibiting only desired or exemplary behaviors. In the case of students with disruptive behaviors, such as aggression, all instances of these behaviors would be edited out of the intervention tape, leaving only desired and exemplary behaviors. In addition to resultant imitative learning, the student's efficacious beliefs are also altered to be consistent with the exemplary behavior that is depicted in the edited videotapes (Kehle et al., 1986). The loss of self-confidence and self-esteem frequently seen in children with TBI makes self-modeling a particularly appealing intervention. It is also appealing because it can be adapted so that minimal attentional, initiating, and problem-solving skills are necessary to benefit from it. Even students with problems in learning can benefit from the procedure after repeated exposure.

In several published studies, the results of self-modeling interventions have been quite impressive (e.g., Kehle et al., 1986; Kehle & Gonzales, 1991). The reliability and potency of the self-modeling intervention, however, has been enhanced by incorporating other cognitively and behaviorally based strategies, such as spacing effects, mystery motivators, and self-reinforcement (Kehle, Sutilla, & Visnic, 1994). Following is an example of how self-modeling was used with an extremely noncompliant and aggressive 9-year-old student (Gretchen) who sustained a TBI 1 year ago. First, the professional in charge of the intervention required an edited videotape depicting the child complying with the classroom teacher's requests during ongoing class instruction. In Gretchen's case, the help of the school psychologist was solicited. After the school psychologist's unsuccessful attempt to get Gretchen to respond to the teacher's requests, her father was brought into the class to make the same requests while being videotaped. Gretchen complied with his commands. The tape was altered, however, to show her complying with her teacher's requests, not her father's. A 7-minute tape was shown back to her on five different occasions over a period of 4 weeks, to ensure that the treatment was properly spaced over time. Spacing effects have been heavily investigated and shown to be one of the most remarkable phenomena to emerge in the 100-year history of research on learning (Dempster, 1988). For example, two spaced presentations can be twice as effective as two massed presentations. Surprisingly few interventions, however, incorporate this into their designs (Kehle, Jenson, & Clark, 1992).

Prior to the beginning of the intervention with Gretchen, the school psychologist tacked a manilla envelope to the bulletin board in the front of the class. On the envelope were a big question mark and Gretchen's name. The class was told that the envelope contained a "mystery" motivator, a gift that Gretchen would really like and could have following compliance with the teacher's requests. (As noted earlier, mystery motivators are designed to increase the anticipation and value of a reinforcer.)

During the viewings of the tape, Gretchen was instructed to stop the tape whenever she thought she responded appropriately to the teacher's request. Each time Gretchen stopped the tape, she was allowed to choose from a variety of small reinforcers displayed on a table near the video monitor, regardless of whether her behavior on the tape was appropriate. Charting Gretchen's compliance with teacher commands was also taking place. A minimum daily compliance rate of 80% was set for Gretchen in order for her to receive the mystery motivator. Gretchen received the reward several times throughout the intervention. Just in case students missed the improvement in Gretchen's behavior, with her permission, the edited tape was eventually shown to the rest of the class. This showed classmates that she was capable of behaving appropriately and also served to increase peer expectations for Gretchen's improved behavior.

Use of Reductive Procedures. Time-out is defined as the removal of the student from a reinforcing environment, with subsequent placement in a less reinforcing environment for some period of time contingent on a specific misbehavior (Reavis et al., 1993). Franzen and Lovell (1987) emphasized that the environment from which the child is removed must be relatively more reinforcing than the time-out setting. For students seeking a quiet place where stimulation and demands are reduced, this may not be an appropriate intervention. Time-out, however, is a very potent reductive technique for children with behavior disorders (Rhode et al., 1993). Reavis et al. described a continuum, based on restrictiveness, of nonreinforcing environments that can be employed as time-out settings. These range from leaving the child at his or her desk or in the instructional setting to in-class seclusion to removal from the classroom and placement in a separate secluded setting. Perhaps the least restrictive form of time-out is simply ignoring the student's inappropriate behavior for a specific amount of time. It is only effective, however, if the teacher's attention is reinforcing to the student.

Withdrawal of the misbehaving student's work materials is relatively more restricting than simply ignoring him or her. The work materials are removed without comment and the student is required to sit at his or her desk. With younger children, the teacher can assign a time-out to a valued object belonging to the child—the favored toy or object is removed for a specific period of time contingent on the child's behavior. Rhode et al. (1993) described such an in-class time-out procedure called "Bumpy Bunny Time Out" in their book, *The Tough Kid Book.*

More restrictive is the employment of a time-out ribbon. This procedure, developed by Foxx and Shapiro (1978), is effective with younger children who exhibit particularly difficult behaviors. Ribbons are given to all of the students in the class; the ribbons are required for children to participate in any class activity. The ribbon is removed if the child misbehaves. Without a ribbon, the student is ignored by the teacher and the entire class. For students who have suffered loss in self-esteem or are having problems relating socially, this technique should be used only after careful consideration of other alternatives.

Reavis et al. (1993) also described a contingent observation time-out, whereby a student is placed away from the class; he or she can still observe all of the class activities but is ignored by the teacher and classmates. A slightly more restrictive rendition of the contingent observation time-out is the no-look time-out: The student is instructed to close his or her eyes, place his or her head on the desk for a specific amount of time, or face a wall. The student may also be placed behind a screen.

Time-outs that involve removal of the student from the classroom for a specific amount of time are substantially more restrictive and include the student being seated in the hall, placed in another classroom, put in in-school suspension, or placed in a dedicated time-out room. Although Reavis et al. (1993) found the use of time-out in another classroom to be helpful—for instance, in a class one or two grades above the student's placement—it is unclear what impact this would have on the student with TBI who has academic problems and who may feel self-conscious. Placing the student in a classroom where students are well behaved and engaged in academic work, however, may be helpful and needs to be considered.

Behaviors that necessitate the use of a dedicated time-out room should be relatively serious, such as physical aggression, destruction of property, and severe noncompliance. The amount of time the student spends in time-out is generally 1 minute for each year of the student's age. Depending on the cognitive level of the child with TBI, this may have to be altered. Reavis et al. (1993) outlined numerous procedures for the correct implementation of time-out in a dedicated room, and these seem appropriate for the student with TBI: The staff should be knowledgeable about, and have allegiance to the correct implementation of, the procedures; they should themselves have experienced being in time-out; the student's parents must support the use of time-out, and the procedures must be part of the student's Individualized Educational Program; the procedure should be described to the student prior to its implementation; and conversation with the student should be suspended after he or she is instructed to go to time-out.

The use of a dedicated time-out room necessitates the continuous observation of the student by a professional, or paraprofessional, during such placement. This can be accomplished by having a 180-degree peephole installed in the door. Reavis et al. (1993) also suggested that the door to the room be designed so that the adult on the outside must hold the door handle in a locked position. If the student refuses to go to time-out, two things may be necessary: One minute of time for each request to go to time-out is added; and/or the previously acquired skill of manual guidance is employed by whoever is in charge of the intervention. If there is a possibility of physical aggression, additional staff may be required.

Overcorrection. Another effective but relatively intrusive reductive technique is overcorrection. Overcorrection is the enforced practice of behaviors incompatible with the inappropriate behavior after that behavior occurs (Franzen & Lovell, 1987). For example, if the student complies with the teacher's request to sit down but emits a verbally inappropriate response while doing so, the teacher may require the student to practice an appropriate response (e.g., "Sure I will") for a specific period of time. Overcorrection is designed both to eliminate undesired behavior and to teach appropriate behavior (Franzen & Lovell, 1987). For students who have memory problems, this will certainly provide them with the opportunity for repeated practice. Again, one of the critical issues with these students is that their self-esteem not be damaged in the process. Some students may find this procedure to be humiliating.

Pharmacologic Treatments

Pharmacologic treatments that alter central nervous system (CNS) functioning have been useful in reducing emotional outbursts and aggressive behaviors (Yudofsky, Silver, & Schneider, 1987). Pharmacologic treatment, in fact, has become an increasingly important therapeutic option for the management of postinjury behavior disruptions (Rose, 1988). This should not be too surprising, given the impact that brain injury has on the mechanisms that control emotions and behavior. Medications that have been used to increase attention and reduce aggression in children who have sustained brain injuries include anticonvulsants (e.g., Tegretol and Depakote); benzodiazepines (e.g., Clonidine and Valium); neuroleptics (e.g., Haldol); antidepressants (e.g., Tofranil, Prozac, and Zoloft); stimulants (e.g., Ritalin and Dexedrine); and lithium salts.

Research has demonstrated the effectiveness of a number of these medications (e.g., Clark, Baker, Gardner, Pompa, & Tait, 1990; Glenn, 1987a; Haas & Cope, 1985; Siassi, 1982). Clark et al., for example, showed that stimulant medication can be effective in improving the attending behavior of children who sustain a TBI. The overall number of studies, however, are few (Cope, 1987). Given the fact that various neurochemical mechanisms can be involved in the development of disruptive and aggressive behaviors in individuals who have brain injury, it may be more difficult to determine an effective medication protocol. Consequently, the use of pharmacologic treatment by medical personnel for individuals with TBI needs to proceed with caution (Glenn, 1987b). Glenn (1987a) stated that the best way to begin pharmacological management of aggressive and disruptive behaviors is by withdrawing sedating drugs and administering stimulant medications, such as methylphenidate. These medications not only improve alertness, attention, and initiation, but also have a calming effect on many of these children. Being even more cautious, Cope (1987) stated that "unless a true behavioral emergency exists, the primary approach to disordered activity in TBI should be environmental or behavioral" (p. 4). He presented three arguments for this advice. First, the behavioral approach establishes baselines that the physician can use to judge the effectiveness of neuropharmacologic intervention if it becomes necessary. Also, Cope claimed that neuropharmacologic agents appear to be successful in that they function to depress the patient's state of arousal. Therefore, control of maladaptive behavior is gained at the expense of dampening the patient's adaptive behavior. Finally, the nosology of TBI is inadequate and, therefore, accurately predicting which individual will respond to a particular neuropharmacologic agent is impossible (Cope, 1987).

CONCLUSIONS

Behavioral disturbances, like cognitive impairments, can be quite disabling and cause considerable distress for the individual who has sustained the injury and his or her family. If not properly treated, problems that develop following injury can persist for months, even years. It has been well documented that persistent cognitive and behavior problems can negatively affect a student's chance of achieving academically and socially. Unfortunately, little research that looks at the effectiveness of various interventions with this population has been conducted. Although Michaud, Duhaime, and Batshaw (1993) concluded that data are not presently available to allow the design and implementation of effective school-based intervention programs, the present authors disagree.

There are scant data to support the use of specific interventions with TBI populations, but behavioral research has yielded a substantial amount of scientifically based information regarding the management of children who have similar behavior problems. Besides, the interventions that are currently available are not precise enough to treat students who exhibit behavioral disturbances as a result of TBI differently from those who exhibit such behaviors due to other causes. The use of behavioral treatments that address both antecedents and consequences of behaviors and take into consideration a student's cognitive strengths and weaknesses may be a reasonable first step. This may mean that cognitive interventions have to be implemented at the same time that other behavioral management strategies are being used. If behavioral and/or cognitive strategies prove to be ineffective, then the next step would be to consider use of adjunctive medication therapies.

9. Management of Attention and Memory Disorders Following Traumatic Brain Injury

CATHERINE A. MATEER, KIMBERLY A. KERNS,

AND KAREN L. ESO

Advances in acute medical treatment technology have led to an increase in survival rates for individuals with traumatic brain injuries (TBI). Children, adolescents, and young adults (birth to 24 years) constitute the group at highest risk for brain injury, and survival rates for this population are higher than for their adult counterparts (Ylvisaker, 1985; Fletcher, Ewing-Cobbs, McLaughlin, & Levin, 1985; Goldstein & Levin, 1987; Levin, Benton, & Grossman, 1982). As more children survive once-fatal head injuries, clinicians are faced with the challenge of understanding and meeting the special needs of this ever-increasing population.

Although much is known about the effects of injury on the mature adult brain, knowledge of the effects of such injuries on the developing young brain is still limited. Traditionally, researchers and clinicians alike have hypothesized that the "plastic" nature of a child's developing brain protected it from permanent damage due to injury, and, thus, children were thought to recover more rapidly and more completely than adults (Kennard, 1942). It is well documented that children recover physically at a faster rate than adults following brain injuries; however, recent research has demonstrated that, like adults, children often show persistent cognitive

153

and behavioral deficits despite a resumption of normal daily activities (Fay et al., 1994; Fletcher, Ewing-Cobbs, Miner, Levin, & Eisenberg, 1990; Knights et al., 1991; Levin et al., 1988). In fact, Levin et al. (1993) compared children and adolescents with head injury and found that cognitive impairment was more consistently present in the children who were injured at a younger age.

Deficits in attention/concentration, memory, and executive functions are the most frequently reported cognitive sequelae following traumatic brain injury in both adults and children (Beers, 1992; Binder, 1986; Donders, 1993; Kaufmann, Fletcher, Levin, & Miner, 1993; Levin et al., 1988). As memory and attention are critical for successful functioning in even the most basic aspects of everyday living, deficits in these cognitive processes often contribute to significant disability following TBI (Ewing-Cobbs, Fletcher, & Levin, 1985; Glisky, Schacter, & Tulving, 1986a; Klonoff, Clark, & Klonoff, 1993). Although children and adults with brain injuries show similar types of cognitive deficits, the long-term effects of these deficits, superimposed on an active developmental process, produces a very different pattern of recovery in children than in adults (Boll & Barth, 1981; Gulbrandsen, 1984; Thompson et al., 1994).

Studies looking at long-term recovery in children with brain injuries have found that age at onset of injury has a significant impact on the ultimate extent of recovery in this population (Levin, Ewing-Cobbs, & Benton, 1984; Thompson et al., 1994). Age at time of injury has been shown to affect long-term recovery in two ways: First, the predominant causes and the severity of brain injury have been shown to vary as a function of age. For example, in very young children (< 5 years), falls are the most common causes of brain injury. With increasing age, the likelihood of having a brain injury increases, as does the chance of having a more severe injury due to higher probability of involvement in more high-speed and high-risk activities (e.g., sports- and recreation-related injuries; bicycle, pedestrian, and motor vehicle accidents). While severity of initial injury has an obvious impact on recovery of function at any age, the child's developmental stage at the time of injury has also been found to affect overall recovery in both mild and more severe types of injury (Gulbrandsen, 1984). Trauma to the well-established adult brain tends to produce static deficits, whereas trauma to the developing young brain results in deficits that may change in quality and severity over time.

Brain injury in children not only disrupts established functions but also affects those functions that are in the process of developing and those that have yet to begin development. Disruption of primary skills may result in changes to the order, rate, and/or level of learning in the child

(Beers, 1992; Dennis, 1988; Fay et al., 1994). Higher order skills, which depend on established primary skills, may later develop incorrectly, incompletely, or not at all. In many cases, children initially appear to have fully recovered from their injuries (with no apparent residual deficits) but, over time, begin to demonstrate deterioration in cognitive, behavioral, and socioemotional functioning (Beers, 1992; Mateer & Williams, 1991; Eslinger & Grattan, 1991). This process is sometimes referred to as "growing into a deficit." Problems may appear weeks or even years after the initial injury, as greater academic and social demands are placed on the child's already compromised learning abilities, or when abilities dependent on damaged brain regions fail to develop (Barth, Gideon, Sciara, Hulsey, & Anchor, 1986). Knowledge about the interaction between the effects of the brain damage and the ongoing process of development is crucial to understanding brain injury in children, but this interaction is currently not well understood.

The long-term cognitive and behavioral effects of injury to the developing brain constitute a barrier to treatment, rehabilitation, and education in pediatric populations (Bigler, 1987). Individuals designing pediatric cognitive rehabilitation programs are faced with children whose brains not only are recovering from injury but also are in the process of maturation. Conflicting conceptions about the nature of cognitive systems (Flavell, Miller, & Miller, 1993), varied explanations about cognitive development (Kail & Bisanz, 1982), and insufficient information regarding the nature of brain–behavior relationships in children serve to compound the difficulties of pediatric rehabilitation programming (Rutter, 1981; Telzrow, 1987).

Over the past decade, there has been a dramatic increase in clinical and research interest in the area of cognitive rehabilitation, and as a result, many rehabilitation programs for adult survivors of brain injury have been developed. Fewer rehabilitation programs exist for children with brain injuries, and those that have been developed tend to be modifications of methods used with adults with brain injury or are applications of treatments used with children with learning disabilities. Although the use of these programs with children with brain injuries has only recently begun to be systematically evaluated, the success of similar programs with adults with brain injuries and children with learning disabilities provides an optimistic rationale for their application in this population.

The remainder of this chapter will discuss the nature of cognitive rehabilitation and review treatment methods designed to remediate or circumvent deficits in memory and attention, with reference to their application in a pediatric brain-injured population.

APPROACHES TO THE REHABILITATION OF INDIVIDUALS WITH COGNITIVE IMPAIRMENT

Approaches to management of acquired cognitive impairments generally fall into one of three broad categories. One category of interventions includes externally focused approaches, which do not attempt to change the person's underlying cognitive abilities or behaviors but, instead, attempt to alter aspects external to the individual. Included in this category are environmental modifications, changed expectations for the individual, and the use of specialized teaching strategies. These strategies do not assume that any change will occur in the individual's abilities or that there will be generalization of improved functioning in other contexts or settings. The second category of intervention involves procedures designed to actually improve or restore cognitive abilities. Finally, the third category involves the training and implementation of procedures or strategies that the individual with cognitive impairment can use to compensate for or lessen the functional impact of cognitive deficits. The latter two approaches can be considered more internally focused interventions, in that they are designed to directly change the individual's abilities and/or behaviors. Each of these approaches will be discussed in greater detail below.

Externally Focused Interventions. An example of such an approach would involve *modifying the environment* by, for example, decreasing distractions or organizing the workspace. These modifications can be undertaken by parents, teachers, or caregivers and do not necessarily require specific action on the part of the individual with TBI. Another way to alter the environment is to provide external cues, such as checklists, or other devices that serve to remind or cue the individual. Although the caregiver, parent, or teacher may be responsible for implementing these cues, the injured individual must be trained to attend to, understand, and respond to them appropriately if they are to be of practical use.

A second, somewhat related approach is to alter the demand or need for certain skills or abilities. This approach takes the injured individual as he or she is and *alters expectations* for his or her functioning. If, for example, a school-age child is having difficulty with recall of information, exams might instead be set up in a recognition or multiple-choice format.

A third approach that focuses on external factors rather than internal ones involves the use of *specialized teaching strategies* that are known to facilitate learning, memory, or behavioral change. Certain forms of training or teaching, for example, make use of the principle of "errorless learning" (described later in this article) to facilitate learning of new information in individuals with memory impairments.

Internally Focused Interventions. These interventions include both restorative and compensatory approaches. Restorative strategies attempt to change the injured individual's cognitive capabilities. This approach has probably engendered the most controversy. It involves implementing exercises that facilitate practice on tasks requiring specific cognitive abilities or processes in an attempt to improve/restore those abilities, as well as other higher order abilities that depend on those processes. This *process-specific* approach has yielded some positive results for certain cognitive areas, such as attention, but not for others, such as memory (Sohlberg & Mateer, 1989a).

Another approach involves teaching the individual to use techniques or strategies that will allow *compensation* for underlying cognitive impairments. These can range from simply learning to refer to and follow a checklist for some behavioral routine, to learning to use quite intricate external memory or organizational systems. There is little or no expectation that use of such compensatory strategies will alter the individual's underlying cognitive ability, only that he or she will be better able to function through systematic use of the device. This approach requires a well-thought-out design for the compensation, a commitment to training its use, and a plan for ensuring generalization of the compensation to functional environments.

Many of the techniques that attempt to improve underlying skills or to teach the active use of compensatory strategies rely, in part, on the use of *behaviorally based training strategies.* These approaches involve an analysis of behaviors, their antecedents, and the consequences that serve to reinforce or weaken the behavioral response. Implementation of these approaches requires an understanding of behavioral principles and a systematic plan for implementing a behavior modification program. It also requires identification of appropriate rewards or motivators, and a commitment to adhering to the program by everyone working with the individual in the settings in which the behaviors are desired. Although cognitive abilities are not always thought of in behavioral terms, many cognitive abilities have behavioral correlates, and there is a strong historical precedent for treating a broad range of cognitively based skills, including expressive language and social skills, through behavioral techniques.

In learning new actions or behavior patterns, individuals with brain injuries rely on particular aspects of learning and memory, including both *procedural memory* and *implicit memory.* For example, systematic recording in, and drawing upon, a memory system involves procedural memory in the development of new habits and behavioral sequences. Similarly, implicit memory has been utilized in some rehabilitative approaches. It is not clear in children, however, how and when these different forms of memory develop or how much memory capacities may be affected by acquired injury. Thus, little is known about how or if these techniques can be utilized in rehabilitation for children.

Another aspect of working with individuals who demonstrate cognitive impairments involves the facilitation of insight and self-awareness with regard to their cognitive abilities, and instruction in the use of self-instructional and metacognitive strategies. Without sufficient insight into the presence of cognitive difficulties and some recognition of their practical impact, it is often difficult to establish the use of many of the compensatory aids and strategies that have been found to be useful for many individuals with cognitive impairment. Although several authors have discussed the importance of working on insight and addressing the psychological impact of acquired impairment (Prigatano, 1991; Prigatano, O'Brien, & Klonoff, 1993), this area frequently is not addressed in treatment.

Regardless of which approaches or specific strategies are utilized in remediation, some general principles of intervention should always be considered. First, it is important to undertake a comprehensive neuropsychological evaluation of the injured child's cognitive and behavioral profile and to determine how his or her strengths and weaknesses are affecting, or are likely to affect, various aspects of real-world functioning. In the case of children, cognitive impairments often have a primary impact on education and learning potential, as well as continued social and emotional development. The selection of strategies must be individually tailored and take into account not only the child's profile, but also the educational and family setting and resources available. Treatment programs should be designed to meet specific goals and frequently evaluated for efficacy. Generalization plans must be implemented and evaluated at multiple levels to ensure real-life applicability. Finally, the impact of the intervention in terms of improved adaptive functioning should be evaluated realistically. In the following sections we will discuss the literature to date on the efficacy of these various approaches to the treatment and management of attention and memory disorders.

Remediation of Deficits in Attention

A discussion of the efficacy of various approaches to rehabilitating impairments in attention in children is complicated by three major factors: first, a lack of clear, accepted theory regarding the notion of attention as a cognitive ability; second, a limited research base on the development of attention; and, third, a limited number of studies that have systematically described or evaluated treatment of acquired attention disorders in children. What is known about working with attentional abilities comes largely from the clinical research on adults with acquired disorders of attention and from the literature on management of children with developmental disorders of attention, particularly attention-deficit/hyperactivity disorder (ADHD). At present, it is not clear how applicable the findings in these fields of research are for children with acquired disorders of attention.

The term *attention* has been used in the literature to refer to a broad collection of states, processes, and abilities, only a few of which have been specifically evaluated in either adults or children with acquired injuries. The literature suggests that the great majority of even patients with severe brain injury recover the most basic aspects of attentive behavior, including normal sleep/wake cycles and "tonic" arousal (e.g., emergence from coma). Problems may persist, however, in higher levels of attention, including integrity of orienting responses to novel stimuli. Problems are also often seen with the maintenance or duration of attention (vigilance) over long periods of time. Another difficulty frequently reported following brain injury is slowed speed of information processing and/or slowed speed of responding. It has been suggested that speed of processing is a limiting function of attentional capacity (Case, 1992; Case, Kurland, & Goldberg, 1982). Problems with working memory have also been described following injury to frontal systems secondary to traumatic brain injury. Many investigators consider problems with working memory an impairment of attentional control. Some studies have also reported problems with inattentive behaviors, such as distractibility and inability to inhibit responses to irrelevant information, as well as a tendency to overprocess redundant stimuli. There is also support for problems with higher levels of attentional control, including difficulties with set shifting (cognitive and behavioral flexibility) and with dual task processing or divided attention (see Van Zomeren & Brouwer, 1994, for a review). Given the broad scope of problems that have been considered to be attentional in nature, it is perhaps not surprising that the literature on remediation is inconsistent.

Environmental Modifications. Perhaps the simplest approach to helping a child with attentional problems is to implement modifications that reduce distractions. This can include preferential classroom seating, selective amplification, use of carrels or study rooms, or allowing a student to wear earplugs or a headset during independent study. Changes in the teaching approach used with a child, such as keeping presentation of information short and concise, providing repetitions, and allowing the child to take frequent breaks, can also be helpful. Additional techniques include making sure the child is focusing on the instructor, allowing the child to work in small groups in order to minimize distractions from other students, and cuing the child to pay attention.

Behavioral Approaches. Some of the earliest reports of successful intervention with adolescents and adults with brain injuries who demonstrated severe problems in maintaining attention were those of Wood and Fussey and their colleagues in Great Britain (Fussey & Giles, 1988; Wood & Fussey, 1987). In a series of well-controlled case studies utilizing behavioral techniques, these authors demonstrated improvements in a wide variety of adaptive behaviors, including maintenance of attention to task.

A number of studies have looked at the use of behavioral approaches for increasing attentive behavior in children with ADHD. Though cognitive behavioral treatments have been successful in reducing impulsivity (Kendall & Braswell, 1993), which is one of the major symptoms of ADHD, in general these treatments have been less successful at remediating the inattention associated with this disorder (Kendall & Panichelli-Mindel, 1995). Other behavioral approaches aimed specifically at improving attention and on-task behavior in ADHD children have utilized response–cost contingencies. The "attention training system" described by Gordon, Thomason, Cooper, and Ivers (1991) makes use of a response–cost program to increase attention to task (on-task behavior). These investigators demonstrated that their attention training program significantly increased on-task behavior in children with ADHD; however, these positive training effects were shown to dissipate upon cessation of training. Behavioral techniques have been demonstrated to be effective in decreasing specific problem behaviors, but their generalizability and stability over time tend to be limited. For example, when a classroom-based contingency program was used, reductions in behavioral inattention were not maintained when the contingency was removed, and did not generalize to other, similar situations (Barkley, 1988).

Direct Retraining Approaches. There has been a growing literature regarding the effects of interventions designed to improve different aspects of attention in *adults*. A number of researchers have reported significant posttreatment improvement on standard measures of attention following treatment programs that provided repeated opportunities to practice and exercise a variety of attention-dependent skills or processes (Ben-Yishay, Piasetsky, & Rattock, 1987; Diller, Ben-Yishay, Gerstman, Goodkin, Gordon, & Weinberg, 1974; Gray & Robertson, 1989; Gray, Robertson, Pentland, & Anderson, 1992; Niemann, Ruff, & Baser, 1990; Sivak et al., 1984; Sohlberg & Mateer, 1987; Sturm, Hartje, Orgass, & Willmes, 1993). These studies incorporated a variety of specific procedures that included both auditorily and visually based tasks. Some utilized computer-based activities, whereas others relied on paper-and-pencil materials, other manipulatives, audiotaped materials, or some combination thereof.

Sohlberg and Mateer (1987) reported improvements on measures of attention following work with tasks included in their Attention Process Training (APT) program. The APT materials are a group of hierarchically organized remediation tasks based on the author's clinical model of attention. This model of attention was derived by examining cognitive theories of attention in concert with clinical observations from the assessment and rehabilitation of individuals who had sustained TBI. In this model, attention is considered to be a multidimensional cognitive capacity that directly affects new learning, memory, communication, problem solving, perception, and all other dimensions of cognition. Attention is divided hierarchically into five dimensions: focused attention, sustained attention, selective attention, alternating attention, and divided attention (Sohlberg & Mateer, 1989a).

Focused attention is defined as the ability to respond to specific sensory information, generally presented in a visual, auditory, or tactile modality. This type of attention is disrupted in metabolic disorders affecting level of consciousness, in the early stages following some types of brain trauma, and during emergence from coma, when an individual may initially be responsive primarily to internal stimuli and only gradually regain the ability to respond to specific external events.

Sustained attention refers to the ability to maintain a consistent behavioral response for a period of time, doing a continuous and repetitive activity. Sustained attention incorporates the notion of vigilance and involves both persistence at an activity over time and consistency in maintaining that behavior. Patients with a disruption in sustained attention may be able to focus on a task for only a few seconds or minutes, or may dramatically fluctuate in the accuracy of their performance over even brief periods of time. Sustained attention, at perhaps a higher level, also includes the construct of "mental control," or "working memory," which involves the ability to maintain and manipulate more than one piece of information in one's mind at a time.

Selective attention is described as the ability to maintain a behavioral or cognitive set in the presence of distracting or competing stimuli. It incorporates the idea of "freedom from distractibility" and the ability to ignore irrelevant information. Individuals who have deficiencies in this area are easily drawn off task by extraneous or irrelevant stimuli, including both external sights and sounds (the "cocktail party phenomenon") and internal distractors (worries, ruminations, sensations, or thoughts). Clinical examples include individuals who are unable to perform tasks in noisy environments, such as a homemaker who, after a brain injury, is unable to prepare a meal if her children are playing in the kitchen, or the child who, following an injury, has problems attending to a teacher's lecture when others are whispering in the classroom.

The construct of *alternating attention* refers to the mental flexibility that allows individuals to shift their focus of attention. Alternating attention involves switching between tasks having different cognitive demands or requiring different behavioral responses. For example, a student must shift between listening to the lecture and writing notes. The individual must monitor which information will be attended to and/or which responses are appropriate. Individuals with difficulty in this area have problems changing tasks quickly or shifting their attention to new stimuli. They may continue with an old behavior that is no longer appropriate, or may need extra cues to initiate a new task.

Divided attention is described as the ability to respond simultaneously to more than one task or stimulus. Either more than one behavioral response is required or more than one stimulus needs to be monitored. Divided attention is required whenever multiple, simultaneous demands must be managed (e.g., driving a car while drinking coffee). Some tasks that require divided attention involve overlearned behavior patterns and thus are easily accomplished by most individuals (e.g., walking and chewing gum). Other tasks require higher levels of attentional capacity, such as driving a car while trying to find your way on a map, and are not as easily accomplished.

The APT materials are based on this hierarchical model of attention. Many of the tasks included in the APT materials rely on audiotaped stimuli that are used in a continuous performance design. At easy levels, patients respond to single target numbers or words. As the level of difficulty increases, greater demands are made on working memory. For example, patients may have to respond to stimuli presented in a particular sequence (e.g., numbers ascending or descending), or restate in alphabetical or reverse order words presented in increasingly longer sentences. In selective attention activities, distracting background sounds are incorporated. Shifting and divided attention tasks require attentional control abilities and mental flexibility.

Adults with acquired attention deficits subsequent to a variety of etiologies (e.g., traumatic brain injury, CVA, etc.) have demonstrated improvements on measures of attention after training on the materials. Gains have been demonstrated not only in individuals with moderate to severe injuries, but also in individuals with mild cognitive impairment (Mateer, 1992; Mateer, Sohlberg, & Youngman, 1990). Mateer followed up her study with several additional reports indicating positive effects of attention training not only on attention, but also on measures of memory function (Mateer, 1992; Mateer & Sohlberg, 1988; Mateer et al., 1990). It was proposed that for some individuals with brain injury who experienced memory problems, improvements in attention had a facilitatory effect on memory abilities. Niemann et al. (1990) also reported an improvement in both attention and memory following attention training but found no such differences in either attention or memory following memory training.

There is a small but growing body of information regarding the use of direct retraining of attention deficits in children. One promising intervention has been the use of the previously described APT materials (Sohlberg & Mateer, 1987) with children. Williams (1989) conducted an initial study using this approach with a group of children diagnosed as ADHD. Williams used APT materials in a small-group treatment study involving 6 children with ADHD (ages 8 to 13 years). Williams evaluated changes in performance on training tasks, as well as pre- and posttreatment changes on independent psychometric measures of attention, on measures of arithmetic and reading efficiency, and on a parent-reported measure of attention. His results revealed significant improvements on specific training tasks and on independent measures of attention, with some gains on academic efficiency (though they were not statistically significant); however, no changes were seen in parental reports of children's attention abilities. The lack of change in parent report may have been due to the parents' being more focused on behavioral features of ADHD. Alternatively, it may have been that improvement in cognitive attentional processes were not as readily observed by parents.

Semrud-Clikeman, Teeter, Parle, and Connor (1995) reported changes on measures of auditory and visual attention in children with ADHD following administration of the APT program. In that study, children ages 6 to 12 were administered tasks from the APT in small groups of 5 to 7 for 60 minutes, twice a week over a period of 18 weeks. Pre- and posttesting revealed significant changes on both the D-2 test (a measure of visual cancellation; Brickenkamp, 1981) and the Brief Test of Attention (BTA; a measure of auditory attention requiring the child to focus on and count letters or numbers over increasingly longer trials; Schretlin, Bobholz, & Brandt, in press). On the D-2 measure, the ADHD group performed more poorly than controls prior to treatment but did not differ from controls after treatment. On the BTA there was a significant improvement in the performance of the ADHD group following treatment, whereas no changes were seen in the control group. The authors commented informally that the children off medications appeared to make better gains than those taking medications during the treatment. Additionally, qualitative interviews with teachers revealed that ADHD children seemed to be more attentive and showed improvement in completing tasks in class (M. Semrud-Clikeman, personal communication, June 10, 1996).

Thomson (1994) completed a preliminary study assessing the efficacy of attention training using the APT in children who had sustained traumatic brain injury. In her study, 6 children, ages 14 to 17, who had sustained moderate to severe brain injury at least 12 months previously were trained using the APT materials. The children were seen individually within their school setting for approximately 6 weeks. Utilizing a single case study design, Thomson reported notable gains in several psychometric measures of attention (the Children's Paced Auditory Serial Addition Test [Johnson, Roethig-Johnston, & Middleton, 1988], the Trail Making Test–Part B, and the Arithmetic subtest of the WISC-R), as well as on tasks of academic efficiency (timed mathematics worksheets). Thomson noted that most of the gains made on the training tasks occurred within the first 3 weeks of training, with improvement leveling off considerably after that time. Again, improvement was not seen on reports of attentive behavior in the classroom (Attention Deficit Disorders Evaluation Scale–School Version; McCarney, 1989), as reported by the classroom teacher.

Although additional data are certainly needed, the literature does provide some support for direct attention training approaches in children. However, some problems are evident with the use of attention training materials currently available. When using attention training tasks with adults, there is an assumption that the basic cognitive requirements of the task are well within the person's capabilities. Tasks depend on manipulation of automatic or overlearned abilities, such as number sequencing, simple mathematical operations, alphabetizing, and ordering operations. Many of these abilities have not yet been learned or may not be well established in young children or elementary-age children. Therefore, the use of these tasks may be impossible, or the tasks may not affect underlying attentional abilities. The authors, in conjunction with several other colleagues, have begun to modify attention training tasks to make them more applicable to a younger population.

Thomson and Kerns (in press) described the use of attention training activities, and modifications to the training regimen, with two children with acquired attention deficits secondary to mild traumatic brain injury. One of the authors modified the materials for use with a 12-year-old boy who had sustained a very severe traumatic brain injury secondary to blunt left-cranial impact (this child was in coma for 4 months and inpatient rehabilitation for approximately 1 year). The child had sustained his injury at age 9; his academic skills were found to be at preinjury levels (approximately third grade). He was unable to use many of the attention training materials due to his limited academic skills. For example, when it was found that the child was unable to alphabetize a string of words, the author generated word sets that required ordering increasingly longer strings of items by size—a task within his cognitive ability. Other modifications to the materials included easier identification tasks and visual attention materials that were of more interest to younger children. Modifications of this type have recently been made to the APT materials, such that there is now a set of tasks appropriate for children ages 4 to 10 years that the authors are currently using in pilot testing (Thomson & Kerns) to assess outcome efficacy.

Biofeedback Training. Yet another approach to the remediation of cognitive deficits in attention has been the use of electroencephalographic biofeedback. This approach has been used primarily with children who have ADHD, but the approach may warrant investigation for use with children who have acquired attention deficits. Studies have shown that many children with ADHD differ from nondisabled children on measures of brain electrical activity (EEG) and in their event-related potentials (ERPs). For example, many individuals without attention deficits demonstrate slower theta range EEGs during rest but shift to faster beta range activity with increasing alertness. Some children with ADHD have not shown this shift, suggesting that a reduction in electrophysiological alerting may be an underlying feature of ADHD. In some cases with this profile, EEG biofeedback has been used as a method to increase beta activity. Lubar (1991) reviewed a number of studies utilizing EEG biofeedback in children with ADHD that have supported not only significant improvement on psychometric measures of attention and general ability, but also improvement in academic skills, duration of on-task behavior, and sustained attention (Lubar & Lubar, 1984; Tansey, 1985, 1990). Despite reported success with biofeedback training in children with ADHD, there are some negative findings and some reported difficulties with interpreting the studies (Cobb & Evans, 1981; Lee, 1991). A more detailed review of this literature is beyond the scope of this chapter.

Although EEG changes have been identified in some adults with acquired attention disorders secondary to TBI (Unsal & Segalowitz, 1995), there is only limited research regarding the nature of such changes and even less available regarding possible posttraumatic EEG changes in pediatric populations. The authors were not able to locate any research that utilized a biofeedback approach to improving attention in children with acquired deficits. Given the reports of improvement in some children with ADHD, this seems to be an area that deserves more attention as a possible means of remediation for attention deficits in children with TBI.

Megacognitive and Self-Regulatory Strategies. Another approach to working with children with attentional problems involves specific training in self-regulatory or self-monitoring strategies. These strategies stress goal setting, performance monitoring and evaluation, and self-regulation, and have been investigated in children with developmental attention deficits as a possible means of improving attentive behavior, decreasing impulsive behavior, and increasing use of active learning strategies.

Loper (1982) described two types of metacognitive training. The *mechanical approach* involves a routine recording of behavior and is characterized by regularity and repetition. For example, at randomly signaled points, the individual might be instructed to ask himself or herself, "Am I paying attention?" and record his or her response on an answer sheet. Barkley, Copeland, and Sivage (1980) demonstrated increases in observable attention in children with hyperactivity using this approach. The *elaborative approach* is a self-interrogatory scheme whereby the child asks a set of open-ended questions, the responses to which will vary with the material under consideration. For example, after reading a paragraph, the child might ask himself or herself, "What was the main idea of that paragraph?" These open-ended questions structure the child's thinking so that he or she is able to better encode and store material. This structure also ensures that the child is attending to the material.

Despite some reports describing the positive impact of these procedures, there has not been a general consensus that these approaches (alone or in combination with medication) are effective in improving behavioral and/or academic functioning in children with ADHD (Abikoff, 1987, 1991). In addition, studies of both spontaneous and trained use of self-monitoring strategies suggest that a student's awareness of learning outcomes is critical to continued strategy use. Monitoring of strategy effectiveness and learning outcome has been seen as a complex metacognitive activity that involves directed attention and sophisticated reasoning processes (Ghatala, Levin, Pressley, & Goodwin, 1986; Zimmerman, 1990). Because these abilities are often disrupted in children with acquired disorders of attention, these children may be limited in their use of such strategies or may need very intensive training in their use. Despite these possible limitations, self-regulatory management strategies are helpful for some children.

Borkowski, Peck, Reid, and Kurtz (1983) attempted to teach the acquisition, maintenance, and generalization of organizational strategies in grade-school children identified as impulsive or reflective. Strategy scores were higher for reflective children than impulsive children during transfer but not training, suggesting a relationship between these personality/behavioral variables and the ability to use strategies in new contexts. In 1987, Reid and Borkowski reported on the effectiveness of training metacognitive strategy use in a group of children with hyperactivity. The children received either self-management training in rehearsal strategies or the same self-management training plus attribution training designed to enhance beliefs about the importance of effort in improving performance. The addition of attribution training contributed significantly to not only the reduction of hyperactivity, but also enhanced beliefs about the importance of effort and, in general, a more mature knowledge about memory.

There is little information to guide clinicians in the use of such strategies in children with TBI. The problem is further complicated by a limited research base with record to fostering metacognitive abilities and self-management of cognition and behavior in nondisabled children (Flavell et al., 1993). Metacognition relevant to strategy use develops with age and experience (Garner & Alexander, 1989); there is only limited research examining how aspects of metacognition development are affected by acquired injury. Some researchers have identified problems with insight and awareness in children with TBI (Grattan & Eslinger, 1992), consistent with work documenting limitations in self-awareness in adults with TBI (Prigatano, 1991). Such problems might contribute to the problems that children with TBI have in learning to use metacognitive strategies in new environments.

Dennis, Barnes, Donnelly, Wilkinson, and Humphreys (1996) investigated the metacognitive skills of knowledge appraisal and knowledge management in children with head injuries and in normally developing children. The deficits of children with head injury on the tasks presented seemed to arise less from a deficient knowledge base than from problems in the sustained application of cognitive appraisal skills. The authors suggested that deficits in basic skills, such as attention and memory, would predude acquisition of an information base on which metacognitive processes might act. Alternatively, they suggested, a fundamental lack of metacognitive processing due to deficits in core metacognitive skills could produce a range of problems in other cognitive domains or skills. For example, inability to reflect on one's own memory could limit the use of memory strategies, resulting in poor memory for what is being learned.

Crowley and Miles (1991) reported on the use of a cognitive intervention in a 16-year-old male who had sustained a severe TBI $1\frac{1}{2}$ years earlier. The student was failing algebra. This appeared to be due not to a lack of conceptual knowledge, but to incompleteness of work, a failure to detect and perform operations in a given problem, and transient inattention. There was also a pattern of intermittent, random math fact mistakes, calculation errors, transpositions, and oversights. These errors seemed to be due to poor self-monitoring, lapses in concentration, perseverative tendencies, and inflexibility in set shifting. Thus, the functional academic-skill goal in Crowley and Miles's study was competence in mathematical computations. The intervention utilized a goal-directed approach, charting of competence on each goal, and use of behavioral principles. Several specific compensatory strategies were developed to increase self-monitoring, including self-executed written cues, use of reference sheets, and a strategy for self-checking of answers. Training was provided in 40 sessions over an 8-week period. After training, the subject's performance of algebra processes per se had not shown improvement, but he demonstrated improved self-monitoring. In particular, there was an absence of omissions, perseverations, and erroneous operations when compared to pretraining measures. This finding suggested improved self-monitoring, and some generalization of skills obtained to a math domain that was not the major focus of the remediation attempts. This case study provided an excellent example of a behaviorally based and individually tailored approach to working with some of the cognitive and self-regulatory deficits that often interfere with academic performance.

In summary, there are several approaches to working with children who demonstrate disorders of attention. Although refinements and further research are clearly needed, and new approaches will likely emerge, several of the approaches described show promise for limiting the impact of attentional problems in this population.

Remediation of Deficits in Memory

Memory impairments are among the most frequent and disruptive neuropsychological sequelae of traumatic brain injury in children (Dalby & Obrzut, 1991; Telzrow, 1987). These impairments can hinder the ability to recall previously learned information or experiences, to remember recent events, or to acquire new information and skills. Given that one of the major "tasks" of the developing child is learning a vast amount of new information, these deficits can have a major impact on the child's academic and social adjustment. Although problems with memory may be seen early after injury, their devastating impact is often realized only years later.

Direct remediation of memory deficits, through restoration of memory ability, has been attempted through the use of repetitive exercises and drills or through training in the use of visual or verbal mnemonic strategies (Crovitz, 1979; Gianutsos & Gianutsos, 1979; Wilson, 1982). Though these strategies have demonstrated very limited efficacy in adult clinical samples, they have remained popular in clinical practice. Evidence from a number of studies suggests that the effects of these "practice" approaches are highly specific to the training tasks and do not readily generalize to new contexts or materials (Ericsson & Chase, 1982; O'Connor & Cermak, 1987). Similar findings have been demonstrated with elaboration strategies. These strategies include training in the use of verbal elaboration or other encoding strategies, as well as such techniques as visual imagery. Research has suggested that new information can be learned utilizing these strategies, but that the strategies are rarely utilized spontaneously and are often difficult to apply in real-world settings (Cermak, 1975; Glisky & Schacter, 1989; Harris, 1992; Wilson, 1987).

There is a small body of research involving children both with and without learning disabilities regarding the effectiveness of memory training strategies. Mullin and Lange (1974) reported that nondisabled kindergartners demonstrated a better ability to retain auditory and visual stimuli after 25 fifteen-minute sessions in which they were trained in specific strategies to remember pictures, geometric shapes, and numbers. However, there were no measures of generalization of this approach. Wang and Richarde (1987) reported that elementary-school-age children who received training in self-monitoring with regard to memory were more likely to use a successful elaboration strategy on a paired associate learning task than children who did not receive the training. The authors also stated that, by fourth grade, most children engaged in such elaborations without explicit memory-monitoring training.

In a recent study by Brady and Richman (1994), children with reading disabilities received mnemonic training in either a visual elaboration or a verbal rehearsal strategy. Children who demonstrated a concomitant memory disorder benefited from verbal rehearsal but not visual training, whereas children with concomitant language and memory disorders made greater gains in the visual mnemonic training condition. These data suggest a relationship between children's cognitive strengths and deficits and their ability to employ a given memory strategy effectively. These findings have important implications for work with children with traumatic brain injury, as these children often demonstrate a broad range of cognitive and linguistic problems in addition to their difficulties with memory and learning. As almost all of the literature on memory strategy training has focused either on nondisabled children or on children with developmental delays, the applicability of such approaches with children with traumatic brain injury is unknown.

Training Use of Compensatory Memory Aids. Given the dearth of support for direct retraining approaches to remedy memory impairment, much of the focus in memory rehabilitation in adults has turned to the training of external compensatory memory aids (Franzen & Haut, 1991; Glisky & Schacter, 1986; Sohlberg & Mateer, 1989b). External memory aids are devices or systems that can be used to store and retrieve information. They vary from extremely sophisticated to very simple systems; examples include computer-based systems, paging systems, electronic watches, electronic organizers, memory notebooks, and posted checklists. The systems can be designed to store both previously known and new information (e.g., names, telephone numbers, birthdates). They can serve as a record of specific experiences through use of a diary or daily log, to assist individuals who have impaired episodic memory. Systems can be designed to cue or prompt behavior through auditory or visual signals. They can provide a guide for future behavior through the use of "To do" lists and calendars. Systems can be individually designed to meet very specific needs and support many aspects of everyday living, work, and school environments.

Regardless of the type and components of the external memory system selected, it is always necessary to train the individual to use the system effectively and to use it in the real-world situations in which it is needed. It is often difficult to train new skills necessary for using compensatory memory aids in an individual who has impairments in memory and new learning. Learning may be further compromised by the difficulties with initiation, abstraction, and problem solving often seen following traumatic brain injury. Even individuals without these deficits require time and motivation to learn to record in and refer to external memory systems, and to spontaneously utilize them. Despite widespread clinical use of memory systems, there has been little research regarding how to best teach individuals with memory impairment to use such systems.

Sohlberg and Mateer (1989b) described a three-stage behavioral training method for teaching the use of an external memory system. That study provided data on a young man who was severely amnesic and suffered other cognitive impairments following a traumatic brain injury. This individual required approximately 6 months to (a) develop consistent recall of the sections and purposes of the system, (b) consistently record in the system, (c) accurately monitor the system, and (d) use the system in a range of complex settings. This individual returned to independent living and was able to work in a structured setting with the assistance of this aid, although, as expected, he demonstrated no improvement on standardized laboratory measures of recall. Individuals with less severe cognitive and memory deficits may learn to use a system more quickly, but almost all individuals we have worked with have needed some assistance with system development and training.

In a recent study by Schmitter-Edgecombe, Fahy, Whelan, and Long (1995), 8 subjects with traumatic brain injury received 9 weeks of either specific memory notebook training or supportive therapy. The notebook training utilized both behavioral learning principles and educational strategies for individualizing instruction. Following treatment, the group receiving notebook training reported fewer memory failures on a daily checklist measure than the group receiving the supportive therapy. Although there was a trend in the same direction, this finding no longer reached statistical significance at a 6-month follow-up. These findings suggest the need for regular monitoring of system use following the initial training period.

Research on memory-system use in adults is limited, and there is even less information available regarding the use of external memory systems with children. As with adults, it is not enough to provide a child with an assignment sheet and assume this will be sufficient for remediating problems in remembering class assignments. It is important to train children in the use of the memory systems, and to modify the system to meet the children's needs.

Kerns, Thomson, and Youngman (1993) presented data on the use of such a system with a 14-year-old with severe memory deficits secondary to brain tumor and consequent treatment. In this single case report, a memory book system was designed after sufficient task-analysis and behavioral data were collected regarding the type of memory failure this child experienced, as well as the type of information that was most important for her to access. A three-pronged approach similar to the one previously described, including acquisition, application, and adaptation, was utilized. Training in use of the system was provided to the young girl by a school counselor (in consultation with the investigators). Following implementations of the memory system, reports from teachers and parents indicated that the client made significant improvements in completing and turning in assignments and was better able to manage academic demands and access extracurricular activities (e.g., remembering events happening after school, meetings for clubs she belonged to, etc.). It is important to note that though this system had a direct impact on the child's ability to organize her behavior (such as turning in assignments and remembering materials for class) and consequently affected her grades, it did not directly affect her ability to learn new academIc material. This report additionally emphasized the importance of involving school personnel and family in instruction in the memory book system to ensure that it was properly utilized in all settings.

Recently, a number of new electronic devices have become available that could be used as external memory aids for children. Specifically, a line of electronic organizers designed for children is now available in retail stores. These organizers, like their counterparts for adults, have functions for storing phone numbers, appointment dates, and activities; simple diary functions; and calculators. Unlike the adult versions, they are icon based, typically store less information overall (8 kilobytes vs. 64 to 128), and offer a number of functions popular among children (e.g., being able to transmit information to other systems, daily fortune features, etc.). These systems are also typically much less expensive than adult systems and are designed to be more attractive to children (bright colors, additional child-oriented features, etc.). Though the authors know of no formal studies utilizing such systems, they would seem to hold potential for some purposes and have the advantage of being attractive to children and young adults. This could be important, as the authors have found, clinically, that many adolescents dislike using memory notebooks because they are cumbersome and mark them as different from their peers. As with memory book systems, it is imperative that a child be trained to utilize an electronic memory system and that parents and educators commit to assisting the child in its use. It is unrealistic to expect a child to use a system like this without specific acquisition and application training.

Additionally, some features, such as setting alarms, may initially be better tended to by parents, with children being trained to respond to information presented when the alarm rings.

Specialized Instructional Strategies. Another direction that the field of memory rehabilitation has taken is identifying training or instructional techniques that result in improved learning in individuals with memory impairment. Glisky (1992) described a computer-assisted instructional approach to teaching domain-specific knowledge to adults with traumatic brain injury. This specific training approach, called the "method of vanishing cues," was based on empirical studies demonstrating that amnesic patients can acquire a variety of motor, perceptual, and cognitive skills although they may not remember the actual learning episodes (Brooks & Baddeley, 1976; Charness, Milberg, & Alexander, 1988; Cohen & Squire, 1980). Many amnesic patients also exhibit normal priming effects, such that they produce previously encountered information in response to partial cues even though they fail to recall the prior encounter (Warrington & Weiskrantz, 1968, 1974). Squire (1987) described these phenomena as indicating spared skill learning or procedural learning relative to factual or declarative learning in amnesics. Graf and Schacter (1985) suggested that "implicit" memory, which does not rely on conscious awareness of past experiences, is intact, whereas "explicit" memory, which requires conscious retrieval of prior events, is impaired. Glisky proposed that individuals with memory impairment would be able to use preserved implicit memory to acquire new declarative knowledge as well as new skills. Indeed, Glisky demonstrated that both amnesic individuals and brain-injured patients with severe memory impairments could learn a vocabulary of computer-related terminology and a series of basic computer operations (Glisky & Schacter, 1987, 1988, 1989; Glisky, Schacter & Tulving, 1986a, 1986b). Issues of transfer and generalization and the constraints of this procedure have more recently been discussed (Glisky, 1992).

Similar to Glisky's (1992) report of successful training using this method of vanishing cues, Wilson and colleagues (Wilson, Baddeley, Evans, & Shiel, 1994; Wilson & Evans, 1996) reported the use of "errorless" learning in individuals with severe memory disorders. An awareness of the existence of preserved implicit memory in many amnesic patients has had little impact on memory rehabilitation practices. Even with the method of vanishing cues, learning tends to be slow and limited. Baddeley (1992) suggested that implicit learning may not occur at normal levels in individuals with memory impairments, and that individuals who depend on this type of learning are poorly equipped to deal with errors during the learning phase. Indeed, prior studies (e.g., Brooks & Baddeley, 1976) have shown that preserved learning in amnesic subjects was most evident when few errors were made during the training of a new procedure. In the Wilson et al. (1994) study, six separate experiments were conducted. In each, individuals with memory impairment were presented with information for later recall or recognition in either an "errorful" or an errorless condition. For example, in the errorful condition, participants were instructed to make multiple guesses at naming a staff member from a picture, prior to being provided with a correct response and writing it down. In the errorless condition, participants were not allowed to guess but were immediately provided with the correct name and instructed to read this correct response and write it down. In later recall or recognition trials, learning was superior in the errorless learning condition. The relative effectiveness of errorless learning was shown in such tasks as memory for a list of words; programming of an electronic aid; and learning of names, facts, and orientation information.

It is interesting to note that teaching strategies such as these have actually been described previously by educators working with children who have intellectual handicaps or specific learning disabilities. There is actually a substantial body of literature describing techniques for facilitating acquisition of both information and skills in individuals who have developmental learning and memory problems (Sidman & Stoddard, 1967; Terrace, 1963; Touchette, 1968). It seems ironic that professionals involved in memory rehabilitation are often unaware of, or are not trained in, the use of these techniques for enhancing learning.

Direct instruction is a formalized teaching approach in which instructional communications are presented logically and unambiguously. It utilizes such behavioral techniques as task analysis, modeling, shaping, reinforcement of appropriate responses, and continuous assessment to ensure learning. Student engagement is maintained through high response and success rates, and skills are sequenced to build upon previous learning. As with errorless learning, behavioral fading is utilized, minimizing the number of errors made in the learning process. Direct instruction also utilizes high mastery criteria, similar to those suggested for training external memory systems. Direct instruction has been successful with a wide range of learners with special needs (Colvin, 1990; Engelmann & Carnine, 1982; White, 1988).

Glang, Singer, Cooley, and Tish (1992) reported on the use of direct instruction techniques for teaching academic skills to 3 children with brain injuries. In this study, students who had sustained a severe brain injury at least 1 year earlier participated in a 6-week tutoring program for 2 hours of instruction per week. All 3 students made substantial academic progress in targeted instructional areas (reading, language, math, and keyboarding). Although some acquired skills were ones lost after injury, some of the gains made by these children represented new learning. In one case a direct instruction approach was also used to teach a self-management technique that reduced aggressive outbursts during instruction and increased academic engagement. The positive results of this study suggest that this approach holds promise for children with TBI.

In summary, the literature regarding rehabilitation strategies for individuals with memory disorders strongly suggests that memory deficits are not amenable to restoration techniques. Instead, the use of external memory aids in combination with specialized instructional strategies appears to hold the most promise for rehabilitation of memory, in both children and adults.

SUMMARY AND DIRECTIONS FOR FUTURE RESEARCH

A severe brain injury can leave a previously healthy child with significant handicaps. Cognitive deficits resulting from brain injuries have been shown to affect a child's ability to learn new information and to develop new skills and behaviors. A disruption in the ability to learn is of particular concern in pediatric populations, who are required to learn large amounts of new information and for whom many years of development still lie ahead. It is therefore critical that early, effective rehabilitation of cognitive deficits in children with brain injuries be implemented to enhance new learning and promote subsequent functional adaptation.

Although recent research has demonstrated that certain cognitive deficits (i.e., attention and memory) seen in brain-injured adults are amenable to rehabilitation, these positive findings must be evaluated critically to determine their real-world applicability. Because the ultimate goal of any rehabilitation program is to facilitate effective and independent functioning of the individual within his or her environment, the issue of generalizability of treatment effects is critical. A treatment that is useful in improving cognitive functioning only within a clinical setting cannot be considered an effective treatment; although the treatment was effective in changing the individual's performance on some task, it did not benefit him or her in terms of coping with the demands of the real-world environment. To achieve generalizability of treatment effects, cognitive components to be trained must be integrated into functional tasks and practiced in real-life situations/contexts that are relevant to the individual undergoing treatment.

In addition to generalizability, the issue of maintenance of treatment effects upon cessation of rehabilitation must also be addressed. In school-age populations, the transition from hospital (rehabilitation center) to home and school has been considered one of the greatest challenges of pediatric rehabilitation. To ensure that treatment effects are maintained outside the context of formal rehabilitation, a cooperative relationship must be established among rehabilitation providers, educational services, and parents. Parents should receive formal training in the special needs of their brain-injured child, the services available to help them meet those needs, and both their own legal rights and the legal obligations of others in the provision of such services. In this way, parents become able to effectively monitor the rehabilitation process and advocate for appropriate educational and rehabilitation services. Continuity of care is a critical aspect of the rehabilitation process because rehabilitation is only effective if its benefits can be maintained. Parents must also be provided with information and support.

Though still in its infancy, cognitive remediation in children with brain injury has begun to demonstrate positive results, and there is cautious hope that these early findings may lead to more effective interventions. It will continue to be useful to examine the efficacy of remediation approaches developed for use with adults with brain injuries as well as for children with learning disabilities. However, future research in cognitive rehabilitation for children with traumatic brain injury should emphasize the development of treatment approaches designed to meet the special needs and characteristics of this population. If remediation programs are to be successful with this population, they must be designed to meet the changing needs of the brain-injured child as he or she grows and develops.

10. Pediatric Traumatic Brain Injury: Challenges and Interventions for Families

JANE C. CONOLEY AND SUSAN M. SHERIDAN

Traumatic brain injury (TBI) is a serious threat to the health and welfare of children and adolescents in the United States (Eiben et al., 1984; Frankowski, 1985; Goldstein & Levin, 1987). A substantial number of injured children will exhibit mild to severe physical, intellectual, emotional, or behavioral difficulties for indefinite periods following the injury (Brooks & McKinlay, 1983; Lezak, 1986; Mauss-Clum & Ryan, 1981). In recent years, educational agencies have turned more attention to responding to the needs of children and youth who have suffered a traumatic brain injury. Creating and maintaining effective educational programs for survivors of injury is a daunting task for a host of reasons associated with the injury itself (Ben-Yishay & Prigatano, 1990).

When planning programs for learners with head injuries, care providers must keep in mind that the TBI survivor is only one member of an injured family system (Brooks, 1991a). A growing literature of research and clinical reports documents not only the massive effects the injury can have on parents, siblings, and extended family, but also the critical role a well-functioning family plays in the survivor's eventual adjustment (Jackson & Haverkamp, 1991; Kaplan, 1988; Kreutzer, Marwitz, & Kepler, 1992; Martin, 1988; Rivara et al., 1992; Rivara et al., 1993; Testani-Dufour, Chappel-Aiken, & Gueldner, 1992).

Families of TBI survivors may experience major psychological, financial, role, and relationship risks due to a child's injury. Difficulties for the family stem from both objective and subjective burden. *Objective burden* refers to objectively observable symptoms and conditions of the child with TBI, such as language, speech, and memory impairments. *Subjective burden* is concerned with the level of distress experienced by family members that is related to both severity of the injury and features of the relative himself or herself. This may be mediated by social variables, such as the presence or absence of support networks, or the change in the relationship between the relative and the head-injured child as a function of the injury (Brooks, 1991a; Brooks, Campsie, Symington, Beattie, & McKinlay, 1987). In general, female caregivers of persons with brain injuries report higher levels of burden. Subjective burden is more highly related to the presence of social aggression and cognitive disability in the child than to factors associated with physical disability. Further, the extent of the child's emotional and behavioral difficulties appears to be more important than the severity of the injury in predicting family members' levels of burden (Allen, Linn, Gutierrez, & Willer, 1994). According to Lezak (1986), the behaviors of individuals with head injuries that are most likely to cause problems for family members include impaired social perceptions and awareness, impaired control, dependency, and inability to learn from experience. Indirect consequences that affect the family include the injured individual's feelings of anxiety, paranoia, and depression.

The difficulties experienced by the families of individuals with brain injury are usually long-lasting, and some may actually increase over time (Bigler, 1989; Bragg, Klockars, & Berninger, 1992; Hall et al., 1994), especially those associated with subjective burden (Brooks, Campsie, Symington, Beattie, & McKinlay, 1986, 1987). Divorce, family conflict, substance abuse, and social isolation are possible outcomes. According to research by Mauss-Clum and Ryan (1981), the most frequently reported maternal reactions to closed-head injuries are frustration, irritability, arrogance, depression, anger, and feeling trapped. Other common responses include denial (albeit sometimes functional or misunderstood denial), anger, and overprotection (Brooks, 1991a).

It is of some importance that what families report to be valuable as they adjust to the injury of their son or daughter is valid information from caring professionals. Although the brain injury of the child cannot be undone, families benefit from consultation about an array of issues pertinent to coping with the child, health and educational systems, and community agencies (Miller, 1993). Consultation can greatly assist families in their continuing efforts to reorganize around the sometimes catastrophic effects of a brain injury in the family (Katz & Deluca, 1992).

Much of the research literature concerned with traumatic brain injury is based on adult male participants (e.g., Allen et al., 1994). Often the reports of family reorganization after injury relate the experiences of wives and children coping with the injury of a husband, or of parents (especially mothers) coping with the injury of their unmarried adult child. Results from these studies may not be directly comparable to those of families with pediatric TBI survivors, given the different role expectations for children in contrast to adults. There is a compelling need for more empirically derived information about the effects of pediatric TBI on families and about designing interventions helpful to families (Lehr, 1990; Waaland, 1990; Waaland & Kreutzer, 1988).

The objectives of this chapter are to outline (a) what families report to be their experiences in coping after an injury occurs, and (b) the tasks families must navigate in order to promote positive family life. Special attention is paid to effective and efficient education, advocacy, counseling, and consultation strategies that a school-based consultant might offer. The special role the psychologist plays in meeting family needs, coordinating school and family interventions, and contributing to the cohesiveness and effectiveness of the school-based team will be highlighted (Barry & O'Leary, 1989).

THE INJURED FAMILY SYSTEM

Parents of children and adolescent survivors of TBI report an array of difficulties following the injury and a sequence associated with their experiences. Both the difficulties and the sequence are instructive for care providers (Brooks et al., 1987; Leaf, 1993; Lezak, 1988; Livingston & Brooks, 1988; Livingston, Brooks, & Bond, 1985a, 1985b; Slater & Rubenstein, 1987).

Recovery Milestones

After serious injuries, parents report that their initial concern is the survival of their child (Rosenthal & Young, 1988). If the child is in a coma, parents focus almost exclusively on assisting the medical team in rousing the child from coma. This process may be brief or may take many months.

When survival seems assured, parents turn their attention to acquiring information about the possible long-term consequences of the injury. Although many parents report high satisfaction with the acute care their child received, they often become dissatisfied with the vagueness of the information received from medical professionals about the effects of the injury. Understandably, parents want a specific listing of symptoms to expect and a timetable for recovery. Medical professionals tend to share the entire range of possible recovery outcomes, from the most serious to the most trivial, and they resist giving rigid recovery schedules (Bond, 1983; Panting & Mercy, 1972).

Parents report other early concerns that relate to the physical disabilities their child may suffer because of the injury. This concern abates as they either access information on how to accommodate the physical challenges, or realize that their child shows few or no obvious residual signs of the accident. Later in the recovery process, parents discover that the psychological, behavioral, and emotional changes in their child are far more disturbing than the physical changes (Allen et al., 1994; Chadwick, 1985; Fletcher, Ewing-Cobbs, Miner, Levin, & Eisenberg, 1990; McGuire & Rothenberg, 1986).

Some pediatric recoveries from even moderate or serious injuries occur rather quickly at first. Parents are euphoric at the obvious improvements in their children's language, attention, and motor skills (Gardner, 1973; Romano, 1974). They may, in fact, deny the extent or permanence of likely disabilities (Martin, 1988). The optimism associated with early signs of rapid recovery may give way to sadness as recovery progress slows down significantly 10 to 12 months postinjury. When the injury has been severe, parents begin to experience what some have called "partial death" and "mobile mourning" (Rosenthal & Muir, 1983): Their child is alive but is not the child they knew before the injury. Although they thought they had grieved at the time of the accident, they tend to grieve again and again as their son or daughter misses usual developmental or social milestones. These may include starting school, playing sports, going to a prom, or graduating from high school. When the injury has been rather minor, leaving no physical sequelae, the children can suffer the pressures of being what might be termed "almosters"—they can *almost* learn like they used to, or they are *almost* as agile as they used to be (Jackson & Haverkamp, 1991).

In addition, the relief associated with improvement is often marred when parents find they must find alternative placements for their son or daughter. Short- and long-term residential care is not easily accessible to many families, because of either its cost or its distance from their home Jackson & Haverkamp, 1991). Such inaccessibility puts enormous stress upon a family. Many families experience both challenges; that is, they must find ways to fund the rehabilitation process *and* travel long distances to be with their child during the first stages of rehabilitation (Brooks, 1991b). Even when a child can come home (or parents experiment with home placement), the young person's special needs may force one parent to give up a job or have to build some network of support that includes medical care, supervision, and rehabilitation (Hall et al., 1994).

Family coping resources are taxed because they must attempt to accomplish a wide array of tasks (Bragg et al., 1992). Financial strain due to injury costs is common (Hall et al., 1994). These include both medical and often legal costs, as well as ongoing rehabilitation costs (e.g., assistive and augmentative devices, residential or partial hospitalization costs, respite care) and costs related to modifying their home environment (e.g., ramps for wheelchairs). Although families may be eligible for some insurance or state or federal (Social Security) financial assistance, accessing these funds can be difficult and time-consuming.

Other family members, especially siblings of the TBI survivor, may vie for some of the attention lavished on the survivor (Dyson, Edgar, & Crnic, 1989; Simeonsson & Bailey, 1986). These attempts are tinged with guilt about their resentment toward their injured sibling, and with a sense of futility. They report knowing that they will never do anything as significant as surviving from a traumatic brain injury. It has been suggested that siblings of individuals with severe head injuries experience psychological distress for up to 5 years postinjury (Orsillo, McCaffrey, & Fisher, 1993). As siblings grow older, they also report realizing that the burden of care for their injured brother or sister may fall upon them. This is an anxiety-producing and sometimes anger-producing realization (Rivara et al., 1992). Although not a great deal is known about the relationship between psychopathology and having a sibling with a head injury, some studies have documented that siblings of children with other handicaps are at risk for developing behavioral problems (Breslau, 1982), anxiety (Breslau, 1983), social withdrawal (Lavigne & Ryan, 1979), feelings of guilt and anger (Chinitz, 1981), reduced self-esteem (Ferrari, 1984; Harvey & Greenway, 1984), and feelings of inferiority (Taylor, 1980). Generally speaking, siblings who are young, male, and close in age to the child with a handicap experience the greatest difficulty. It should be noted, however, that positive and constructive reactions to the presence of a disabled sibling are possible (Parke, 1986).

Friends and extended family tend to be helpful in the first few months following a trauma, but their attention and support drift as the long-term recovery process continues. They may add stress to the nuclear family by offering irrelevant advice or even criticism to the family caretakers (Miller, 1993).

The family's skills in managing the various interfacing systems that make up their world become critical. Parents often report disillusionment with medical and rehabilitation teams, and adversarial relationships are a constant threat to treatment progress. This adversarial stance, often developed during the medical and short-term rehabilitation stages of recovery, can set the stage for difficulties between families and schools (Martin, 1988).

The premorbid functioning of the family is a strong predictor of its members' success in coping with their TBI survivor. Well-functioning families are especially helpful in promoting growth in the survivor's emotional and behavioral skills (Rivara et al., 1992; Rivara et al., 1993).

Summary

Following their child's injury, a family experiences a dramatic swing of emotions, from fear to happiness to bewilderment to anger to discouragement, through depression, mourning, and, finally (it is hoped), reorganization. Family members move from being relieved that their child will live to finding the child somewhat difficult to sometimes blaming the child for not trying hard enough to recover, not compensating, or being irresponsible. Anger may also be turned toward therapists or medical personnel if the child's condition fails to improve or worsens. Accepting that their child may remain forever childlike and/or different (in skills and personality) is very difficult. The family must shift their expectations from hopes of full recovery to accepting that little or no change is likely. Parents have many dreams associated with their children. These must sometimes give way to new goals that involve a lifetime of dependency on the part of the survivor (Allen et al., 1994).

WHAT FAMILIES NEED

Families with head-injured children have many needs, including education, family support/advocacy, behavioral family therapy (Livingston et al., 1985a, 1985b; Miller, 1993), and home-school consultation.

Education

Families must receive clear information about the nature of the injury their child has sustained. This information should be repeated several times if necessary and in terms that make sense to nonmedical personnel and a manner that is sensitive to the family's vulnerability. Care should be taken not to overwhelm the family with too many facts and details early on. The amount of information first presented should be limited, to allow family members sufficient time to process the newly acquired knowledge (DePompei & Zarski, 1989). Throughout the educative process, certain key points should be conveyed to families (Lezak, 1978, 1986); these are summarized in Table 10.1.

Families report not knowing enough about the rehabilitation process—for example, their role and appropriate expectations. They benefit from a rather formal introduction to the rehabilitation unit and from becoming part of the process with a plan for specific family involvement (Martin, 1988).

Table 10.1

Key Points to Include in Family Education and Counseling

1. Anger, frustration, and sorrow are natural reactions of family members when a relative experiences a brain injury.

2. Caretakers should preserve their own emotional health, physical well-being, and sanity in order to be of benefit to the child with a head injury.

3. Families should be informed and helped to process details surrounding the child's injury and organic limitations to recovery.

4. Recovery is not a continuous and reliable process. A child may show rapid recovery in some areas and during some phases of rehabilitation; in other cases, recovery may be slow or absent. These realities can help families resist blaming treatment staff, medical facilities, or school personnel when recovery is halted.

5. Conflict and disagreements with the individual with a head injury are inevitable. Caretakers must rely on their own judgment in making decisions regarding care.

6. The family role changes that are concomitant to a member sustaining a brain injury can be stressful to all.

7. Real limits exist pertaining to what family members can do to change the head-injured individual's behaviors and personality. Feelings of guilt or ineptitude are normal but not realistic.

8. The family ultimately may be faced with decisions about alternative living or care arrangements for the member with a head injury.

9. The family should review legal documents and financial arrangements concerning the care of the individual with a head injury.

Note. Adapted from Lezak (1978, 1986).

Prognostic indications should be kept to a minimum during this phase of the recovery process to the extent that family members can accept realistic expectations. It is possible that family members have not yet fully dealt with the complex emotions associated with the injury and may not be psychologically equipped to deal with long-term issues, particularly if they are negative.

The development of a plan is a good basis for introducing critical information, for example, how to structure their child's leisure time, what to expect in terms of sexuality from their adolescent survivor, or how to deal with externalizing behavior problems (Asarnow, Lewis, & Neumann, 1991; Black, Jeffries, Blumer, Wellner, & Walker, 1969; Slater & Rubenstein, 1987). In schools, the IEP development process can serve this purpose. Psychologists should be active and instrumental in helping the team (including parents) to develop appropriate educational goals and acquire the necessary information to adequately address each child's unique difficulties.

Family members often neglect the needs of the siblings of the survivor as well as their own need for leisure time. Siblings of children with head injuries have been shown to display inadequate problem solving and dysfunctional attitudes (Orsillo et al., 1993). They benefit from education about the possible negative effects of prolonged caretaking on themselves and on the rest of the family, as well as effective problem-solving and support strategies.

Depending on the severity of the child's injury and his or her degree of recovery and developmental/cognitive level, including the TBI survivor in educational sessions may be warranted. Some guidelines for this practice have been offered by DePompei and Zarski (1989) and include (a) covering no more than two new topics in a session, (b) repeating main points on several occasions (and encouraging family members to do the same) and asking the child with TBI for verification, (c) reviewing the same information in more than one session, and (d) modeling responses toward the child with TBI for the family.

Family Support and Advocacy

Parents face new and frightening burdens following an injury and need information about the legal and financial situations they face. They benefit from direction regarding insurance, other funding sources, and the legal help they may need to manage personal injury or compensation suits. Ongoing assistance throughout the rehabilitation period is often necessary.

Families often require a case manager to assist them in identifying and accessing all the community and educational services for which they qualify. Case managers may be effective advocates responsible for educating parents about the scope of their child's rights under the Individuals with Disabilities Education Act. Similarly, they may serve as mediators to assist families in the securement of necessary services. Because service needs change with the age of the child (e.g., from preschool early intervention programs to vocational rehabilitation), it is important that case managers be knowledgeable about child development and transition programs, and available to families over time. Case managers are especially helpful if they also know physicians, lawyers, and rehabilitation professionals who are well-informed about TBI.

Linking families with local or national organizations, such as the National Head Injury Foundation (see Note) is also a very helpful way to give them access to information about their child's injury. Further, such linkages can help families cope via their own actions and through more systemic efforts, such as legislation, advocacy with school districts, or regulations affecting disabled people (National Head Injury Foundation, 1985).

Local organizations are a source for self-help or parental support groups. Almost all families feel guilt, sadness, loss, anguish, and anger associated with their child's injury. Although there seems to be no empirical research associated with self-help groups of this type, family groups can play an important role in offering support and normalizing these emotional states, thus preventing the development of more serious family dilemmas (Rosenthal & Young, 1988).

Family Counseling

Many families report significant role strain or overload following their child's injury. The stresses of accomplishing all the challenges associated with caring for their injured child can precipitate negative emotional reactions among family members, especially depression, blame, and anger (Zarski, DePompei, & Zook, 1988; Zarski, Hall, & DePompei, 1987). Family counseling is thus often initiated late in the recovery process, after the family has attempted (and possibly failed) to assimilate the behavioral, cognitive, language, and other changes in the head-injured child into the existing family structure.

It is not unusual for the mother and father to differ in the ways they react to their injured child. These differences (e.g., one parent is concerned and anxious while the other parent is demanding and aloof) may be the source of considerable conflict among family members as the rehabilitation process goes on (Miller, 1993). If these patterns become apparent in counseling sessions, the clinician can focus on reframing the family members' reactions.

Family members may be separated for significant periods of time in order to assist in the rehabilitation process. This separation also contributes to role strain in remaining family members, as well as to potentially significant role changes. For example, older children may have to take on major responsibilities for childcare and homemaking tasks.

If the family has difficulty supporting each other during these stressful times, depression, substance abuse, and even divorce are possible outcomes (Hall et al., 1994). Family counseling is both a preventive and a remedial strategy to consider, especially if it focuses on fostering emotional resources and coping skills and if the therapist can also teach the family strategies for dealing with their injured child. For example, during a rather rapid initial recovery phase, families recall that they were in a "honeymoon" period, believing that their lives would soon be back to normal (Miller, 1993). Many find, however, that they need to acquire new skills, especially ones related to teaching and goal-setting strategies, to work with their injured son or daughter. They may have to teach their adolescent how to use the toilet and brush his or her teeth. They may have to be involved in language training. Of some special importance is the family's need for strategies to cope with aggressive outbursts from the TBI survivor, as aggressiveness is a significant stressor on families (Brooks, 1984).

Siblings of the child with head injuries pose special challenges in family counseling. Siblings use coping strategies such as wishful thinking, self-blame, and avoidance at least as often as more effective, problem-focused or social support coping strategies. Depending on their age, they may not be verbally or emotionally mature enough to express their feelings and confusions. If this goes unrecognized, the sibling may endure significant psychological hardship. Therefore, counseling for siblings is often recommended.

It may also be useful to involve the child with TBI in family counseling sessions to the greatest extent possible. Therapeutic indications for involving the child will likely be related to his or her developmental status; level of injury; and degree of physical, cognitive, and behavioral functioning. Specific therapeutic goals might focus on helping all family members, including siblings, express thoughts and concerns regarding the injury, and exploring alternative effective coping skills.

An important counseling goal with the family members of a head-injured child is encouragrng and supporting their attempts to reorganize their family system. It is important for family members to recognize that the trauma the child experienced caused a significant alteration in the entire family system, and reorganization of all aspects of the system (e.g., parents, siblings, extended family members) is necessary for family recovery to occur. In other words, simply "treating" the injured child's problems will not address the internal changes that are required of all family members, and of the family system.

Home–School Consultation

A key element of family coping and involvement in their child's recovery is a strong link between families and schools. Reentry into the school setting following an injury may pose significant challenges for the child, the family, and the school (see Clark, chapter 11). Families need the continued support of experts who can provide them with information, skills, and emotional support. Educators must rely on parents to continue educational programs in the home to improve their students' chances for optimal recovery. Cooperative consultative relationships between families and educators become essential to maximizing a child's education and treatment program.

Establishing supportive, conjoint teams of parents and educators is a complex task. Education, medical, and rehabilitation experts often disappoint parents because the professionals simply lack the solutions the parents want so much. Professional teams often report that parental dissatisfaction with their work leads them to blame each other and weakens the team's functioning.

Well-informed school psychologists can be the critical link between families and school personnel. The families and the schools must engage in a mutual process that leads to a reorganization around the child who has the injury. An *empowerment* model is preferred over one that provides families with "solutions" for challenges the child may encounter upon school reentry. In such a model, there is a focus on the strengths and problem-solving abilities of the family as a unit. Parents are considered an active and central component of educational programming for their child (including programs to meet their child's academic, social–emotional, behavioral, and vocational needs). For example, in a conjoint consultation model (Sheridan & Kratochwill, 1992; Sheridan, Kratochwill, & Bergan, 1996), parents and school personnel share equally in the identification and prioritization of issues to be addressed through individualized intervention. Parents, teachers, and school specialists work together to develop and implement a strategy or set of strategies to deal with the most pressing issues facing the child. Further, they continue with this dialogue as interventions are implemented, and monitor the need for modifications, to ensure the best possible treatment regimen for their child.

There are four stages in conjoint consultation. Three of the four stages involve structured interviews wherein the child's parents, the teacher, the school psychologist, and other relevant individuals come together to address prominent concerns. In the first stage of consultation, *problem identification,* participants identify specific academic, behavioral, or social–emotional issues to be addressed. In the Problem Identification Interview (PII; Kratochwill & Bergan, 1990; Sheridan et al., 1996), participants work together to focus on one or two specific concerns. These concerns become the behavioral priority for consultation. Relevant goals are established for the child, and strategies for collecting behavioral data are determined. In general, specific data should be collected to determine the actual severity of the injured child's behavioral changes upon school reentry, and to assess possible environmental conditions that may be contributing to the child's difficulties (e.g., seating arrangements, group size and expectations, classroom transition schedules). To obtain a comprehensive picture of the child's behaviors, data should be collected at both school and home.

The second stage of conjoint consultation is *problem analysis,* during which the team (including the parents, teachers, school psychologist, and others) reconvene in a Problem Analysis Interview (PAI; Kratochwill & Bergan, 1990; Sheridan et al., 1996) to discuss the data that have been collected, as well as conditions that may be related to the behavioral occurrence (i.e., antecedents and consequences). An intervention plan is then developed, with all team players contributing their ideas and expertise. Specific tactics are determined for addressing the injured child's difficulties at both home and school. It is imperative that all key individuals involved with the child be knowledgeable about and active in the implementation of the intervention. This will ensure consistency among care providers and maximize the child's chances for success.

During *treatment implementation*, the third stage of conjoint consultation, the intervention is put into place. All individuals who play an active part in the plan should be familiar with their specific roles and responsibilities. The school psychologist consultant is in a good position to monitor each aspect of the program to ensure that the plan is being implemented as intended across home and school. In some cases, direct training or modeling of some of the treatment components will be necessary for consultees who are unfamiliar with certain strategies. It is also important that data continue to be collected during this stage, to assess the child's responsiveness to the intervention and movement toward consultation goals.

Finally, the last stage of conjoint consultation, *treatment evaluation*, involves evaluating whether the child is making progress on the specific behaviors or concerns targeted for consultation. In the Treatment Evaluation Interview (TEI; Kratochwill & Bergan, 1990; Sheridan et al., 1996), all consultation participants meet to review the data collected prior to and during the implementation of the treatment plan. It is often the case that the intervention program will require some modification; indeed, in some situations an entirely new plan will be generated. If the initial goals for the child have been met, team members will typically recycle back through the consultation stages and address another concern facing the child. This stage is especially critical when a child's recovery level and rate are variable. Continuous evaluation of the appropriateness of goals for the child, and of progress or regression surrounding those goals, is critical. It is very important at this stage to ensure that strategies be put into place to help the child maintain treatment gains that have been made.

Summary

Involving parents in educational programming is a logical extension of the other family-based approaches (i.e., education, support/advocacy, and family counseling). Parents are often the persons most knowledgeable on issues regarding their family and their child's condition, particularly if they have been active in the recovery process. They have firsthand information about their child's temperament, motivation, responsiveness, tolerance levels, and degree of adaptation. They can provide necessary background information on the nature and course of the injury, adjunct services being provided, family adjustment, and child strengths.

Parents can also be advocates for their child and help establish meaningful goals for treatment. Family members who have received adequate education, support, and counseling should have a realistic vision of what is in store for their child and what can be expected regarding rehabilitation. Parents' adjusted hopes and aspirations for their child should be validated and respected as educational teams establish treatment objectives. To do this sincerely, parents and educators must be actively and cooperatively involved in home–school consultation and partnership activities.

AUTHORS' NOTES

1. Jane Close Conoley acknowledges the financial and technical help and clinical experiences offered in support of this chapter from the leadership, staff, and clients of Quality Living, Inc., Omaha, NE.
2. The order of authorship is alphabetical; both authors contributed equally in the preparation of this chapter.

NOTE

The toll-free number for the National Head Injury Foundation is 800/444-NHIF.

11. Children and Adolescents with Traumatic Brain Injury: Reintegration Challenges in Educational Settings

ELAINE CLARK

Each year as many as a million children and adolescents sustain a traumatic brain injury (TBI), many serious enough to require hospitalization (Kraus, Fife, & Cox, 1986). Although children with such injuries are by no means new to the educational system, the growing number of more severely injured students may be. Advances in technology have resulted in faster and more sophisticated medical care (Carney & Gerring, 1990); therefore, more children and adolescents are surviving their injuries, even the most serious ones. Current estimates are that 95% of all children and adolescents with TBI can be expected to live, and 65% of those with more severe injuries survive the insult to the brain (Michaud, Rivara, & Grady, 1992). Because recovery often takes months, or even years, schools are an important extension of the rehabilitation that begins in the hospital. Given the structure that schools provide, and the variety of specialties represented on their staff, schools may be in one of the best positions to provide service to these students (Mira & Tyler, 1991). Educators' lack of knowledge as to how TBI can affect a student's academic and social functioning, however, can be an obstacle in providing this service (Blosser & DePompei, 1991; Mira, Meck, & Tyler, 1988; Savage, 1985). The purpose of this chapter is to inform educators about some of the challenges that school-age children with TBI face and about ways to facilitate the reintegration of students back into the classroom. For many students with TBI, this is a very significant hurdle to overcome.

Federal Law Mandating Service

Recognizing the important role of the schools in meeting the unique needs of this population, federal legislators passed P.L. 101-476 in 1990 to include TBI as a special education category. According to this law, titled the Individuals with Disabilities Education Act (IDEA):

> Traumatic brain injury means an acquired injury to the brain caused by an external physical force, resulting in total or partial functional disability or psychosocial impairment, or both, that adversely affects a child's educational performance. The term applies to open or closed head injuries resulting in impairments in one or more areas, such as cognition; language; memory; attention; reasoning; abstract thinking; judgement; problem-solving; sensory, perceptual and motor abilities; psychosocial behavior; physical functions; information processing; and speech. The term does not apply to brain injuries that are congenital or degenerative, or brain injuries induced by birth trauma. (Definition from 57 Fed. Reg. 189 (1992), p. 44802)

Despite the fact that this law has been in existence for more than 4 years, a recent study conducted at the University of Utah showed that professionals working in the schools do not know which students are eligible for services under TBI and which are not (Anderson, 1995). This is not surprising, as many states have not established guidelines to serve this population. In fact, according to a study by Katsiyannis and Conderman (1994), 16 of the 34 states surveyed were still in the process of writing their guidelines. Further, despite the fact that the guidelines in the majority of states that had established them closely paralleled federal law, several states' eligibility criteria were different. Utah, New York, and Wisconsin, for example, include "internal" causes of TBI. According to the federal law, only students who have injuries caused by "external force" to the brain, that is, children with open- or closed-head injuries, or who experienced near-drowning, are eligible for services under TBI. Children whose injuries are caused by "internal" events, such as brain tumors, stroke, central nervous system infections, and exposure to toxic substances can be served under other special education categories (e.g., Other Health Impaired, Learning Disabilities, Behavior Disorders, and Intellectual Disabilities) but are excluded under TBI.

The reasons for the decision by the federal government to exclude these students are unclear, given the fact that they share many of the same characteristics as students with "externally" caused injuries, have many of the same educational, emotional, and social needs, and are likely to benefit from the same interventions (i.e., interventions that focus on reintegration and frequent monitoring of progress). The rationale is even less clear when one considers the fact that children with hypoxic encephalopathy from near-drowning are included but children who suffer the same brain injury from electrocution, cardiac arrest, or anesthetic accidents are excluded.

CONSEQUENCES OF TBI

Motor Problems

Problems with gait, coordination, spasticity, and speech are commonly seen in children with TBI (Levin, Benton, & Grossman, 1982). The fact that motor function is the first function to recover, and rather quickly at that (DiScala, Osberg, Gans, Chin, & Grant, 1991; Ylvisaker, 1986), means that most students with TBI will be walking and talking by the time they return to school. Educators may interpret this as the child being "back to normal," when this is not necessarily the case. And, for the child and family, rapid recovery of motor function may set the unrealistic expectation that other functions will recover at a similarly fast rate.

Language Problems

Although speech deficits recover at nearly the same rate as motor skills, receptive language and higher level communication problems are more persistent and can interfere with learning (Blosser & DePompei, 1989; Ylvisaker, 1986). Language problems such as pragmatics, verbal fluency, word finding, concept formation, and verbal comprehension are more likely to parallel the recovery of cognitive skills (Michaud, Duhaime, & Gatshaw, 1993) and are more difficult to detect.

Cognitive Problems

Common cognitive problems that result from injury include difficulties with the following: attention; memory; language comprehension; concept formation; integrating, organizing, and generalizing information; problem solving; and judgment (Blosser & DePompei, 1989; Michaud, Duhaime, &

Gatshaw, 1993). Research by Jaffe and his colleagues at the University of Washington (Jaffe et al., 1993) has shown that children who sustain moderate or severe head injuries are at greater risk for these types of problems than are mildly injured children. This is consistent with the literature that shows negligible cognitive deficits in children with mild TBI. Bijur, Haslum, and Golding (1990) showed that on cognitive measures, children with mild injuries were indistinguishable from their noninjured peers.

Behavioral and Emotional Problems

More severely injured children are also more likely than their less severely injured peers to evidence persistent behavioral and emotional disturbances (Bijur et al., 1990; Jaffe et al., 1993). Like cognitive problems, behavioral and emotional problems can result from injury to the brain and can interfere with students' academic and social success. Families actually rate behavior disturbance and personality change as the most troublesome and persistent problem following injury (Thomsen, 1984). Although educators often fail to attribute behavior problems to injury, research has shown that children with TBI are three times more likely than the general population to develop serious behavior disorders (Michaud, Rivara, Jaffe, Fay, & Dailey, 1993). Common behavioral sequelae from injury include increased aggression, poor anger control, and hyperactivity (Bijur et al., 1990; Filley, Cranberg, Alexander, & Hart, 1987). These behaviors also happen to be the most common reason for referral to special education, regardless of the etiology of the problem (Morgan & Jenson, 1988). Although externalizing behaviors may be more apparent than internalizing problems (i.e., anxiety, depression, emotional lability, social withdrawal, and somatization), internalizing symptomatology can also interfere with the child's ability to function in school (Begali, 1992). Savage and Wolcott (1994) provided some excellent ideas for interventions with these children.

Behavioral and emotional problems are caused not only by neurophysiological disturbance from the injury, and a reaction to it, but by other factors as well. Constitutional factors, prior predisposition to psychological disturbance, secondary physical handicaps, cognitive problems, and psychosocial stresses can all contribute to the child's psychological status following injury (Rutter, 1981).

Health Problems

Other TBI-related problems that have been shown to interfere with learning are medical. One of the most common physical complaints following injury is headache. Headaches are estimated to affect around 20% of children within the first 6 months of their injuries (Lanser, Jennekens-Schinkel, & Peters, 1988). Some children continue to complain of headaches 6 years out; however, there is no clear evidence that in these cases the injury is causally related (Lanser et al., 1988). Children with TBI are also at greater risk for developing seizure disorders, especially children who sustain penetrating head injuries (Levin et al., 1982). Seizures can have significant implications for learning and social relationships and future work. Vision and hearing can also be affected by injury, as can sense of smell and taste (Michaud, Duhaime, & Gatshaw, 1993). Some of these children will also have dysphagia, or problems swallowing (Ylvisaker & Weinstein, 1989).

Achievement Problems

More than a quarter of the subjects in Klonoff, Clark, and Klonoff's (1993) study reported that they had failed a grade or been retained, and nearly a third of the parents in Greenspan and MacKenzie's (1994) study reported that their child was in special education 1 year after injury. Granted, a number of children with TBI experienced academic problems before their injuries; in fact, about half of the children Greenspan and MacKenzie studied who were in special education after injury had been receiving services before. Problems with academic achievement, however, may not be apparent for a year or more after injury (Chadwick, Rutter, Brown, Shaffer, & Traub, 1981), and when they are detected, they may not be attributed to the injury. Like behavior problems, the longer the interval from the time of injury to the detection of achievement problems, the less likely an attribution will be made to the prior injury (Michaud, Duhaime, & Gatshaw, 1993). Even if correctly attributed, however, improvements in academic achievement are often slow.

One year after injury, the children with moderate or severe injuries in Fay et al.'s (1994) study had made modest gains in spelling, which were attributed to recovery of motor skills, and some very small improvements in reading and math since the initial testing (see Jaffe et al., 1993). When these children were retested 2 years later, there was negligible change in mean test scores, and the children with moderate or severe injuries continued to perform significantly below the control group on tests of reading, math, and spelling. Although increased severity was associated with lower test scores, it should be noted that the mean scores for all groups (mild, moderate, and severe injury) were within the normal range for the standardized test. This longitudinal cohort study highlights the importance of making appropriate group comparisons. Curriculum-based academic measures may, therefore, be particularly relevant for these children.

Predicting Outcomes and Providing Services

Studies estimate that 20% of head injury survivors are left with some degree of disability (Kraus, Rock, & Hemyarai, 1990). The range of impairments, however, is quite broad. Deficits in reasoning, memory, language, visual–spatial and motor skills, and behavioral areas have been documented by a number of researchers (Ewing-Cobbs, Levin, Eisenberg, & Fletcher, 1987; Goldstein & Levin, 1985; Jaffe et al., 1993; Thompson et al., 1994; Winogron, Knights, & Bawden, 1984). Although the literature is fairly consistent in showing that the impact on cognitive functioning from mild injury is rather negligible—that is, these children tend to be indistinguishable from their noninjured peers (Bijur et al., 1990; Jaffe et al., 1993)—it is not always easy to assess severity and thus predict which children will have what problems, and for how long.

Whereas severity of injury is commonly used to predict the outcome from TBI (Filley et al., 1987), not all severity indicators are equally useful (Costeff, Groswasser, & Goldstein, 1990). Duration of coma (a state of unconsciousness in which the person cannot be aroused and/or does not respond) and posttraumatic amnesia (PTA; loss of memory occurring immediately after injury that may continue for hours or days) have been shown to be relatively good predictors of outcome (Klonoff et al., 1993; Michaud et al., 1993). Factors other than the injury itself, however, have been shown to confound predictions based on coma and PTA. For example, many of the extracranial injuries that children with TBI sustain that produce increased physical and psychological stress (i.e., shock, hypotension, hypoxia, and metabolic disruption) result in an underestimation of the severity of injury to the brain; thus, the outcome from injury may be less favorable than initially predicted (DiScala et al., 1991). In a recently published follow-up study of 95 children with TBI, Greenspan and MacKenzie (1994) found that whereas severity was associated with physical limitations caused by the brain injury, behavioral problems were not associated with severity (with the exception of hyperactivity).

Although knowing what to expect in terms of impairments is difficult, educators can expect that children who have moderate to severe injuries will evidence their unique problems during the first year, and especially in the first 3 months (Thompson et al., 1994). The subjects in Greenspan and MacKenzie's (1994) study were still having significantly greater problems with physical health and behaviors than the general population 1 year after injury. Costeff et al. (1990) found that none of their more severely injured subjects had improved significantly in cognitive functioning after 1 year, and nearly half of the 31 children studied were still experiencing significant social and behavior problems at that time. When Fay and her colleagues (Fay et al., 1994) retested their moderate and severely injured subjects 3 years after injury, they also found that a significant number were exhibiting cognitive and behavioral problems when compared with a control group of same-aged peers. Their subjects performed worse than controls on 40 out of 53 neuro-behavioral measures.

Despite the fact that research has documented persistent problems in a large number of children following brain injury, discharge from hospitals is often equated with a return to normalcy. Surprisingly few children receive any follow-up care once they are discharged from the hospital. Data obtained from the Pediatric Trauma Registry (DiScala et al., 1991) show that children who sustain traumatic injuries are more likely to be discharged to their homes than to rehabilitation facilities. Even the more severely injured children are unlikely to receive any follow-up care once they are discharged from the hospital (Carney & Gerring, 1990). For the less severely injured child, the situation may even be worse—not only does the return home come much sooner, but so does the return to school. In many cases, children with milder injuries are never even admitted to the hospital (Bijur et al., 1990). Educators may never be notified of the child's injuries, thus obscuring the potential for problems (Savage, 1991). It is not surprising that teachers often end up being the first persons to raise concerns about the student's progress.

ISSUES RELATED TO EDUCATION

Not all students with TBI require special education. However, most children with moderate to severe injuries will require some additional educational assistance. Depending on the degree and nature of the student's deficits, services can range from accommodations in the general education classroom to one-on-one assistance. Figure 11.1 provides a suggested guideline that takes into consideration the continuum of placement and service options that needs to be considered in order to provide the student with the least restrictive environment. Even in cases where the student is already receiving special education assistance, those services should be carefully reviewed to determine if any changes are required, including changing classification to TBI. Students who need support for their educational programs but do not qualify for special education may be able to receive services through general education under Section 504 of the Individuals with Disabilities Act of 1973. Section 504 requires that reasonable accommodations be made for students with disabilities so that they will be able to access education. Referrals for these services are typically brought to the attention of the

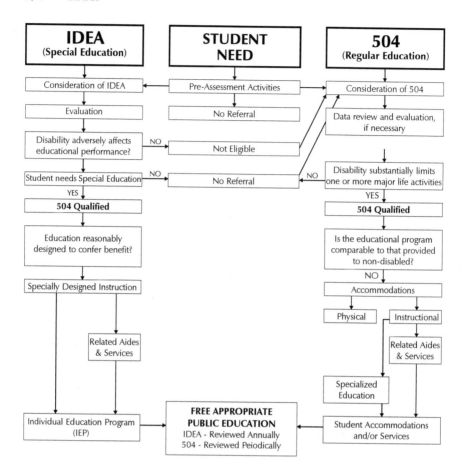

Section 504 coordinator, although in some cases special education personnel may be involved. The act requires that school districts evaluate the student before making any change in his or her programming or placement. When significant changes are necessary, a 504 conference committee should be convened to consider what the student's unmet needs are, the evaluation results and 504 eligibility, and the service needs based on eligibility (USOE, 1993). Staff inservice may also be a component of 504 services and may also alleviate the need to make programmatic changes or further accommodations.

Regardless of the type of service that is provided, that is, whether it is through general or special education, it is important to recognize that students with acquired traumatic brain injuries are often very different from their peers with other kinds of special learning needs, because those differences have important implications for educational programming. Unlike their peers with learning disabilities, students with TBI typically experienced success in school before their injury (Blosser & DePompei, 1989). These students are initially more likely to view themselves the way they were, not the way they are. Returning to school forces them to confront newly acquired deficits or, in some cases, a worsening of prior problems. This causes considerable frustration, as does the fact that these deficits appear suddenly and recover at such an uneven and unpredictable rate. Dramatic changes in the first 3 months, followed by a slowing in recovery rate (Chadwick et al., 1981: Knight et al., 1991), often set unrealistic expectations for the student and school. Educators who understand these differences in students with TBI can help to set realistic goals and plan more appropriately for them.

Another problem that needs to be considered when making educational plans for this population is the fact that providing services can create a fiscal crisis for the school. As Lash (1994) pointed out, schools cannot anticipate the costs for these services as easily as they can the costs for the traditional special education student already in the system. Schools have a variety of specialists who could potentially work with students who sustain brain injuries; however, the small number of TBI students in a particular school makes it difficult to divide resources and costs among them. Optimal service for the student with TBI, however, is interdisciplinary (Michaud, Duhaime, & Gatshaw, 1993).

Team Approach

A thoughtfully composed and well-informed team is critical for ensuring that services are provided, and are done so in a timely manner. Because successful transition from the hospital or rehabilitation to the school is enhanced by planning early for the student's return, the team, headed by a carefully selected case manager, should be organized before the student returns to school. Communication lines set up in advance ensure that school personnel are apprised of the student's condition and helps to prevent gaps in service. Scheduling regular team meetings will provide an opportunity for the exchange of ideas and creative problem solving.

The needs of the particular student often dictate the composition of the team, but typically it consists of a case manager, classroom teacher, special education teacher, school psychologist, speech and language pathologist, parent, and student. Students and parents offer an invaluable perspective on the problems and provide information that would otherwise be unavailable. Other potential team members who can provide important perspectives and professional knowledge include physical and occupational therapists, counselors, adaptive physical education teachers, administrators, neuropsychologists and rehabilitation specialists. The extent of these members' involvement will be determined by the student's disabilities (e.g., emotional adjustment problems, language impairments, and motor skill deficits). Other, less likely members include physicians and nurses. Other than providing information that can be used for TBI diagnosis (a requirement for special education in some states), physicians' participation is generally limited to consultation. Few schools have nurses in-house; however, when the health-care needs of the student cannot be managed by other school personnel (e.g., dealing with tracheotomies and catheters), nurses are important team members and direct service providers to the student.

The case manager, perhaps the most critical team member other than the classroom teacher, is often assigned by the administrator because of his or her knowledge about TBI or willingness to learn. It is important for this person to be in a position to see the student often, preferably daily, to coordinate services. Coordinating services may also go beyond the boundaries of the school. To maximize community resources, such as state head injury associations and health service organizations, team members need to be aware of, and tied into, these agencies. These agencies are valuable resources not only for school personnel, but also for students and their families. In addition to general education teachers, support staff, such as clerical and cafeteria workers, bus drivers, and paraprofessionals, benefit from receiving information about these students.

Inservice Training

One of the primary services of the team is inservice training for other key school personnel. Tyler and Mira (1993) stressed that inservice training should include both general information about head injury and its impact on behavioral, cognitive, and physical functioning, and specific information about the particular student's deficits and educational needs. Training should also include information about strategies that will assist students as they return to the classroom, including ways to modify the environment (i.e., adapting schedules, instruction, and behavior-management methods).

Inservice training serves another very important function, that is, alerting staff to the possibility that some of their other students who are experiencing cognitive, behavior, or social problems may have had an earlier head injury (Michaud, Rivara, Jaffe, et al., 1993). Although they may never have been identified for any service, especially special education, this does not mean that they did not need it. Some may even be eligible for additional help under IDEA or Section 504.

SCHEDULE FOR REINTEGRATION PLANNING

A thoughtful plan for reintegrating the student into the classroom is highly dependent upon the cooperation of a number of individuals, both inside and outside the school. Communication with hospital staff is especially important in the early stages; parent contact is essential throughout the period of time the student needs special assistance.

Immediately Following Injury

Planning for reintegration should actually begin at the time the child is admitted to the hospital. If the school district or region has a TBI representative, he or she should be notified about the injury. This person should be able to assist in determining what resources are available, as well as the appropriate person to serve as the case manager. At this stage, contact is made with the family and a hospital representative. In some circumstances, hospital personnel will contact the schools, but school personnel need to be prepared to take responsibility for this. It may be necessary to obtain a release from the parents before making contact, especially if information about the student is provided to the hospital. Figure 11.2 provides a suggested checklist for these and other activities.

Information regarding the severity of injury needs to be obtained from the hospital, as this has been identified as a primary factor in recovery and long-term prognosis (Klonoff et al., 1993). Information as to how certain behaviors (in particular, agitation and aggression) have been managed in the hospital is also important, as it may be helpful in planning for the student's return. Ineffective management of difficult behaviors in acute care settings increases the risk for continued problems with behavioral control (Papas, 1993). In addition to obtaining information about the student's health status, rehabilitation staff may also call on the school to be of assistance by providing them with information about the student's preinjury strengths and weaknesses and supplying them with school texts and assignments, if needed. Rehabilitation staff may be able to use this information to conduct ecologically relevant assessments of the child's functioning and develop individualized treatment plans. Setting up situations that are similar to those that the student will face upon returning to school can be particularly useful.

A number of students with TBI will require ongoing medication management for behavior problems, as well as for medical concerns, such as headaches and seizures. Given the impact that medication alone can have on behavior and learning, educators need to have a basic understanding of the intended effects and unwanted side effects (e.g., sedation, excessive thirst and restroom trips).

Student: _____   School/Grade: _____

Date of Injury: _____   Parent Name/Phone #: _____

IMMEDIATELY FOLLOWING INJURY
A school representative will be assigned to the case by administrator.
The school representative will:

    Contact parent(s) to:
      • inquire about their child's condition
      • obtain release for hospital contact (get release to and from school)

    Contact the child's case manager at the hospital to:
      • inform them of the school's concern

    Meet with the child's classroom teacher(s) to:
      • inform them of the child's condition
      • obtain/review current educational records

AFTER STUDENT'S CONDITION HAS STABILIZED
The school representative will:

    Arrange a meeting with the hospital case manager to:
      • obtain information regarding the child's condition
      • determine if/when to send school work

PRIOR TO DISCHARGE
The school representative will:

    Visit with student and rehabilitation staff
    Obtain copies of hospital evaluations (psychological, educational, PT/OT, speech)
    Conduct inservice in school to:
      • provide specific information about the student's condition
      • provide more general information about TBI
      • discuss potential modifications (ramp, wheelchair, lighting)

IMMEDIATELY AFTER HOSPITAL DISCHARGE
The school representative will:

    Contact parent(s) to:
      • determine if the child will be getting post-acute rehab. care
      • set a tentative date for return to school, if no further rehab. is being provided

    Follow-up with hospital case manager
      • get update on discharge condition/special needs (i.e., tracheostomy, ambulation)

    Establish a TBI team and designate a case manager (if different from representative)
      The team will:
      Develop a tentative plan for school reentry (consider need for environmental modification, special education, 504 and related services)

ARRIVAL AT SCHOOL
The team will:

      • Assign personnel to conduct initial evaluation and give feedback to teachers and parents
      • Further modify classroom environment to meet student's needs

AFTER FIRST WEEKS AT SCHOOL
The team will:

      • Reassess the student's needs and modify educational plan accordingly
      • Maintain contact with parents and teachers

Figure 11.2. Suggested school reintegration checklist.

After Stabilization

After the student's condition has stabilized, a meeting needs to be arranged with the hospital representative, or case manager. This will be a good time to determine if schoolwork needs to be sent, and what special medical needs the student is likely to have upon return to school. A visit to the rehabilitation unit at the hospital not only will allow the educator to get information, but also will give students information about what is going on in school and an opportunity to talk about their feelings about returning. If a visit with the student is not possible, perhaps, the rehabilitation staff can provide a videotape that will demonstrate the student's progress. During the student's hospital stay, educators also need to prepare for other physical concerns, including the student's need for assistive devices, continuing rehabilitation, and assistance with health-care needs. Despite the relatively fast rate of recovery of motor skill function, it still may be necessary to modify the school environment to accommodate these students (e.g., wheelchair access). Speaking with parents right before the student returns, and even visiting with the student at home, will provide an update on information about these and other problem areas (e.g., vision, hearing, fatigue, headache and other pain complaints).

An inservice should be conducted that provides general information about TBI, as well as specifics on the student's condition. Although inservices such as these will be unnecessary as educators build their knowledge base about TBI, at the present time they are important. In-class meetings may also be arranged to provide information to peers about the student's condition and to prepare them for his or her return, thus hopefully reducing the odds of the student with TBI being abandoned by peers who cannot adjust to the changes (e.g., in personality, social behavior and skills). The student with TBI, however, should be consulted about what information to share with his or her peers (Ylvisaker, Hartwick, & Stevens, 1991).

Upon Hospital Discharge

At the time of discharge, parents and hospital representatives should be contacted by the school's designated case manager to obtain updated information about the child's condition. Copies of progress reports and pertinent hospital records (e.g., neuropsychological and psychoeducational evaluations, reports from physical therapists, occupational therapists, and speech pathologists) should be obtained. Special needs, such as speech or physical therapy, can also be assessed. At this time a tentative date for return to school can be set and a tentative plan developed for school reentry. Any modifications to the school environment will need to be made at this time.

The timing of the student's return to school can be a factor in a successful transition. Preferably, before returning to the general classroom, the student should demonstrate capability in interacting within the school environment and an ability to respond to instruction. Mira and Tyler (1991) recommended that the student be able to tolerate multiple stimuli in the classroom and work unassisted for at least a half-hour. The exact criteria for returning to school will depend on the age of the student, as well as the school situation, but generally students should demonstrate that they can benefit from being back in the classroom (i.e., acquire new information and behave appropriately in social interactions).

Arrival at School

Upon the student's return to school, the appropriate team members should conduct an initial evaluation. In many cases, this will be the responsibility of the school psychologist and/or speech–language pathologist; depending on the individual needs of the student, however, the special education teacher may also be involved. At this time, a reassessment of the student's educational needs must be made and any tentative educational plans modified as needed. Feedback needs to be provided to teachers and parents about the student's functioning. Parents may also need information about available services in the schools, and, when needed, special education laws (e.g., P.L. 101-476) and procedures (e.g., the assessment process, Individualized Education Programs [IEPs], right to due process). Some parents will also benefit from basic information about head injuries, including problems that can be expected and what they can do to manage their child's behavior at home and improve his or her performance in school (Zasler & Kreutzer, 1991).

In the Months Ahead

Monitoring of school progress should not cease after the first few weeks. These students often require monitoring months and even years after their return to school. Some of these students do quite well once they settle into the routine of the classroom again, and receive additional assistance, but then begin to have difficulties at various junctures of their education, such as graduating from high school. Although issues that pertain to students' transition out of high school are beyond the scope of this chapter, it is important to recognize that these students are likely to need extra help and preparation when making that transition. A study by Baer (1992) showed that only 16% of high school students with disabilities received any postgraduate training or education, compared to 56% of students without any known disability.

Educators also need to keep in mind that progress monitoring should not be restricted to academic performance. The student's adjustment from a social and behavioral standpoint also needs to be considered, given the fact that problems in this area are often the most troublesome (Levin, 1987) and have the potential to interfere with later success.

ASSESSMENT

Ensuring that a student receives appropriate services requires that assessments, like interventions, be aimed toward maintaining suitable levels of performance throughout the student's education. In order to do this, a student's prior level of functioning needs to be assessed. In addition, frequent assessment of progress after injury is necessary. Routine probing helps to determine what deficits are resolved and what changes are needed in terms of interventions. Because students with head injuries can recover considerable function in relatively short periods of time, specific interventions are often short-term compared to other disability categories, and so are the IEPs.

The IEP

Federal law requires that the IEP address the current level of educational performance in the areas affected by the disability. Unlike with most other special education students, the dramatic changes seen in students with TBI during the first several months after injury (Michaud, Duhaime, & Gatshaw, 1993) often require that their goals and objectives be more frequently reviewed to reflect the recovery process. This means that flexibility in programming is essential and that the IEP is an evolving program. A review of the IEP should be done once during the first 3 months, and periodically thereafter. Scheduling an IEP review in the spring of each school year will provide an opportunity to troubleshoot for difficulties encountered the previous year, and to plan for the next. Plans that might be considered to achieve continued progress include summer school or an extension of the student's regular school year, as well as the provision of a tutor or personal aide. Ongoing assessment is critical for ensuring that the IEP addresses problems that are interfering with the student's progress.

Nature of Assessment

Because a traumatic brain injury can cause a wide variety of problems that interfere with a child's learning, many of the standard educational assessment tools are not adequate for evaluating the impact of injury. Tests such as the Wechsler scales and the Woodcock-Johnson can be useful but are most beneficial when used in conjunction with other neuropsychological measures. Table 11.1 provides a list of several tests that are typically found in a neuropsychological test battery. Many of these are familiar to school psychologists and educators, although some may not be. Neuropsychological assessments are generally conducted by means of a fixed or flexible battery of standardized tests. The two most widely used fixed batteries are the Halstead-Reitan (Reitan & Wolfson, 1993) and the Luria-Nebraska Neuropsychological Battery (Golden, Puisch, & Hammeke, 1985). These batteries contain a number of tests that measure cognitive, language, sensory, perceptual, motor, and attentional functions. Some tests measure memory functions, but supplementary memory tests, such as the Tests of Memory and Learning (Reynolds & Bigler, 1994), are recommended.

Regardless of the specific battery or tests that are selected, it is important that both a quantitative and a qualitative analysis of the child's test performance be made. Research has repeatedly demonstrated that children with TBI, even the more seriously injured, may fall in the "normal" range when their test scores are compared to those of the standardization group; however, the way in which they earned their scores is apt to be quite different (Fay et al., 1994). Assessing this difference is critical for designing interventions that maximize the student's learning style and strengths. Although it is preferable that testing be completed in the school, there may be occasions when testing needs to be done outside the school. For example, there may be cases where there is no professional in the school district or region who has adequate knowledge or experience with TBI to conduct an appropriate evaluation. In this case, a referral to an agency outside the school would be necessary.

Breadth of Assessment

To further ensure that the assessment lends itself to the development of an appropriate educational plan, school staff should collect a thorough developmental, medical, family, and educational history. It is critical that the student's prior functioning (e.g., academics, social interactions) be assessed. This information, typically obtained from educational records and from talking with parents and teachers, will allow for the modification of the educational program to meet the student's needs. Many of these children have prior learning and behavior problems that can interfere with postinjury progress (Michaud, Rivara, Jaffe, et al., 1993).

Informal assessments in a variety of situations, including one-on-one, small group, and large group interactions, can also provide important information about the child's functioning in settings that are less structured and more distracting, and that require more self-initiation. Informal assessments may also be useful for gathering information about other environments in which the child interacts, such as the home. Neither the child nor the child's brain operates in a vacuum; rather, the student with TBI functions in an environment that

---

Table 11.1
Neuropsychological Test Instruments

Intelligence
Wechsler Intelligence Scales (WISC-III, WAIS-R, WPPSI-R); Kaufman Assessment Battery for Children; McCarthy Scales of Children's Abilities; Differential Abilities Scale

Achievement
Woodcock-Johnson Achievement Tests, Wechsler and Kaufman Achievement Scales, Gray Oral Reading Tests, Woodcock Reading Mastery Test, Key Math

Language
Clinical Evaluation of Language Fundamentals–Revised, Peabody Picture Vocabulary Test, Aphasia Screening Test, Token Test, Verbal Fluency Test, Test of Oral Language Development, Test of Written Language, Preschool Language Scale–Revised

Memory
Tests of Memory and Learning, Wide Range Assessment of Memory and Learning, Wechsler Memory Scale–Revised, California Verbal Learning Test, Rey Osterrieth Complex Figure Test, Tactual Performance Test

Attention
Continuous Performance Test, Conners Ratings Scales, Attentional Deficit Disorders Evaluation Scale, Stroop Color and Word Test, Speech Sounds Perception Test, Seashore Rhythm Test

Mental Flexibility and Concept Formation
Wisconsin Card Sorting Test, Trail Making Test B, Category Test, Stroop Color and Word Test

Visual Functions
Rey Osterrieth Complex Figure, Motor-Free Visual Perception Test, Visual Motor Integration Test, Raven's Progressive Matrices

Motor Functions
Finger Tapping Test, Grooved Pegboard Test, Purdue Pegboard Test, Grip Strength, Bruininks-Osteretsky Test for Motor Proficiency

Social and Adaptive Behavior
Achenbach Child Behavior Checklist (parent, teacher, and youth forms); Vineland Adaptive Behavior Scales; Scales of Independent Behavior; AAMD Adaptive Behavior Scales (school and parent versions)

Personality
Personality Inventory for Children–Revised, Personality Inventory for Youth, Minnesota Multiphasic Personality Inventory–Adolescent

---

Note. Readers can locate these tests in *Tests in Print* (Murphy, Close-Conoley, & Impara, 1994).

consists of a family, a school, and a community. Assessment should focus on the demands that are placed on the student by these various environments and determine how well the student is responding to them. Assessment is also valuable in terms of divining how well each of the systems is functioning. In some cases, one or more of the environments is not functioning adequately enough to provide the services and support these students need. Assessing family functioning is especially important because the sudden onset of impairments and the uncertainty of outcome make it difficult for some families to cope (DePompei & Blosser, 1991). Once the child is discharged from the hospital, families are often left without the support network they have come to depend on. At the same time, other children in the family begin to demand attention and parity with their siblings (e.g., household chores). Parents often find themselves with less time and fewer financial resources (DePompei & Blosser, 1991). Financial problems following injury can be due to a number of factors, including added costs for medical care and parents taking more time off from work to care for the child (Max, MacKenzie, & Rice, 1991).

Timing

The timing of assessments, like interventions, is also an important consideration. Although formal assessments that are conducted during a more stable period of the student's recovery will typically be more helpful than those undertaken during periods of dramatic change (e.g., shortly after injury), it is also important that the child be evaluated as early as possible after injury, as postinjury IQ has been found to be one of the two best predictors of outcome (Klonoff et al., 1993). Regardless of when the student with TBI is tested, it is important to consider factors that may influence performance, such as physical problems, fatigue, and medication effects. These same factors can interfere with any planned interventions.

Many students will not be able to participate in a full-day program immediately after returning to school. In some cases, brief rest periods may suffice, while in other situations a reduction in the school day or class assignments will be necessary. Because children with TBI typically have more difficulty later in the day, more difficult subjects should be scheduled early in the school day. Pull-out services by specialists such as speech pathologists and occupational therapists, as well as in-class side-by-side teaching, should also be timed to occur when the student is at the peak of her or his performance.

Scheduling also plays a key role in increasing academic productivity by reducing distractions and excessive stimulation. Some students will require early class release to avoid the congestion and chaos in hallways during class period changes. This may also benefit the student who has problems with balance and orientation by providing extra time to navigate the hallways and get to the next class safely. Aides can also help in this regard, by assisting the student to move about the school and access various facilities, including the lavatories. Although a peer tutor can assist these students with homework assignments and time management, caution needs to be taken when using peers in areas of hygiene.

CASE STUDY: FRANK

While traveling over the Thanksgiving holiday, Frank, a 10th-grade student, was ejected from the family's car when it spun out of control and rolled over. As a result of the accident he suffered a severe brain injury. He was unconscious at the scene and remained in a coma for 1 week. He spent 2 weeks in intensive care and an additional 4 weeks in the hospital's rehabilitation unit. Two days after the accident, the school principal contacted Frank's parents. After determining that the injury was quite serious, the principal asked the school psychologist to serve as the school's representative and Frank's case manager.

The school psychologist phoned the rehabilitation unit and was put in touch with the speech therapist who was serving as Frank's hospital case manager. The school psychologist imparted details about Frank's prior school performance, including the fact that he was receiving LD services at the time of the accident. Two weeks before discharge, the school psychologist visited Frank at the hospital and met with the speech therapist and other representatives from the rehabilitation team. The team provided copies of their evaluations at that time and also discussed their recommendations. Given the fact that Frank was continuing to be aggressive and noncompliant, the hospital team recommended that he spend some time in a postacute rehabilitation facility that specialized in behavior management. Frank was subsequently transferred to that facility. During the time he was at the facility, the school psychologist conducted an inservice training session at the high school to discuss issues pertaining to head injuries in general, as well as to Frank's particular case.

Although the school psychologist maintained biweekly contact with Frank's parents throughout Frank's 3-month rehabilitation stay, the school psychologist did not have any contact with the rehabilitation facility staff until 3 weeks prior to Frank's discharge. At this time the school psychologist met with the staff at the facility to obtain information about Frank's progress and current problems. An IEP meeting at the school was immediately arranged and held before Frank returned.

Because Frank did not exhibit any residual motor or language problems by the time he was discharged from the rehabilitation facility, the only school personnel at the meeting besides the school psychologist were the LD resource teacher who had worked with Frank before the accident, the school guidance counselor, and the principal. Frank and his parents also attended the meeting, along with one of the rehabilitation specialists from the facility. At the IEP meeting, the parents were given information about additional services the school could provide besides the LD services he was already receiving. A decision was made to change his diagnosis to TBI, although he was to continue to receive resources from the LD consultant. In addition to this, counseling services were added to his IEP and biweekly meetings scheduled. There was unanimous agreement that Frank would have to gradually reintegrate into school by attending only half days for a couple of weeks and receiving home teaching the other half. As a result of fatigue and headache, it was actually 4 weeks before Frank was able to tolerate a full day.

Throughout the remainder of the year, the school psychologist monitored Frank's progress by maintaining weekly contact with the school counselor. IEP meetings were also held every 3 months to ensure that the services were adequate. Although there were no instances of physical aggressiveness in school, his teachers continued to complain that he was argumentative and noncompliant. He did not complete or turn in his homework on a regular basis and refused to participate in certain classroom activities. As a result of this, Frank was assigned a study buddy. Testing at the end of the year showed that Frank was achieving at a rate quite similar to the one before the accident. The decision was made to continue his LD services but keep him classified as TBI. To ensure that transition planning would be addressed by the age of 16, at the beginning of Frank's 11th-grade year a transition plan that included vocational education was added to his IEP. Frank acquired some mechanical skills while in the program and ended up graduating on time. Following graduation he got a full-time job with the forest service.

CONCLUSIONS

Frank is a good example of a student who benefited from early and appropriate reintegration planning. However, not all adolescents who sustain a traumatic brain injury have as positive an outcome as Frank. Although recent changes in federal legislation have paved the way for students with TBI to receive this type of service, educators often feel unprepared to address the unique needs of these students. Most educators are not well informed as to what TBI is all about and do not know what to do for these students.

Given the range of problems that occur as a result of TBI, this is not surprising. Because recovery often takes months, or even years, schools are an important extension of rehabilitation that begins in the hospital. In order to provide the service that these students need, school personnel must be prepared in advance to help them as they return to school. A well–thought-out, comprehensive plan for services that takes into account the student's strengths and weaknesses, both before and after injury, is critical if the student is to succeed academically and socially. Frequent reassessment of the plan and modification of goals and objectives that reflect the student's recovery are essential in order to provide all the academic and social support that is needed, when it is needed. Even the most creative and flexible educational plan, however, does not guarantee that reentry into school will be easy. Reentry is challenging for students with TBI regardless of the circumstances (Savage & Wolcott, 1988). Educators who are aware of this and have some knowledge of what to do to assist these students as they return to the classroom will have the best chance at helping the student meet these challenges.

12. How Education Should Respond to Students with Traumatic Brain Injury

RIK CARL D'AMATO

AND BARBARA A. ROTHLISBERG

Each year, over 1 million children and adolescents experience an acquired, or traumatic, brain injury (TBI) because of an accident or abuse. Unlike most medical conditions that affect school performance, TBI can cause long-term variations in a child's ability to think, move, and interact with others (Bigler, 1990a, 1990b). However, it is only recently that TBI and its consequences for educational attainment have been addressed in a concerted fashion (e.g., Harrington, 1990; Lehr, 1990; Reynolds & Fletcher-Janzen, 1989; Savage & Wolcott, 1994), with changes in public law for the provision of special education services acknowledging this sizable school-age population. School districts may take the position that students with TBI can be served by present school staff in existing classroom settings. However, this requires the provision of specialized training for school personnel so that the unique needs of the students with TBI will be met. The purpose of this chapter is to consider how the silent epidemic (Russell, 1993) of TBI among youngsters affects assessment efforts and provision of educational interventions that promote learning.

CONCEPTUAL ISSUES INVOLVING TBI

History of Educational Service

P.L. 94-142 (Federal Register, 1975, 1990) furnished a mechanism for the provision of educational services to individuals with exceptional needs. However, although many classifications of educationally handicapping conditions were acknowledged, traumatic brain injury was not listed as a specific diagnostic category in that law (Harrington, 1990). Students with TBI could be designated as learning disabled, emotionally disturbed, other health impaired, or physically handicapped and receive services under those categories. Unfortunately, individuals with TBI may not show patterns of deficit that qualify for such alternate identification, and they may not benefit from the programming offered for those diagnoses (Waaland & Kreutzer, 1988). The exclusion of TBI was partially remedied by applying Section 504 of the Rehabilitation Act of 1973 to this population—ensuring modifications of the student's educational plan. With the reauthorization of P.L. 94-142 (now P.L. 101-476, IDEA, 1990), the category of traumatic brain injury was officially recognized (Russell, 1993). The educational definition of traumatic brain injury, in 34 Code of Federal Regulations Part 300 (1993) reads as follows:

> An acquired injury to the brain caused by an external physical force, resulting in total or partial functional disability or psychosocial impairment, or both that adversely affects a child's educational performance. The term applies to open or closed head injuries resulting in impairments in one or more areas, such as cognition; language; memory; attention; reasoning; abstract thinking; judgment; problem-solving; sensory, perceptual and motor abilities; psychosocial behavior; physical functions; information processing; and speech. The term does not apply to brain injuries that are congenital or degenerative, or brain injuries induced by birth trauma. (p. 14)

Definitional Questions

Brain damage is often understood from an evaluation of the cause of the damage. Documented trauma to the brain after birth from accidents, assaults, and abuse are usually defined as *traumatic brain injuries,* whereas injuries stemming from infections, tumors, metabolic disorders, toxins, and anoxic injuries are seen as *nontraumatic brain injuries* (Savage & Wolcott, 1994). *Open*-head injuries result from a penetrating missile (such as a bullet); *closed*-head injuries follow internal damage with the skull uncompromised (from a fall or shaking). The definitions of these terms are not universally accepted. Some practitioners see all injuries as falling under the term *acquired brain injury;* others see all injuries as falling under the nomenclature of TBI (Bigler, 1990b; Savage & Wolcott, 1994). The term *acquired* offers some clarity in that it differentiates between children born with a disability and those who are afflicted with brain injuries later. Definitional disputes should not be surprising, given the scope of possible injuries, and they mimic the history of disagreement over the definition of learning disabilities (Gaddes & Edgell, 1994).

Whatever the term used in an educational context, exclusions for congenital and degenerative brain injuries and birth trauma are usually made in accordance with the federal definition. Therefore, children with congenital and degenerative disorders are not seen as part of any educationally related TBI designation. These students may qualify for special education services under the "other health impaired" diagnosis.

Differences in Relation to Other Educational Disabilities

Developmental Concerns. Understanding the consequences of head injury in childhood is complicated by the development of the central nervous system and the changing nature of the traumas to which children are exposed. For instance, rapid growth and changes in brain structure caused by myelination and neuronal formation mark the first 2 years of life, during which head injury due to abuse (e.g., shaking) and falls is most common. Later, when the ability to handle and plan more abstract activities is evolving, vehicular accidents are the most common causes of damage. Therefore, the nature and timing of the insult may cause unpredictable consequences, as the trauma disrupts the normal progression of cerebral development (Haley, Cioffi, Lewis, & Baryza, 1990).

Much of what is understood about brain–behavior relations has been based on adults who have experienced brain damage. Studies of the changes in performance from premorbid (before injury) levels due to open- and especially closed-head injuries have begun to unlock the mysteries of lateralization of function, generalized location of language and memory ability, and the prognosis for focal versus generalized brain damage (Bruce, 1990). Unfortunately, when considering the expectations for improvement for children who have experienced TBI, there are limitations in generalizing findings from adult models (Fletcher & Taylor, 1984; Rutter, 1983). Injury incurred during the development of the nervous system can have more extensive consequences for the child's prognosis than it can for the adult's (Lehr, 1990). Many neuropsychologists have expressed frustration over the lack of predictability between severity of damage and long-term recovery. Some children with generalized, apparently severe damage have few residual difficulties, while other children with seemingly small lesions experience profound academic and adaptive difficulties (Fletcher & Taylor, 1984). Moreover, early damage can disrupt the acquisition of more complex cognitive behaviors—thereby increasing the potential for delayed onset of deficits as the child matures (Lehr, 1990; Russell, 1993; Waaland & Kreutzer, 1988). The inherent uncertainties about the effects of damage complicate our understanding of TBI and the development of long-term plans for recovery.

Designations of TBI From Mild to Severe. The educational treatment of children with TBI demands special attention because of the variability this type of injury can impose. Impairment resulting from cerebral insult can be viewed along a continuum of consequence, from lethal damage to effects so mild they cannot be distinguished from normal functioning (Fletcher & Taylor, 1984; Russell, 1993). Two related prognostic indicators of cerebral impairment are coma (depth and duration) and posttraumatic amnesia (PTA), the time between injury and recovery of continuous memory (Hynd & Willis, 1988; Lezak, 1983). Individuals who are injured but do not experience a coma, or who remain comatose for only a short period, usually display less brain damage than individuals who sustain lengthy comas or PTA. Instruments administered by medical personnel to screen in these areas include the Glasgow Coma Scale (GCS; Teasdale & Jennett, 1974), the Rancho Los Amigos Scale of Cognitive Levels (Los Amigos Research and Educational Institute, 1990), and a review of PTA severity levels (Bigler, 1990b). Importantly, however, adult measures must be adapted for children because adult norms are inaccurate with children (see Hynd & Willis, 1988). Other meaningful prognostic indicators include age, intracranial pressure, premorbid intelligence, psychiatric history, and neuroradiological and neurological findings (Bigler, 1990b; Lezak, 1983). Although school personnel will not evaluate students in these areas, they should have an understanding of the meaning of such factors for expected prognosis.

The high degree of individual variability within the category of TBI means that educational programming must be tailored to each student's needs. Depending on the severity and type of injury, the child's premorbid adjustment, the age at which the injury occurred, the length of time since the injury took place, and the student's current medical regimen (Medical Economics Data, 1993), cerebral trauma may result in pronounced consequences (Bigler, 1990a, 1990b). The challenge for school personnel comes in acknowledging the changes in behavior while planning for continued progress in learning (Utah TBI Task Force, 1994).

Common Characteristics of TBI. An understanding of TBI can be gained only by a recognition of the relationship between brain status and behavior. One's ability to attend to information, organize a plan of action, and solve problems is dependent on the quality of sensory inputs, and the system's capacity for perceiving, integrating, and responding purposefully to the environment. It is difficult to detail common characteristics of children and adolescents who have suffered an injury, but certain patterns are often discernible across sensory, motor, cognitive, academic, social, emotional, and personal modalities (Begali, 1994; Utah TBI Task Force, 1994). Although no two students are alike, changes in how the student learns, thinks, and feels are common. Various deficit patterns have different degrees of impact on the individual's functional domains (Adams et al., 1991; Taylor, 1987). Such patterns and the impact that they have in the areas of learning/school, peer/community, self (i.e., self-awareness), and family/home are displayed in Table 12.1. Most changes will affect all areas of the student's life, although disturbances in self-awareness are not well understood (Crisp, 1992). School staff have the potential to play a crucial role in helping the student adjust to what will most likely be a changed relationship to his or her environment.

Rapid Change in Functioning. Expectations for learning are based on normal child development and on the premise of a child's relatively steady course in the acquisition of academic and social skills. Students add to their fund of information, understand more complex information and relationships, and apply and plan for more complex problem-solving strategies as they grow older. Children who have received diagnoses under other, traditional special education categories may experience difficulties in one or more of these areas, but they tend to do so in a consistent fashion. That is, once identified, behavioral expectations (cognitive, social, and psychological) follow relatively predictable patterns. For example, a child with mental retardation will require modifications in curricula to allow for increased time to learn material, a greater emphasis on functional skills, and repeated exposure to subject content despite grade level. Educational planning can be long-term, with goals and objectives based in part on the educators' experience with other learners displaying similar characteristics.

Students with TBI differ from others with disabilities in that they do not experience well-defined progress and vary widely in their levels of learning difficulty. Instead of yearly progress reports and triennial reevaluations, students with TBI require more frequent evaluation and planning. Initially, education plans might be revised every grading period, and assessment might be called for as frequently as 6-month intervals (Cohen, 1986; Lehr, 1990). To use the

Table 12.1
Common Difficulties Reported Following TBI

Behavior	Learning/school	Peer/community	Self	Family/home
Functional domain involved				
Sensory/motor				
Attention	√	√	√	
Clumsiness	√	√	√	√
Depth-perception difficulties	√	√	√	√
Difficulty shifting attention	√	√		√
Decreased impulse control	√			√
Loss of sensation	√	√	√	√
Olfactory confusion	√		√	√
Decreased organizational ability	√	√	√	√
Physical difficulties or losses	√	√	√	√
Change in self-monitoring	√			√
Task orientation difficulties	√		√	
Visual problem/impairments	√	√	√	√
Sensory overload	√		√	
Cognitive/academic				
Decreased ability	√	√	√	√
Group activity difficulties	√	√		
Learning style changes	√		√	
Math difficulties	√		√	√
Memory difficulties	√	√	√	√
Change in motor speed	√	√	√	√
Poor/reduced judgment	√			√
Problem-solving difficulties	√			√
Reading difficulties	√	√	√	√
Reduced frustration tolerance	√	√	√	√
Spatial reasoning difficulties	√	√		
Verbal expression problems	√	√	√	
Emotional/social/personal				
Cooperation problems	√	√	√	
Denial and immaturity	√	√	√	√
Difficulties with nonverbal cues	√	√		
Dressing difficulties	√		√	√
Frequent mood changes	√	√	√	√
Inappropriate behaviors	√	√		√
Irritability/anxiety/depression	√	√	√	√
Personal hygiene problems	√	√	√	√
Personality inconsistencies	√	√	√	√
Reduced stamina and endurance	√	√		
School attendance problems/tardiness	√	√	√	
Sleep difficulties	√	√		√
Social awareness	√	√	√	

Note. Adapted from Bigler (1990a), D'Amato & Rothlisberg (1992), Hynd & Willis (1988), Kaufman (1990), Lezak (1983), Reynolds & Fletcher-Janzen (1989), Sattler (1992), Savage & Wolcott (1994), and Wedding et al. (1986).

standard annual–triennial period with this group of youngsters might mean that significant psychological and physiological changes would be missed.

To meet the needs of students with brain injuries, educational specialists, such as school psychologists, must adjust their usual procedures for identification and treatment to accommodate the changes associated with recovery. Indeed, Lehr (1990) argued that "these children may require the most complex array of combined services that a school system has been expected to deliver, and they may require them throughout their school years" (p. 191).

ASSESSMENT OF TBI

Unlike some educational diagnoses that depend on assessment data to validate their use, assessment of function in TBI is less a case of proving brain injury than of translating that medical condition into educational services. Although injuries can be medically classified from mild to severe, the behavior sequelae, or manifestations, will depend on the individual student. Consequently, to prepare students for a return to school, the education professionals involved must form a partnership not only with the student and his or her parents, but also with the medical/rehabilitation staff.

As required by law and ethical practice, a *multimethod, multisource, multisetting* evaluation should be conducted (Adams et al., 1991; Merrell, 1994). Although the focus of assessment is the individual with the injury, it must be recognized that the student does not exist in isolation from his or her environment. Home, school, and community reactions to the changes in the youngster caused by the brain trauma will factor into the child's adaptation (Blosser & DePompei, 1991). Consequently, an ecologically oriented assessment and intervention scheme will best serve educational needs (Leu & D'Amato, 1994). Assessment should consist of direct observations, administration of behavior rating scales, interviews with the student and family members, a review of medical and school records, and a collection of the student's work samples (Sattler, 1992). A variety of self-report measures, including objective and projective tests, should be used as well. Indeed, multiple sources of information, such as parents, family members, and the student, should be included in the evaluation; and multiple settings, incorporating information from the home, school, and community, should be considered (Sachs, 1991; Utah TBI Task Force, 1994). All areas that should be weighed in the evaluation can be found in Table 12.2.

A unique assessment procedure used with TBI that may be foreign to school personnel is the contrasting of *current* data with *premorbid* informa-

Table 12.2
Areas to Be Assessed Formally or Informally in TBI Evaluations

Perception	Concentration/attention
Visual	Basic academic skills
Auditory	
Tactile–kinesthetic	
Integrated	**Styles of Processing**
	Auditory/verbal processing
Motor functions	Visual/spatial processing
Strength	
Speed	
Coordination	**Personality/behavior**
Lateral preference	Adaptive behavior/daily
	Living
Intelligence/cognitive abilities	Development
Verbal functions	Play
Language	Environment/social
Reasoning	Parental
Memory/learning	Sibling
Integrative functioning	Family
Numerical ability	Community
Nonverbal functions	Student coping/tolerance
Perceptual organization	
Reasoning	
Memory/learning	**Educational/classroom environment**
Integrative functioning	Learning environment
	Peer/community reactions
Academic achievement	Student competencies
Language/communication skills	Teacher/staff knowledge
Memory	Teacher/staff reactions

Note. Adapted from Begali (1994), Bigler & Nussbaum (1989), Dean & Gray (1990), Lau & D'Amato (1994), Whitten et al. (1992).

tion (D'Amato, Rothlisberg, & Rhodes, in press; Lezak, 1983). When analyzing information, it is imperative that decisions be based on a clear review of current, not previous, functioning. Thus, although it is important to review information about the student's abilities before the accident, that information should not supersede the skills the child currently displays. Schools that save work samples from previous grade levels have an advantage when evaluating TBI students, because such samples constitute a ready-made database from which to compare current abilities to earlier skills. Such a comparison is necessary to fully understand the uniqueness of each student with TBI. For example, this information is extremely useful when attempting to chart the course of the child's brain injury and develop recommendations regarding prognosis and interventions.

The multidisciplinary team format already in use in the schools helps in the data collection and review process. The school psychologist may be the logical person to coordinate the evaluation and work as a liaison with medical staff, as social and behavioral difficulties as well as academic challenges result from injury. Every effort must be made to establish premorbid status and understand the extent of injury so that the qualitative changes in performance can be better understood.

Developmental History

Parent interviews are a key component in the assessment of TBI, because they provide parents' perceptions of their child's academic skills as well as his or her social and emotional characteristics (D'Amato et al., in press). Preexisting difficulties can be discussed apart from the student's current status. Parents often report that children who have experienced TBI seem to behave in a less mature manner than they did before the injury. Emotional outbursts and difficulty dealing with frustration can be pronounced (Waaland & Kreutzer, 1988). Continued communication with the parents can provide essential information to the school staff for educational planning and help establish the cooperative relationship so necessary to family systems attempting to cope with the changes in their children (Sachs, 1991; Wedding, Horton, & Webster, 1986).

Medical Issues

As the child makes the transition from hospital or rehabilitative setting to home, the school's collaboration with medical staff can provide valuable information for charting the child's progress. Medical staff can provide the school with information on the extent of impairment and the course of recovery. Because rehabilitative services (i.e., physical, occupational, and/or speech therapy) may continue as part of the school placement, the knowledge gained about a child's individual characteristics from acute care staff could save the school valuable time in trying to develop the most appropriate plan for the child's educational needs. It is also important to know whether the child or adolescent is receiving medication for his or her injury, because many drugs have side effects. Understanding what to expect from the medication, and deciding who will administer it in school, should be clarified before school reentry (Medical Economics Data, 1993).

Perceptual and Motor Skills

Although most practitioners assess basic perceptual and motor competencies (e.g., adequate hearing, arm–hand use), this area is especially important with TBI referrals (Adams et al., 1991; Dean & Gray, 1990; Sattler, 1992). This is due to the great inter- and intraindividual variability that students with this type of injury display in perception and movement. A first step, then, is to evaluate whether the student possesses any physical manifestations of cerebral injury, such as difficulty in hearing, seeing, walking, or completing hand movements. These skills are often overlooked, and subtle changes should be carefully evaluated. For example, students who once could write well may now have difficulty with writing speed, letter formation fluency, and coordination; such eye–hand coordination problems are common in children with brain injuries (Jaffe, Brink, Hays, & Chorazy, 1990). Unfortunately, school staff may view slow writing and sloppy letter formation as a reflection of poor motivation, not realizing that these behaviors are related to the child's primary disabling condition.

While neurological–medical evaluations assess for sensory–motor abnormalities, it is also important to evaluate higher level integrative functions (Lezak, 1983). These functions dictate that the student concurrently use visual, auditory, and tactile systems to perceive, understand, and process information, such as when visual or auditory information must be encoded and written down. Data on the student's ability to consolidate material can be gleaned from medical reports, classroom observations, and teacher or parent interviews, or secured through more formalized assessments of vision, hearing, verbal understanding, visual perception, tactile functions, and planning.

If after a careful review of medical reports questions still remain regarding a student's competencies, it may be helpful for the school psychologist to conduct a mental status examination (see Sattler, 1992; Wedding et al., 1986). This quick examination establishes the student's basic competencies in orientation, memory, judgment, oral reading, writing, and spelling. It is not uncommon for a student to be able to perform certain activities on one day and not the next, thus warranting a repeated assessment of skills. Observing the child in transitional movements and working on familiar and unfamiliar tasks can reveal whether poor motor planning or related deficits exist (Haley et al., 1990). Instruments frequently used to evaluate perceptual and motor abilities are listed in Table 12.3.

Intellectual/Cognitive Ability

In most definitions of educational disability, the assessment of intellectual performance is a central component in diagnosis. In cases of TBI, ability is less a diagnostic indicator than it is a descriptor of the degree of trauma

Table 12.3
Common Instruments Used in Evaluation

Motor (fine and gross)
Bender Gestalt Test of Visual–Motor Integration
Bruininks-Oseretsky Test of Motor Proficiency
Detroit Tests of Learning Ability (3rd ed.)
Developmental Test of Visual–Motor Integration
Finger Oscillation Test
McCarthy Scales of Children's Abilities
Strength of Grip Test

Intelligence/cognitive
Battelle Developmental Inventory
Bayley Infant Intelligence Test (2nd ed.)
Das-Naglieri Cognitive Assessment System
Differential Ability Scales
Kaufman Assessment Battery for Children
McCarthy Scales of Children's Abilities
Stanford-Binet Intelligence Scale (4th ed.)
Wechsler Intelligence Scale for Children (3rd ed.)

Attention/concentration/memory
Children's Auditory Verbal Learning Test
Detroit Tests of Learning Ability (2nd or 3rd ed.)
Goldman-Fristoe-Woodcock Test of Auditory Discrimination
Mental Status Examination
Test of Memory and Learning
Wechsler Memory Scale–Revised
Wepman's Auditory Discrimination Test
Wide Range Assessment of Memory and Learning

Academic achievement
Differential Ability Scales
Kaufman Assessment Battery for Children
Kaufman Test of Educational Achievement
Key Math Diagnostic Arithmetic Test–Revised
Peabody Individual Achievement Test–Revised
Wechsler Individual Achievement Test
Woodcock Reading Mastery Test–Revised
Woodcock-Johnson Psycho-Educational Battery–Revised: Achievement
Wide Range Achievement Test (3rd ed.)

Styles of Processing
Auditory/Verbal (see also Communication and Intelligence/cognitive areas)
Detroit Tests of Learning Ability (3rd ed.)
Peabody Picture Vocabulary Test–Revised
Seashore Rhythm Test
Sensory–Perceptual Exam
Speech Sound Perception Test

(table continues)

(Table 12.3 continued)

Visual/spatial processing (see also Intelligence/cognitive area)
  Aphasia Screening Test
  Detroit Tests of Learning Ability (2nd or 3rd ed.)
  Matrix Analogies Test
  Motor-Free Visual Perception Test
  Test of Nonverbal Intelligence (2nd ed.)
  Visual Acuity Screening

Communication/language skills (see also Academic achievement)
  Bracken Basic Concept Scale
  Mental Status Examination
  Peabody Picture Vocabulary Test–Revised
  Revised Token Test
  Test of Adolescent Language
  Test of Language Development
  Test of Written Language

Personality/emotional/environmental
  Behavioral Assessment System for Children (BASC)
    Parent Rating Scales
    Teacher Rating Scales
    Self-Report of Personality
    Student Observation System
    Structured Developmental History
  Behavior Evaluation Scales
  Burks' Behavior Rating Scales
  Child Behavior Checklist
  Clinical Interview with Child or Adolescent
  Family Adaptability Cohesion Evaluation Scales
  Family Environment Scale
  Home Visit and Interview
  Kinetic Family or School Drawings
  Minnesota Multiphasic Personality Inventory–2
  Personality Inventory for Children
  Revised Children's Manifest Anxiety Scale
  Sentence Completion Tests
  Thematic Apperception Tests
  Vineland Adaptive Behavior Scales
  Wishes and Fears Interview

Educational/classroom environment
  Classroom Environment Scale
  Classroom Observations
  The Instructional Environment Scale
  Piers-Harris Children's Self-Concept Scale
  School Social Behavior Scales
  Sociograms
  Teachers Interviews

Note. Space does not permit listing references for all of the above tests; most are common instruments that can be found in the library. The authors can be contacted for additional information.

experienced. Scores on intelligence or cognitive tests are among the single best predictors of severity of trauma but, because of their standardized structure and format, may not provide the range of information on cognitive processing desired for educational planning (Ylvisaker et al., 1990).

Most commonly used intelligence tests (see Table 12.3) have been criticized as too narrow. Many measures depend heavily on a well-established knowledge base and verbal expression to survey cognitive skills (e.g., Stanford-Binet Intelligence Scale [4th ed.], Wechsler Intelligence Scale [3rd ed.]). Actually, intelligence test scores of children with TBI may show that verbal skills remain relatively robust, whereas perceptual–motor, memory, and spatial skills are adversely affected by injury (Ewing-Cobbs, Fletcher, & Levin, 1986; Ylvisaker et al., 1990). Because verbal skills are often described as the most relevant to educational progress, the stability of the verbal performance in this circumstance may result in an overly optimistic view of students' competence in returning to the classroom (Ewing-Cobbs et al., 1986). Therefore, the evaluator's dependence on standardized test procedures can adversely affect the amount of information gained from ability assessment; instead, for students with TBI, testing the limits and modifying examination procedures may yield a more accurate description of expected classroom performance (Harrington, 1990; Ylvisaker et al., 1990).

The standardized testing format of ability tests can actually help students compensate for their difficulties (Waaland & Kreutzer, 1988). Standardized directions demand that the examiner present a consistent, well-defined task to the student and observe and record the student's answer. Information is meted out in small units in this one-on-one situation. Because assessment conditions are meant to optimize performance, the length of each session and the environmental conditions are also controlled. Unfortunately, such procedures may act to mask the very aspects of TBI most critical to breakdowns in learning, like being unable to select key aspects of a learning situation, plan a method of response, or integrate new information into established knowledge.

Many researchers suggest that much can be learned about the effects of a brain injury by changing the testing format to directly observe areas of suspected difficulty (see Harrington, 1990; Ylvisaker et al., 1990). Traumatic brain injury often causes loss of processing efficiency and difficulties in attention/concentration, organization, reasoning, memory, and planning ability. In the uncontrolled classroom situation, students with such an injury often quickly overload on information and lose the capacity to spontaneously choose strategies to remedy their difficulties. Methods of detecting the child's degree of learning impairment during the evaluation include the following (see also Cohen, 1986; Harrington, 1990; Ylvisaker et al., 1990, for excellent suggestions on the assessment of TBI):

- Modifying instructions to include more clues to the problem's solution to determine learning efficiency;
- Modifying response requirements to determine if alternate modes are more appropriate for the student;
- Assessing attention to novel and/or previously experienced tasks at various times of day and under varying levels of distraction;
- Varying the rate at which information must be processed or tasks completed, to determine the effects on performance;
- Detecting the response to frustration when tasks presented are too difficult or when the examiner adds stressors;
- Assessing the number of trials needed to remember visual or verbal information and the accuracy of recall or recognition over time; and
- Gauging the spontaneous use of problem-solving strategies in attempting different tasks.

Careful observation of formal activities, testing the limits of standardized instruments, or introducing other informally produced items into the sessions can give the examiner insight into not only the student's ability to answer correctly, but also how he or she goes about processing the information.

Academic Achievement

Assessment of academic ability can fall prey to many of the same difficulties seen in the standard evaluation of the student's cognitive ability. Many, if not all, of the standard instruments tap into the knowledge base of well-learned material. The structure of the assessment process presents basic reading, math, and written language problems to the student in the rarified atmosphere of an individualized testing situation. If the student can recall information and respond with these well-learned skills, the achievement test score obtained may overestimate actual classroom performance. Certainly, within the classroom, the child's capacity to attend to, organize, and plan approaches to problems will be taxed to a greater extent than during the testing situation (Ewing-Cobbs et al., 1986; Harrington, 1990). Again, the examiner or the classroom teacher can get a better sense of the student's capacity to deal with scholastic subjects by testing the limits of his or her tolerance for a natural learning setting. Aspects of this could include those listed in Table 12.3 (under Intellectual/cognitive) and the following:

- Gauging the student's response to content questions that are progressively more abstract;
- Determining whether the student can self-initiate to complete a school activity or whether cues are needed;
- Observing test performance when the student is paired with other students compared to when he or she is left to work independently; and
- Contrasting responses when frequent feedback on performance is given or when the length of tasks is modified.

One of the keys to understanding academic performance appears to involve the speed at which a student might overload based on the complexity of the information provided and the response expected. Because the effects of TBI can go undetected for years until more abstract or complicated learning occurs, the problem of processing overload is likely to grow more pronounced as the student progresses through the grade levels (Cohen, 1986; Lehr, 1990).

Processing Styles

Although few authors agree on how to evaluate the student's ability to process information, most recognize that it is an important area (D'Amato, 1990, 1991; Kaufman, 1979b; Sattler, 1992; Wedding et al., 1986). Whatever the paradigm selected, most psychologists consider data from the domains of verbal and nonverbal processing, fluid and crystallized processing, simultaneous and successive processing, associative and cognitive processing, and linguistic and motoric development to be important (Hammill, 1991; Hartlage & Telzrow, 1983; Hynd & Willis, 1988; Sattler, 1992). The emphasis should be on how information is processed, not on the content or subject area under investigation (Kaufman, 1979a, 1979b; Telzrow, 1985, 1990). The typical psychological evaluation covers many of the areas detailed above, but visual–spatial processing and auditory–verbal processing are seen by some as areas that are especially critical because of their relationship to hemispheric-related interventions (D'Amato, 1990; Whitten, D'Amato, & Chittooran, 1992).

Language/Communication

Depending on the location and extent of damage, the student experiencing TBI may evidence speech and language deficits. A speech and language clinician should work closely with rehabilitative staff to determine the degree to which the student's communication skills have been compromised (Harrington, 1990). Although simple receptive and expressive tasks may suggest strong superficial language ability, any evaluation should include an analysis of the child's ability to analyze and integrate information presented in a verbal format. Disturbances in memory might increase word-finding problems; problems with abstraction might interfere with figurative speech and in seeing cause-and-effect relations (Dennis, 1992; Russell, 1993). A common difficulty among children recovering from head trauma involves the social aspects of speech (Russell, 1993). Often, students with TBI will have difficulty in making straightforward, sequentially appropriate responses to questions and difficulties in engaging in social discourse.

Personality/Behavior

As previously discussed, personality changes are common in children who have experienced TBI. In fact, some authors argue that personality changes are the most difficult consequence of the injury as reported by family, friends, and school personnel both during and after rehabilitation (Deaton, 1990; Lezak, 1983; Savage & Wolcott, 1994; Wedding et al., 1986). Thus, a comprehensive evaluation of adjustment must address the student's ability to complete daily living skills, interact socially, and cope with the results of the injury (see Table 12.1). Behavioral information from school staff, parents, and the child himself or herself should be collected (D'Amato, 1990, 1991; Gray & Dean, 1989). Often, the child will show emotional unpredictability and lability that will affect relationships with peers and teachers (Russell, 1993). Decreased tolerance for stress and frustration may present itself as resistance to educational tasks (Deaton, 1990; Harrington, 1990). Depending on the student's degree of impairment, adaptive behavior scales also may be included as part of the evaluation. The child's worldview may be gauged using both projective and objective measures. Particular consideration should be given to the support that is available to the student from family, friends, and school personnel. Sample measures that may be useful in this area can be found in Table 12.3.

Educational/Classroom Environment

Students at school do not exist in isolation; they interact regularly with peers and school personnel. The general education teacher and the special education staff each will have significant influence on the child, and the match between the student and his or her principal teacher is important (Adams et al., 1991; Leu & D'Amato, 1994). The teacher's classroom management style, classroom organization, degree of control, tolerance, level of emotional support, and knowledge of TBI can be key factors in the student's school adjustment (Blosser & DePompei, 1994; Telzrow, 1990). Therefore, evaluation of the student's existing and future placement should be conducted regarding these variables. Much of the information in this area can be collected informally; however, some standardized environmental scales developed for the home can be adapted for the classroom (see Table 12.3).

EDUCATIONAL INTERVENTIONS: AN S.O.S. FOR STUDENTS

Because students who have experienced a brain injury have not been recognized in the past as requiring modified educational services, educational settings have been slow to adjust their expectations and programs for these students. The assumption has been that as the child's outward manifestations of an injury fade, the internal damage is repaired as well. Parents and teachers may presume that the youngster will return to school and continue as he or she did before, whatever the level of brain injury sustained (Russell, 1993). Unfortunately, lack of planning for school reentry can cause untold frustration and confusion for children and adults alike.

Students with TBI vary widely in terms of the scope and severity of their disability. Traumatic brain injury can dramatically transform a child's ability to organize, solve problems, remember, attend, and relate to others. Children who acted competently before the injury may suddenly exhibit inappropriate responses to common academic tasks. The dissonance between previous personality/school performance and current adjustment may cause school staff to misinterpret the student's behavior. For example, teachers may view emotional outbursts or incomplete work as intentional misbehaviors rather than a function of the injury (Deaton, 1990).

Although the exact features of TBI will change with the individual student, certain commonalities in performance have been observed with this group of learners (D'Amato, 1991; Savage & Wolcott, 1994). Teaching staff might benefit by thinking of these commonalities and modify their teaching methods in terms of a well-known acronym— S.O.S.— that stands for broad categories of intervention: Structure, Organization, and Strategies. These categories are interrelated in that they deal with bringing order into the life experiences of students whose injuries have impaired their natural capacity to spontaneously direct aspects of their learning. For the purposes of discussion, *structure, organization,* and *strategies* will be distinguished by the degree of external control required. For example, structure will refer primarily to the physical organization suggested for maximal learning, whereas organization refers to teaching methods used to establish order and relevance in the student's learning. Strategy development refers to attempting to instruct the student in the acquisition of various planning and self-monitoring schemes.

Within each intervention category, certain suggestions for remediation, adaptation, or alternative methods of instruction will be made. It should be noted, though, that few validated treatment options are available that ensure educational success, particularly with the range of individual differences in TBI (D'Amato, 1990; D'Amato & Rothlisberg, 1992). Each student's unique characteristics will have to be considered in fashioning an educational response.

Structure

Traumatic brain injury leads to a sense of disorientation and low tolerance for environmental change, particularly during the initial months of recovery. As the child struggles to make sense out of an altered perception of the world and an altered level of competence, as much structure and stability as possible should be provided (D'Amato, 1991; Utah TBI Task Force, 1994). Minimal distractions, clear expectations for the student, and a basic routine will allow for a growing sense of security and confidence that adaptation is possible (Utah TBI Task Force, 1994). Lessening of structural boundaries could be seen as steps in rehabilitation, but a sure and consistent *safety net* will allow the student to focus attentional resources on the demands of learning, not survival, in the school environment.

Forge a Home–School Partnership. As previously mentioned, parents are an integral link to meeting the needs of a child who is recovering from TBI. Blosser and DePompei (1991) suggested that, unfortunately, grave misconceptions about the consequences of cerebral injury in childhood are typical in parents and school personnel. Initially, to promote effective school entry, it is important to ensure that all parties have a basic knowledge about the injury. This could be accomplished by designating an educational professional as a liaison when cases of TBI occur in the school population. The contact person would communicate with parents to offer support as the child begins his or her recovery and act to facilitate understanding of the consequences of the injury by the child's teachers and classmates. Support for parents can help offset the adjustment difficulties often experienced when children are injured and may promote family adjustment and improve expectations for the child's prognosis (Waaland & Kreutzer, 1988). Such early intervention also can promote consistency between home and school in terms of behavioral programming (Cohen, 1986).

Develop a Work-Release Program. Aside from potential changes in school performance, parents and school staff may also need to plan for transition into the world of work for adolescents with TBI. As the research on employment opportunities for students with learning disabilities shows, students with learning difficulties may find meaningful employment difficult to secure (Rojewski, 1992; Scuccimarra & Speece, 1990). A school's plan for providing transition services to students with disabilities should be extended to those with TBI. Working with vocational educators and adult service providers in the community will likely improve the relevance of the student's individualized educational plan for long-term adjustment—not just to school but to life (Reiff & deFur, 1992; Rojewski, 1992; Sachs & Redd, 1993). Knowledge of the student's strengths and weaknesses as well as motivation for employment will help to shape realistic vocational goals.

Increase Teacher Consistency. Because continuity of programming is essential, a teaching staff trained to work with students recovering from TBI will be optimal for learning. Likewise, students benefit from working with the same teacher or group of teachers for more than 1 year at a time. The extended time together can help to foster trust, friendships, and an appropriate degree of attachment that may be more important than learning the traditional educational content (Leu & D'Amato, 1994; Savage, 1987). Selecting a particular teacher to work with a student with TBI will require an evaluation to maximize the student–teacher match (Hill, Baldo, & D'Amato, 1994; Savage & Wolcott, 1994; Soar & Soar, 1979).

Careful consideration should be given to other students in the classroom, paying close attention to the potential for personality conflicts between the child with a TBI and his or her classmates. School districts have recently recognized the value of an ongoing teacher–student–parent relationship and have begun utilizing multiyear classrooms. For example, a single teacher may teach a group of students for a 2-year period in what is a combined third- and fourth-grade classroom or provide consistency across grade levels in a content area in high school. The multiyear system makes developmental sense and offers much for students with cerebral impairments. However, ultimate success in this area will only happen if a low student–teacher ratio is maintained. Obviously, teachers tend to grow weary of working with extremely difficult students, and a single teacher working with several students with TBI may be problematic.

Augment Behavioral Consistency. Although it is clear that teacher consistency across years is important, behavioral consistency in the classroom is equally, if not more, important. Students who have suffered a brain injury often have a difficult time following directions and making use of independent time; consistency and reliability can help strengthen their abilities and self-control (Adams et al., 1991; Harrington, 1990; Telzrow, 1990). "Activity must continually be defined more narrowly so that each class in the schedule, each activity in the class, and each assignment in each activity reinforce and develop structure" (Rosen & Gerring, 1986, p. 71). Routine is extremely important, as are clear expectations for behavior. Cohen (1986) reported that traditional behavioral techniques may not be effective with students who have experienced a TBI because such techniques require the child to remember cause–effect relations. In addition, these students do not respond to subtle cues. Thus, brief, clear rules and expectations for performance will help eliminate confusion and increase the student's sense of competence.

Control Environmental Stimulation. Some students learn better in quiet classrooms, whereas others need to be stimulated by other active learners. Environmental stimulation should be controlled by the teacher (Begali, 1994; Blosser & DePompei, 1994). Use of study carrels, headphones, ear plugs, and special learning areas can provide the level of stimulation needed for optimal learning to take place. In addition, classmates and/or school staff can monitor and assist students who are poorly oriented to the physical aspects of the school. For example, adolescents with TBI may not react well to frequent class changes or the study halls common in high school. Supervision of behavior will reduce confusion and reinforce appropriate activity.

Environmental structure will also need to be reviewed in career or vocational programming for students with TBI. Recognition of their difficulties and of appropriate workplace accommodations may make the students and their potential employers more comfortable in the job setting because each group's needs are being considered (Sachs & Redd, 1993).

Consider Endurance and Stamina. Because students with TBI may tire easily, the length of the school day may need modification, or a rest time may need to be provided (Begali, 1994). Class selection and assignments may also require revision to allow for simpler class structure or alternate course requirements (Rosen & Gerring, 1986). As the older student begins to experience the world of work as part of career education and monitored practice, productivity levels and work schedules may need to be adjusted (Rojewski, 1992).

Support and Validate Feelings. It is important for school staff to validate the feelings of students recovering from TBI. This can be done by encouraging students to verbalize feelings in safe situations. Counseling and support groups are often needed (Whitten et al., 1992). At later stages in the recovery process, it is appropriate to discuss how behavior relates to feelings, especially with others. Because social behaviors might be impaired by the injury, the development of interpersonal and vocational relationships needs to be addressed (Deaton, 1990; Rojewski, 1992; Russell, 1993).

Organization

Organization, a close ally of structure, can be defined as providing students with TBI with the necessary environmental cues and aids to foster acquisition of new learning and help them to retrieve previous knowledge (Telzrow, 1990). The consequences of TBI may include the student's decreased ability to organize and plan activities and will therefore require organizational modifications (Adams et al., 1991; Utah TBI Task Force, 1994).

Use Instructional Tactics. Traumatic brain injury often interrupts the child's ability to plan activities, complete tasks, and gather information. As a result, teachers must adjust to the fact that a student returning to school with a brain injury may need to reacquaint himself or herself with the procedure of *how* to learn, not *what* to learn (Cohen, 1986). For example, the student may need to be retrained in locating information and selecting what is relevant before the teacher emphasizes content. Consequently, the evaluation should reveal whether the student knows the procedure that will be required to complete a task, and knows what to do at the beginning, middle, and final stages of the task. Not only do students need to learn planning skills, but they also need to learn how to cope if the plan fails, and how to proceed with revisions if changes are needed (Savage & Wolcott, 1994). Planning for and coping with change should be important components in the curriculum.

Teachers can help to simplify the students' struggle with organization by providing them with a clear template of coming activities. A set routine and any organizational cues that the teacher can provide will aid students in detecting important elements of lessons. Teachers may find that providing advance organizers, objective sheets including key words and concepts, clearly specified guidelines for instruction, and multimodal cues can counteract some students' attentional difficulties and consolidate their learning (Ewing-Cobbs et al., 1986; Rosen & Gerring, 1986; Telzrow, 1990). Practice with and repetition of activities, as well as feedback on performance, also can strengthen students' confidence (Prigatano, 1990).

Organize Assignments. Beyond using organizational methods to present information, teachers can also assist students with TBI by allowing modifications to the students' workload. Given the scope of difficulties the student can experience, teachers' expectations for normal performance in the class-room or on the job may need to be adjusted. For instance, note-taking skills may be particularly poor; allowing tape-recording of material or duplication of another student's notes will compensate for difficulties in this area. An assignment notebook or a weekly study plan that can be reviewed by teach-ers and parents may help the student to monitor progress in learning, too. Furthermore, teachers' expectations for assignments and examinations will need to be reviewed. Teachers may need to extend deadlines or break down tasks into smaller units to allow the student additional feedback. The student may also need alternate means of assessment, as recall is typically weaker than recognition of information with this group (Rosen & Gerring, 1986).

Adopt a Life-Skill Curriculum. Although all educational programs should be evaluated for educational relevance, this is especially critical when planning for students with TBI who have particular deficits in functional skills. Whenever possible, activities pertinent to everyday living should be incorporated into the curriculum (Savage & Wolcott, 1994; Whitten et al., 1992). This includes activities like learning to greet others, using a tele-phone, counting change, balancing a checkbook, and reading survival words. At later developmental levels, skills associated with vocational success are especially relevant.

Offer Career Education. Students who have experienced a TBI may have specific needs when moving into postsecondary settings. Transitional pro-grams that stress career education and job training may be particularly criti-cal for students who suddenly find themselves at a different functional level than they anticipated before injury. After determining interest and job-related skills, the student may need the opportunity to practice vocational components in a structured setting with opportunities for observational learning and feedback (Sachs & Redd, 1993). Modeled experiences, job-shadowing, on-the-job training, and/or internships can ease the individual into the vocational setting (Rojewski, 1992). Vocational educators can help students organize their time and practice key skills, as well as work with employers to prepare them for the needs of employees with TBI (see Posthill & Roffman, 1991).

Strategies

In tandem with organization and structure, teachers should consider offering their students instruction in the development of learning strategies (D'Amato & Rothlisberg, 1992). Depending on the age of the student at the time of injury and the severity of damage, the psychological aftermath of trauma may be a persistent disruption to the learning process (Adams et al., 1991). The normal cascade of development from simple to integrated levels of understanding can be blocked, leading the student to stumble not on the factual content of the material to be learned, but on the learning process itself. To complicate matters, memory deficits can exacerbate difficulties in instruction. Unfortunately, much of educational programming focuses on content (e.g., reading, writing, and mathematics) rather than the cognitive underpinnings of learning (e.g., attention, impulse control) that were disrupted by the TBI (Blosser & DePompei, 1991; D'Amato & Dean, 1987; Telzrow, 1990; Waaland & Kreutzer, 1988). Strategy instruction helps students select problem-solving methods and tactics to make learning more efficient.

Consider Methods or Processes. Educators regularly develop student profiles highlighting student needs and strengths; however, most often these profiles reflect academic deficiencies and not strategies for dealing with information. For instance, D'Amato and Dean (1987) found that teachers were quite comfortable with academic content areas (i.e., reading, arithmetic) but did not seem to understand the various methods of information processing at work among the students. Learning styles can relate to visual or auditory modalities (use of phonetic or whole word approaches) and hemispheric processing styles, such as simultaneous or sequential approaches (Hartlage & Telzrow, 1983; Telzrow, 1985; Whitten et al., 1992). Structuring tasks or instructing students in *alternative* approaches to solving problems or completing work will benefit all learners in the classroom (see Harrington, 1990; Telzrow, 1990).

Use Compensatory Methods. Children with cerebral damage may have intractable skill deficits that will not respond to even extensive instruction. A teacher's repeated failure with a child that appears motivated is often a clue that a deficit area is involved. An old neuropsychological adage appropriately states that one cannot teach dead tissue to learn. This is important because extensive practice will never help certain skills to develop in some students with TBI. Thus, it is critical to work with students using competencies that have been maintained. A compensatory approach may act as a method around blocks in the child's learning (Gaddes & Edgell, 1994). For example, visual displays and diagrams may be valuable adjuncts to verbal descriptions if the student is experiencing language comprehension problems. Or, developing a procedure for asking "wh . . ." questions (who, what, where, etc.) may help a student who has difficulty detecting key bits of information in a presentation (Cohen, 1986).

Offer Remediation When Appropriate. Students who have missed or not learned certain skills may benefit from direct instruction in academic areas. Practice in the content area may be enough to bolster confidence, but generalization will be more likely if the student has opportunities to exhibit his or her skills in a variety of situations (Gaddes & Edgell, 1994; Prigatano, 1990). Although remedial approaches can be helpful, students with TBI often will not benefit from this direct, focused, content-based method.

Provide Role Models. Once teachers and peers have established positive relationships with the student who has experienced TBI, it is important to use these relationships to further help the child. Allowing the child to learn from peers, rehearse appropriate educational and social behavior, and receive feedback on the success of responses is invaluable not only to the child with TBI but to others as well. Often, classmates may have a difficult time resolving the differences in the student after his or her injury and display little tolerance for the changes (Lehr, 1990). As mentioned earlier, TBI is not only a personal transformation but a social one as well, affecting all aspects of the child's interactions.

Teach Social Skills. Most students learn how to read significant social cues at an early age. Unfortunately, some students with TBI may need very concrete lessons in appropriate social behavior. Such students' behavior after injury may appear immature and inappropriate. Parents, teachers, and peers can help by providing feedback on the quality of the students' reactions. Because school personnel have the opportunity to observe students throughout the day, they can tailor social skills training groups to discussing and practicing competencies, such as how to start a conversation, selecting topics for conversation, and maintaining interpersonal distance. Devising cues, providing clear expectations and explanations, and offering opportunities for practice will all need to be included in a comprehensive program. Parents and school staff alike should all be responsible for helping in the relearning efforts (Deaton, 1990).

CONCLUSIONS

Traumatic brain injury and its educational ramifications may actually open a new chapter in the relationship among education, psychology, and the medical sciences. No other educational disability demands more of rehabilitative professionals and the resources available for teaching and learning. Traumatic brain injury's variable severity, uneven course, and ecological ramifications will challenge accepted notions of evaluation and intervention based on stable and standard approaches. The pedantic view that the old ways, the slow and steady ways, of studying student responses within legislated time constraints will not meet these students' needs. Many of these children will never be the same as they were before injury. The question then becomes whether education can respond to these unique students' needs. To succeed in this arena will mean that education truly subscribes to the idea of developing individual educational programs and education that is child driven. Traumatic brain injury may represent the greatest challenge that education has yet to meet.

13. Helping Students with Mild Traumatic Brain Injury: Collaborative Roles Within Schools

CHERYL H. SILVER AND THOMAS D. OAKLAND

Traumatic brain injury (TBI) in childhood occurs with sufficient frequency in our country to warrant proactive planning in schools. A recent California epidemiologic study estimated that the annual incidence of TBI resulting in hospital involvement was 185 children per 100,000 (Kraus, Fife, Cox, Ramstein, & Conroy, 1986). Of those children, 88% experienced mild brain injury, 7% experienced moderate injury, and 5% experienced severe injury. The most common causative events were falls, accidents during recreational activities, and motor vehicle accidents.

To some degree, the severity of injury will influence the likelihood that parents seek medical attention for their children after an accident. After serious injury, emergency medical services frequently are summoned immediately. Moderate to severe brain injury manifested in prolonged loss of consciousness usually results in hospital admission. During the course of a child's hospital stay, various professionals (e.g., neuropsychologists and speech, physical, and occupational therapists) may be involved. If extended care is needed, a rehabilitation facility may continue providing appropriate services; this type of facility may also help form a link with the child's school and generate a plan for reintegration.

However, if loss of consciousness is brief or only minor alterations in consciousness occur, children often are taken to emergency rooms, examined,

239

and sent home with simple directions to observe them for changes in behavior. Furthermore, in many instances a child who does not lose consciousness may not be taken for medical treatment. The child often continues to function and the incident is forgotten. However, this type of mild brain injury, also described as a concussion, may have later consequences.

The two purposes of this chapter are to summarize the current knowledge base about mild TBI in children and discuss provision of services in schools when rehabilitation professionals have had little or no prior involvement with the child because of the mild nature of the injury.

SEQUELAE OF MILD TBI

Mild traumatic brain injury usually is defined through the use of the Glasgow Coma Scale (GCS; Teasdale & Jennett, 1974). Scores from 13 to 15 indicate a child has experienced no more than a minor change in responsiveness in one of three categories of behavior: verbal response, motor response, and eye opening. Although not all mild head injuries produce cognitive limitations, a significant number of adults have been reported to experience sequelae that affect their subsequent functioning (Barth et al., 1989; Barth et al., 1983; Boll & Barth, 1983; Eisenberg & Levin, 1989; Levin et al., 1987; Ruff et al., 1989). These sequelae include increased irritability, increased susceptibility to fatigue, reduced concentration, reduced speed of information processing, and memory difficulties. Many of these problems will be noticeable during the early recovery period but may resolve over time (Alves, Macciocchi, & Barth, 1993). However, most individuals who experience mild head injury are not given appropriate information about what to expect and may suffer from secondary emotional distress that produces additional impediments to a successful return to their previous level of functioning (Levin et al., 1987).

After suffering a mild head injury, children may exhibit one or more of the following characteristics: personality changes, reduced attention and concentration, mental inefficiency, and forgetfulness. These qualities might not be recognized as related to this seemingly minor event and may be attributed incorrectly to sources under the child's control. Such attributions may have a detrimental effect on the child's current and future school success (Boll, 1983).

It should be noted that research with children aimed at investigating the potential effects of mild TBI is in its infancy and has yet to provide clear conclusions about the sequelae that might influence school performance. Many early studies produced inconclusive results because of confounding premorbid factors and factors related to age and time since injury (Levin, Ewing-Cobbs, & Fletcher, 1989). Research design issues such as the absence of a control group and small sample sizes plague even current studies. Nevertheless, recognizing that the use of larger samples and assessment of more subtle neuropsychological functions may change future understanding of mild TBI in children, general statements can be made about our current knowledge base.

Most studies have found no long-term IQ deficits in children with mild TBI (Fay et al., 1993; Levin & Eisenberg, 1979). Although Bassett and Slater (1990) found no difficulties on subtests requiring simple information retrieval and use of operations immediately after injury, they reported that impairment was indicated on subtests of the Wechsler Intelligence Scale for Children–Revised (Wechsler, 1974) reflecting verbal and nonverbal reasoning and on the coding subtest, a measure of motor speed and visual encoding. The coding deficiency also was observed at 1-year follow-up (Fay et al., 1993). Impairment in writing to dictation, which has been reported soon after injury (Ewing-Cobbs, Levin, Eisenberg, & Fletcher, 1987), may be related to this finding and may forecast problems in school activities such as copying from the board and taking notes.

Decreases in basic academic skills were not found after mild TBI (Bijur, Haslum, & Golding, 1990; Fay et al., 1993), with the exception of a possible decrease in mathematics functioning (Levin & Benton, 1986). However, little is known about academic functioning beyond 1-year postinjury, a time when the ongoing accumulation of knowledge will be needed in order to perform more challenging academic work. Complex problem solving does not appear to be compromised by mild TBI, either immediately after injury or at 1-year follow-up (Bassett & Slater, 1990; Fay et al., 1993); however, disruption in the ability to organize, prioritize, and solve complex problems in daily living may not be detected in younger children until later, when environmental demands increase (Levin et al., 1989).

Long-term follow-up of language functioning has indicated that children with mild TBI do not demonstrate deficits in broad-based functions such as vocabulary development nor in more complex communication functions such as narrative discourse (Bijur et al., 1990; Chapman et al., 1992). In the first months after injury, however, these children may experience difficulty with word-finding (Bassett & Slater, 1990; Ewing-Cobbs et al., 1987), which has the potential to be frustrating for them and others.

No specific deficits in attention have been reported when measured several months after mild injury (Kaufmann, Fletcher, Levin, Miner, & Ewing-Cobbs, 1993). Studies examining the immediate effects of mild injury on attention and concentration, when children first return to school, have not been conducted. Information about memory functioning appears most confusing. Longitudinal studies generally have reported no residual memory deficits from mild TBI (Fay et al., 1993; Levin & Eisenberg, 1979; Levin et al., 1988). Nevertheless, observable limitations in the ability to acquire information upon initial exposure have been described (Bassett & Slater, 1990; Levin & Eisenberg, 1979). Consistent with much of the literature in pediatric neuropsychology, verbal memory has been evaluated to a greater degree than has visual memory. Conflicting findings do exist: Donders (1993) reported relative weakness in verbal memory, and Levin et al. (1988) noted a relative weakness in visual memory.

Behavioral outcome studies indicate that long-term residual deficiencies in adaptive behavior generally do not occur as a result of mild TBI (Fay et al., 1994; Fletcher, Ewing-Cobbs, Miner, Levin, & Eisenberg, 1990; Papero, Prigatano, Snyder, & Johnson, 1993). Research on short-term outcomes has produced conflicting results, with suggestions of difficulties in some areas of adaptive functioning for children with mild TBI (Fay et al., 1993). Higher levels of hyperactivity also may be found in children who have experienced mild TBI (Bijur et al., 1990). In addition, accumulating evidence suggests that premorbid behavior problems such as hyperactivity may predispose some children to mild head injury; these children may be at particular risk for continuing problems, requiring special monitoring (Goldstein & Levin, 1990).

Most studies provide information about group characteristics of children with head injuries; thus, the results may not be useful when predicting the degree of deficit experienced by any one individual (Fay et al., 1994). Overall, the range of neuropsychological strengths and weaknesses within the subgroups of children with mild TBI in many of the studies described previously suggests that, although they may be considered unaffected as a group, a number of these children have one or more deficits in neuropsychological, academic, or behavioral domains that would merit consideration in school settings. The variability in neuropsychological functioning seen among children included in many published studies indicates the need for individualized assessment of children after TBI, no matter what their level of severity (Ewing-Cobbs et al., 1987; Levin & Eisenberg, 1979).

Thus, although group data appear to provide compelling evidence for relatively minor consequences for learning, caution should be used in applying these findings indiscriminately to the understanding of children with mild TBI. First, although most children with mild TBI may escape serious consequences, some children will require professional attention. Second, because many of these studies did not measure subtle functions (e.g., reduced speed of information processing or multiple aspects of memory functioning), some of the more critical sequelae of mild TBI have yet to be evaluated thoroughly (Barth et al., 1983). Many of the common neuropsychological tests are simply not sensitive enough to detect subtle decrements in cognitive functioning, especially deficits in executive functions (Reitan & Wolfson, 1994). Moreover, the suggestion has been made that, in the presence of normal neuropsychological test findings, actual neurological damage may not be revealed until complex functioning is expected of the child and "the system is stressed" (Gronwall, 1989, p. 161). We may find that these subtle areas reveal the true needs of children with mild TBI. Finally, even if these subtle deficits are short-lived, they may be confusing and frustrating to the child and to the his or her teachers. Unsuspecting or uninformed teachers may fail to make adjustments, creating further confusion and disappointment, and jeopardizing a child's self-esteem. As a consequence, a negative cycle of failure and misunderstanding could extend far beyond the child's actual short-term cognitive deficiencies (Boll, 1983).

LEGISLATIVE VEHICLES FOR PROVISION OF SERVICES

Given that some children who have experienced mild TBI will need special accommodations in the educational setting, plans for provision of services must be in place (see Note). Guidelines under two federal laws can be invoked.

IDEA

Services provided to children with special needs by schools and other public agencies receiving federal assistance often are governed by policies established under the Individuals with Disabilities Education Act (IDEA) Amendments of 1991 (P.L. 102-119) or Section 504 of the Rehabilitation Act of 1973. Some important provisions pertinent to each are summarized below.

Under IDEA, traumatic brain injury is defined as

an acquired injury to the brain caused by an external physical force, resulting in total or partial functional disability or psychosocial impairment, or both, *that adversely affects a child's educational performance* [italics added]. The term applies to open or closed head injuries resulting in impairments in one or more areas, such as cognition; language; memory; attention; reasoning; abstract thinking; judgment; problem-solving; sensory, perceptual and motor abilities; psychosocial behavior; physical functions; information processing; and speech. The term does not apply to brain injuries that are congenital or degenerative, or brain injuries induced by birth trauma.

Although injuries caused by internal occurrences (e.g., infections, tumors, fever, exposure to toxic substances) are specifically excluded in the definition of TBI, children exhibiting brain injury due to these causes may be eligible for services under other IDEA criteria (e.g., learning disabilities, other health impairment). General provisions of IDEA are discussed in greater detail later.

Section 504

Several independent movements during the past 70 years merged to help shape current interpretations of Section 504, including federally authorized rehabilitation services, school law overturning discrimination and establishing equal educational opportunity, federal legislation to remove physical barriers and promote access by persons with disabilities, and Office of Civil Rights activities and initiatives (Farmer, 1992). Section 504 states,

> No otherwise qualified individual with handicaps in the United States, as defined in section 706(8) of this title shall, solely by reason of her or his handicap, be excluded from the participation in, be denied the benefits of, or be subject to discrimination under any program or activity receiving Federal financial assistance or under any program or activity conducted by any Executive agency or by the United States Postal Service. (29 U.S.C. §794(a))

The purposes of the Act and its procedures, in part, are to prohibit discrimination and to assure that students with disabilities from ages 3 through 21 receive suitable educational aids and opportunities to help ensure educational benefits commensurate with those provided to students without disabilities. School districts are encouraged to provide, through general education, services that address educational needs that substantially limit learning. The broad goal is to afford students with disabilities equal opportunities to obtain suitable educational outcomes, to gain educational benefit, or to have equal access to educational programs and activities.

Section 504 neither specifically mentions TBI nor recommends remedies for those persons with TBI; instead, it addresses handicaps in a broad and general fashion. A person is described as having a handicap when he or she meets one of the following three conditions:

1. Has a physical or mental impairment that substantially limits one or more of the following major life activities: learning, performing manual tasks, walking, sitting, hearing, speaking, breathing, or working;
2. Has a record of such impairment; or
3. Is regarded as having such an impairment.

A person is considered to have such an impairment given one or more of three conditions:

1. A service provider treats the physical or mental impairment as a limitation, although it may not substantially limit major life activities;
2. The attitudes of others result in the impairment substantially limiting major life activities; or
3. Despite the absence of impairment, the person is treated by a service provider as having an impairment.

Mild TBI could be classified as a physical or mental impairment under 504.

> The term "physical or mental impairment" is defined as (a) any physiological disorder or condition, cosmetic disfigurement, or anatomical loss affecting one or more of the following body systems: neurological; musculoskeletal; special sense organs, respiratory, including speech organs; cardiovascular; reproductive; digestive; genito-urinary; hemic and lymphatic; skin; and endocrine; or (b) any mental or psychological disorder, such as mental retardation, organic brain syndrome, emotional or mental illness, and specific learning disabilities. (34 C.F.R. §104.3j)

Contrasting IDEA and Section 504

Persons who qualify for services under IDEA also qualify for services under 504. However, given 504's broader parameters, all persons who qualify for services under it may not qualify under IDEA. Differences exist in their general purposes, what they protect, responsibilities for providing an Individualized Educational Program (IEP), educational settings in which services are provided, funding sources, accessibility, procedural safeguards, evaluation and placement procedures, grievance and due process procedures, and enforcement responsibilities (see Table 13.1).

Policies that apply to IDEA are defined more precisely than those that apply to 504. School districts are encouraged to follow IDEA rather than 504

Table 13.1
Comparisons Between IDEA and Section 504

Component	IDEA	Section 504
General purpose	Is a federal funding statute whose purpose is to provide financial aid to states in their efforts to ensure adequate and appropriate services for children with disabilities.	Is a broad civil law that protects the rights of individuals with handicaps in programs and activities that receive federal financial assistance from the U.S. Department of Education.
Who is protected	Identifies all school-age children who fall within one or more specific categories or qualifying conditions.	Identifies all school-age children as handicapped who meet the definition of qualified handicapped person, that is, has or has had a physical impairment that substantially limits a major life activity, or is regarded as handicapped by others. Major life activities include walking, seeing, hearing, speaking, breathing, learning, working, caring for oneself, and performing manual tasks. The handicapping condition need only substantially limit one major life activity in order for the student to be eligible.
Responsibility to provide a free and appropriate public education (FAPE)	Both laws require the provision of a free, appropriate public education, including individually designed instruction, to eligible students covered under them. The IEP of IDEA will suffice for Section 504 written plan.	
	Requires a written IEP document with specific content and a required number of specific participants at the IEP meeting.	Does not require a written IEP document but does require a plan. School districts should document that a committee of persons knowledgeable about TBI and the student convened and agreed upon various services.
	"Appropriate education" means a program designed to provide "educational benefit." Related services are	"Appropriate" means an education comparable to the education provided to nondisabled students, requiring

(table continues)

(Table 13.1 continued)

Component	IDEA	Section 504
	provided if required for the student to benefit from specially designed instruction.	that reasonable accommodations to be made. Related services, independent of any special education services as defined under IDEA, may be the reasonable accommodation.
Special education vs. general education	A student is only eligible to receive IDEA services if the multidisciplinary team determines that the student is disabled under specific qualifying conditions and requires specially designed instruction to benefit from education.	A student is eligible so long as he or she meets the definition of qualified handicapped person; that is, has or has had a physical impairment that substantially limits a major life activity, or is regarded as handicapped by others. It is not required that the handicap adversely affect educational performance, or that the student need special education in order to be protected.
Funding	Provides additional funding for eligible students.	Does not provide additional funds. IDEA funds may not be used to serve children found eligible only under Section 504.
Accessibility	Requires that modifications must be made if necessary to provide access to a free, appropriate education.	Has regulations regarding building and program accessibility, requiring that reasonable accommodations be made.
Procedural safeguards	Both require notice to the parent or guardian with respect to identification, evaluation, and/or placement. IDEA procedures will suffice for Section 504 implementation.	
	Requires written notice.	Does not require written notice, but a district would be wise to do so.

(table continues)

(Table 13.1 continued)

Component	IDEA	Section 504
	Delineates required components of written notice.	Written notice not required but indicated by good professional practice.
	Requires written notice prior to any change in placement.	Requires notice only before a "significant change" in placement.
Evaluations	A full, comprehensive evaluation that assesses all areas related to the suspected disability is required. The child is evaluated by a multidisciplinary team or group.	Evaluation draws on information from a variety of sources in the area of concern; decisions made by a group knowledgeable about the student, evaluation data, and placement options.
	Requires informed consent before an initial evaluation is conducted.	Does not require consent, only notice. However, good professional practice indicates informed consent.
	Requires reevaluation to be conducted at least every 3 years.	Requires periodic reevaluations. IDEA schedule for reevaluation will suffice.
	A reevaluation is not required before a significant change in placement. However, a review of current evaluation data, including progress monitoring, is strongly recommended.	Reevaluation is required before a significant change in placement.
	Provides for independent educational evaluation at district expense if parent disagrees with evaluation obtained by school and hearing officer concurs.	No provision for independent evaluations at district expense. District should consider any such evaluations presented.
Placement procedure	When interpreting evaluation data and making placement decisions, both laws require districts to: (a) Draw upon information from a variety of sources;	

(table continues)

(Table 13.1 continued)

Component	IDEA	Section 504
	(b) Assure that all information is documented and considered; (c) Ensure that the eligibility decision is made by a group of persons that includes those who are knowledgeable about the child, the meaning of the evaluation data, and placement options; and (d) Ensure that the student is educated with his or her nondisabled peers to the maximum extent appropriate (least restrictive environment).	
	An IEP review meeting is required before any change in placement.	A meeting is not required for any change in placement.
Grievance procedure	Does not require a grievance procedure nor a compliance officer.	Requires district with more than 15 employees to (a) designate an employee to be responsible for assuring district compliance with Section 504, and (b) provide a grievance procedure for parents, students, and employees.
Due process	Both statutes require districts to provide impartial hearings for parents or guardians who disagree with the identification, evaluation, or placement of a student.	
	Delineates specific requirements.	Requires that the parent have an opportunity to participate and be represented by counsel. Other details are left to the discretion of the local school district. Policy statements should clarify specific details.

procedures with respect to the provision of services when students are expected to qualify for services under both provisions. Most provisions discussed in this chapter are directly applicable to IDEA because they are defined more clearly. However, many also are assumed to be applicable under 504.

What Schools Are Required To Do

Public schools generally have three important goals: to promote students' academic or educational development, to promote appropriate social behaviors leading to good citizenship, and to help ensure that school attendance is regular and continuous (Webb & Sherman, 1989). Because the goal to promote educational development is most central to a school's unique mission, legislative, administrative, and judicial efforts typically concentrate on ensuring that schools create programs promoting educational development. Although the effects of TBI are wide-ranging and can include adverse physical, social, and emotional qualities, a school's primary efforts are on countering the adverse effects of TBI on educational performance.

Schools are responsible for providing an appropriate public education at no cost to the parents. A specially designed instructional program, one requiring special education and related services, is tailored to the student's individual qualities and educational needs and is provided in an environment that is least restrictive socially. Related services may be provided in one or more of the following 14 areas:

- audiology
- counseling
- early identification
- medical
- occupational therapy
- parent counseling and training
- physical therapy
- psychological services
- recreation
- rehabilitation counseling
- school health services
- social work services
- speech pathology
- transportation

Schools are required to attempt to ameliorate the adverse effects of TBI on educational performance as well as on behaviors and other qualities that have an impact on educational performance through the provision of general and special education services. They are not responsible for improving the injured brain.

TBI is one of 13 disorders recognized under IDEA. Regulations governing the provision of special education services, as stated in the final regulations from the Department of Education (57 Fed. Reg. 189, September 29, 1992), generally are generic to all disorders and are not specific to TBI.

IDEA underscores the importance of the following provisions: evaluation, placement, and reevaluation procedures, personnel development and participation, parent involvement, procedural safeguards and due process procedures for parents and school districts, program options for students, transition services, and assistive technology. With the exception of assistive technology, school districts have become accustomed to providing these services to students with most handicapping conditions, given almost 20 years of work under IDEA.

IMPEDIMENTS TO SERVICE

There are five major impediments to the provision of appropriate services to children with TBI:

1. Schools have little experience with this disability;
2. Few educational personnel are prepared to work with this handicapping condition;
3. Budgetary constraints limit new employment and the provision of ideal services;
4. Existing professionals typically are reluctant to step forward to provide leadership; and
5. Some individuals have the perception that schools, particularly general education, are not responsible for addressing disorders that are primarily medical in nature.

TBI was added as a handicapping condition in 1991; thus, school personnel have less experience providing services to children identified as having TBI-related disabilities. Moreover, programs designed for students with TBI can be offered in either general or special education settings, and few teachers are trained to work with these children. For example, several years ago, only 8% of special educators reported any exposure to TBI during their graduate preparation (Savage, 1985). Fewer general education teachers can be expected to have received exposure. The need for inservice training for both general and special education personnel is critical.

POSSIBLE SOLUTIONS TO PERSONNEL AND PROGRAMMATIC LIMITATIONS

A Six-Step Process

Given these and other impediments to the provision of services to children with TBI, school districts are likely to look to existing staff for leadership. In this section a six-step process that will enable districts to become better prepared to serve the needs of children with TBI.

1. *Survey existing special education and related service provider staff to determine their expertise and interests in this area.* Staff who have been trained as school psychologists, occupational and physical therapists, rehabilitation counselors, and speech–language pathologists are most likely to have some expertise in this area. (Their respective contributions will be discussed in a later section.) Smaller districts and those not employing these specialists may need to form cooperative relationships with nearby districts before conducting this survey.

2. *Form a TBI committee, consisting of those with expertise and interest in TBI who are responsible for providing district-wide leadership.* Identify existing and needed areas of expertise in the provision of direct and indirect services. One committee member should be appointed to coordinate TBI services for the district.

3. *Develop district policies and procedures relevant to TBI-related services.* Such services would include screening and/or prereferral evaluations; referrals; evaluations for determining eligibility: intervention planning, implementation, and evaluation; reevaluations; and consultation. Involve representatives from regional and state education agencies and the district's legal staff in shaping these policies and procedures.

4. *Develop a district-wide inservice program for administrators, teachers, parents, support staff, and others in the community (e.g., child and family agencies, juvenile justice, professional practitioners).* The purpose of such a program would be to acquaint them with proposed district policy and procedures, to elicit their suggestions, and to broaden ownership for meeting the needs of children with TBI. District policies applicable to TBI are likely to require board approval. Once approved, additional inservice programs are likely to be needed to assist in staff development.

5. *Create an advisory board consisting of members of the district's TBI committee together with other professionals within the community or region.* The purposes of this advisory board are to share information and other resources relevant to TBI and to broaden ownership for meeting the needs of children with TBI.

6. *Employ one or more professionals with solid expertise in TBI as part-time consultants to the district.* This work would be managed by the coordinator of TBI services and would be made available to other committee members.

Utilizing Existing Resources

The traditional preparation for many professionals who work in schools can provide a surprisingly robust set of resources to address the needs of children with mild TBI. Several of these professionals are described in this section.

In children with more mild levels of injury, behavioral changes may be the only noticeable sign of injury (Telzrow, 1987). Because of their professional preparation, *school psychologists* typically focus upon observable behaviors that might indicate the presence of changes portending learning problems. One of the most important of these behaviors—particularly when the injury is mild and no overt ill effects can be readily noticed—is that both the children and their teachers may be quite confused about things that are just "not right." Far-reaching difficulties could develop if (a) the teacher is not helped to understand potential effects of the injury, (b) the children are not provided with some understanding of the changes they perceive, and (c) the children are not assisted in making adjustments to the changes. The emotional climate surrounding the injured person has a decided impact upon later functioning, perhaps more than the nature of the actual physical injury to the brain. The school psychologist can assist the teacher in making classroom modifications to enhance learning and the development of healthy, adaptive behaviors.

The *speech–language pathologist* (SLP) can be a valuable participant in efforts to help the child with mild TBI function well upon school reentry. SLPs possess a special understanding of language processes, with the ability to identify subtle dysfunction that has the potential to create serious misunderstandings and many more complex communication problems (DePompei & Blosser, 1987; Russell, 1993). SLPs working in schools also understand classrooms and their unique communication requirements.

The *occupational therapist* (OT) also is in a position to assist the child with mild TBI who has cognitive and psychomotor difficulties. In reference to diagnosis, the orientation and preparation of an OT are particularly suited to the needs of a child with mild TBI because of an emphasis upon a functional approach to assessment (Stahl, 1995). Emphasis is placed on evaluating what children must be able to do and how they can acquire necessary skills. For some children with mild TBI, this approach may be more profitable than the use of a lengthy tabletop test battery.

Additionally, because of the relative shortage of OTs in schools, consultation services provided to teachers are viewed as an effective utilization of limited resources. The OT can help teachers identify mild cognitive and perceptual–motor deficits in the child's classroom performance. The OT also can help the teacher acquire and learn to use or to devise appropriate classroom accommodations, including the development of a more structured environment, which can be a critical element in assisting the child's performance (Hammond, 1995).

The *school counselor* also can assist with the emotional needs of the child with mild TBI. Cognitive changes, even temporary ones, can cause deficiencies in academic and behavioral arenas that had previously been areas of mastery. Children who might have been accustomed to academic success or acknowledged good conduct suddenly may be confused by their own limitations and can find themselves the focus of their teachers' (and parents') frustration. The counselor can be invaluable in providing brief counseling for these children by providing an educational component to help them understand what has happened. Furthermore, the preparation of school counselors enables them to provide group interventions with a child's classmates (Savage & Carter, 1984). Because peer attitudes and influences can greatly affect the child's behaviors and self-image, providing his or her classmates with an orientation to the nature of head injury and suggestions for appropriate responses can pave the way for a smoother transition through the early stages of recovery. Finally, the school counselor often is situated to serve as a liaison between the child's teachers and the parents.

School nurses traditionally have had the closest links to the medical profession. Through their professional preparation, they are likely to be equipped to monitor medical symptoms commonly associated with mild TBI, to help differentiate between those symptoms that have a psychosomatic origin and those that have a physical origin, to counsel with the child and family about the importance of dietary issues and medication use, and to monitor medication use in schools (Creswell, Newman, & Anderson, 1985; Rhodes, Hofen, Karren, & Rollins, 1981).

The *special education teacher or coordinator,* even if he or she has limited knowledge of the cognitive difficulties produced by TBI, is well versed in federal and state regulations and procedures for evaluating a student's needs and obtaining appropriate services. This professional serves a key role and may be a good choice to act as the case manager for the child's total educational plan. The special educator works closely within the guidelines established by the child's IEP, monitors instruction, serves as a resource to the classroom teacher, and may provide some special instructional services directly to the student.

For children with mild TBI who do not need special services or can have their instructional needs met completely in the general education classroom, the general education teacher may be the primary, even the sole, service provider. With preparation and support from collaborators in their schools, general education teachers are likely to be able to modify the standard curriculum and instructional methods so as to offer these children an equal opportunity to benefit from the school environment. The important need to structure and normalize the child's activities, with adjustments as appropriate, can be accomplished best by the classroom teacher. However, as mentioned earlier, few classroom teachers are prepared to work with these children and are likely to require inservice training and continued consultation.

Given the existing resources often found in schools, as just described, collaborative efforts can be expected to provide a solid skills base for addressing the needs of these children. This collaboration should result in the attainment of two primary objectives for the well-being of the student with mild TBI: to promote the professional preparation for all involved in the child's education and to enhance the quality of direct and indirect services provided to the child.

GOALS FOR COLLABORATION

Goal 1: Professional Preparation

The child's readjustment to the demands of the educational setting, together with its associated learning and social challenges, requires school personnel to understand the nature of TBI; the specific mechanisms of the child's injury; and the cognitive, behavioral, and emotional sequelae that commonly occur (DePompei & Blosser, 1993). The question of whether the child "can't" or "won't" follow rules, pay attention, or complete work is particularly thorny. Knowledge about the potential for disruption in functions—including attention span, memory, and organized thinking—can help school personnel understand that "stubbornness" actually may be the child's inflexible, confused thinking and that "laziness" may be due to mental fatigue. This phase of collaboration should focus on helping professionals recognize the possible brain-related etiology of troublesome behaviors and on offering recommendations for addressing behavioral and learning differences.

Some professionals (e.g., the speech–language pathologist) may have the knowledge necessary to offer services to children with TBI and to serve as consultants. However, the professional preparation of many speech–language pathologists and other specialists who work in schools may not have included knowledge about the interface between the symptoms they treat and diminished cognitive functions such as memory (Russell, 1993).

A *pediatric neuropsychologist* may have the most favorable professional preparation for serving the needs of school district staff because of an emphasis on brain–behavior relationships and evaluation techniques to elucidate these relationships. Unfortunately, few school districts have the financial resources to employ a full-time neuropsychologist. One option would be to contract with a consulting neuropsychologist who could work with the district's school psychologist. This consultant could provide training to school personnel about fundamental brain–behavior relationships, the disruption in these relationships brought about by TBI, the cognitive and behavioral changes that might result, and how to work effectively with a child who sustains a brain injury. School districts should ensure their consultant is formally prepared in pediatric neuropsychology and should carefully review the formal preparation of any candidate for the consultant position. The school psychologist may be best able to understand how to identify and select such an individual.

Once a consultant in pediatric neuropsychology has been hired, inservice training should be initiated in a cost-effective manner that suits the structure of the school district. Three modified pyramid approaches are suggested. The first approach might be based upon *disciplines,* with the consulting neuropsychologist working with school psychologists, who in turn work with other school-based specialists, who in turn educate classroom teachers. An alternate approach might be based upon *interdepartment hierarchies,* in which the consulting neuropsychologist educates department heads, who educate their own personnel. Within a *site-based management structure,* the consulting neuropsychologist would educate principals, who in turn educate other personnel in their own schools. The commonality in these approaches is found in the use of a branching format in which an enlarging circle of professionals is targeted.

The primary liaison of neuropsychologist with school psychologist has been suggested for several reasons. Having the same basic education and similar professional preparation, these professionals share common philosophies, approaches, and vocabularies that can facilitate an immediate interface (Oakland & Stavinoha, 1992). Translations from neuropsychological constructs to educational realities will be made more easily. Furthermore, school psychologists and neuropsychologists may function in the same professional community, placing the school psychologist in the best position to investigate neuropsychologists working nearby who claim to be knowledgeable about brain injury in school-age children and to know about the educational environment.

Goal 2: Assessment and Intervention Needs for Identified Children

A specific sequence of events should be incorporated as school policy. First, an appointed school liaison is needed to communicate with parents and the physician (or hospital, if there was a hospital visit) after injury occurs. The school nurse or assistant principal may serve this function well. Relevant information can be transmitted to a central coordinator or case manager, who determines if there is an educational need. This may be accomplished by gathering material from outside sources, family, and teachers; observing the child or arranging for observation; and reviewing the characteristics and demands of the particular school environment to which the child will return. The importance of this case manager has been addressed elsewhere in this book. An interdisciplinary team may need to meet to decide if additional observation or assessment is needed.

Further assessment is the responsibility of various interdisciplinary team members or staff members in their departments. If warranted, the school psychologist can arrange for evaluation by the consulting neuropsychologist. Two options are viable, depending upon the expertise of the school psychologist: The neuropsychologist either personally provides the assessment services or provides supervision to the school psychologist who conducts the assessment. The interdisciplinary team makes various decisions, including the need for special education services; instructional, classroom, and behavioral modifications; and inservice training for local school personnel. As stated previously, intervention may be set up through special or general education.

Auxiliary services may be engaged in the manner prescribed by the departmental structure of the school district. The speech–language pathologist may address needs in the cognitive–communication domain. The school psychologist may assist with plans for cognitive–behavioral needs, perhaps in conjunction with the consulting neuropsychologist. The counselor may address emotional needs. The occupational therapist may be called upon to address cognitive–perceptual and motoric needs. The nurse may be responsible for medications. The teachers most familiar with the injured child are likely to be the most informed about what instructional approaches have and have not worked and can be the frontline service providers.

Perfect approaches may not be found at first. Moreover, the child's needs will change as the effects of the injury resolve. School personnel therefore must monitor the need for ongoing consultation from the interdisciplinary team members. In addition, the potential for later-developing school performance problems as the academic demands increase should not be overlooked. Soon after injury a child may be able to perform age- or grade-appropriate work, but the injury may have produced cognitive dysfunction that will interfere with more complex developmental tasks (DePompei & Blosser, 1993). The case manager or school liaison should be responsible for keeping files active so as to monitor children whose difficulties are not manifested immediately. Changes and additions to school personnel that occur over time will require ongoing attention. The case manager will need to call upon appropriate professionals to provide ongoing inservice training as the child's teachers change, with regard to general education about TBI as well as accommodations for specific children in the caseload.

CONCLUSIONS

Given the greater awareness of the educational needs of children who have sustained TBI, schools have been charged with providing appropriate educational services to them. Children with mild TBI need to be identified and provided with resources that help ensure their continued educational development. The school districts would be wise to devise and implement plans that address the needs of these students, taking advantage of existing school personnel with special areas of expertise and employing a consulting pediatric neuropsychologist to work within a collaborative, interdisciplinary approach.

AUTHORS' NOTE

Portions of the section devoted to Section 504 are based on some material in Oakland (1994).

NOTE

Readers should be alert to decisions at the federal level (e.g., in reference to IDEA, Social Security Services, and the Rehabilitation Act) that may lead to possible restrictions on and reductions in medical and psychological services for children and youth with TBI under these provisions.

PART IV

Conclusions

14. Epilogue: An Ecological Systems Approach to Childhood Traumatic Brain Injury

JANET E. FARMER

The Decade of the Brain has produced significant advances in the study and treatment of childhood traumatic brain injury (TBI). This epilogue will reflect on the state of the field as described in previous chapters and propose some specific directions for the transition into the twenty-first century. As a framework for this review, an ecological systems model will be used to summarize factors that influence child outcomes following TBI (Farmer & Peterson, 1995b; Kazak, Segal-Andrews, & Johnson, 1995; Mullins, Gillman, & Harbeck, 1992; Taylor & Fletcher, 1995; Wallendar & Thompson, 1995). The basic premise of this model is that a child's health-related problems exist in a social and environmental context. The specific behavioral outcome for any given child with TBI is determined by reciprocal transactions between him or her and the immediate environment, both of which change over time and are subject to influences from larger organizational systems. Figure 14.1 presents a schematic of multiple systems, or levels of influence, that affect child outcomes following TBI. Some influences create increased risk of poor outcomes; others offer protection and maximize optimal outcomes. Progress to date and challenges for the future will be discussed in relation to this ecological systems model.

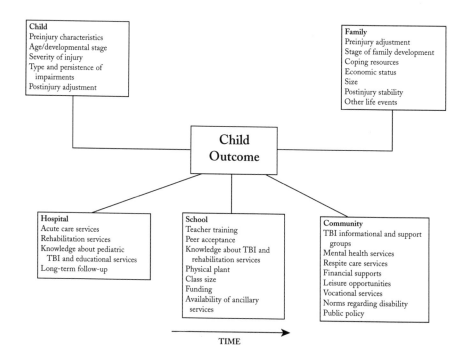

Figure 14.1. Factors that influence outcomes following childhood TBI. (*Note.* From "Pediatric Traumatic Brain Injury: Promoting Successful School Reentry," by J. E. Farmer and L. Peterson, 1995, *School Psychology Review, 24,* p. 232. Copyright © 1995 by the National Association of School Psychologists. Reprinted by permission of the publisher.)

CHILD FACTORS

Age at Onset

A fundamental theme of this book is that, following a TBI, children differ from adults in important ways, including the causes of injury, the impact of injury on subsequent development, and primary systems of care that are available during recovery (i.e., educational settings, family of origin). The idea that young survivors of TBI are spared from cognitive problems has been consistently refuted (Lord-Maes & Obrzut, chapter 6; Mateer, Kerns, & Eso, chapter 9; Wilkening, chapter 5). As noted by Lord-Maes and Obrzut, recent studies have confirmed that younger age at TBI onset is associated with poorer language development; inattention and hyperactivity; slower recovery of motor, visual–spatial, and somatosensory skills; and decreased performance on measures thought to tap frontal lobe functioning (e.g., Tower of London task, word fluency).

However, there is still much to be understood about the interaction between brain injury and the process of development. Preliminary evidence suggests that disruption of primary skills during early childhood results in changes in the order, rate, and/or level of learning, which then produce impairments in later developing, higher order skills. In addition, some research indicates that there can be late effects of TBI, whereby a fully recovered child appears to show marked declines in functioning over time. We do not have an adequate grasp of these long-term effects of TBI on child development or the processes that underlie such changes. Prospective, longitudinal research is needed to expand our knowledge base.

Injury Characteristics

Although the course of recovery may differ based on age at onset, severity of injury is a well-established prognostic indicator for both children and adults. In general, children with mild injuries have few residual problems, and those with more severe injuries have a greater likelihood of persistent functional deficits (in this book see Silver & Oakland, chapter 13; Wilkening, chapter 5). Wilkening pointed out that duration of impaired mental status is now considered an important indicator of injury severity, in addition to the initial depth of coma as measured by the Glasgow Coma Scale (GCS). Although there is a strong correlation between injury severity and child outcomes, studies have often found considerable variability within severity groupings. That is, some children with severe injuries seem to escape significant disability, whereas others with mild injuries are functionally impaired.

Ongoing technological advances may make it easier to resolve these apparent discrepancies and increase our understanding of brain–behavior relationships. For example, Bigler (chapter 2 of this book) described the remarkable improvements in brain imaging that have been made during the 1990s. It is now possible to visualize structural damage in three dimensions, quantify the extent and location of these changes, and relate them to neuropsychological findings. Neuroimaging studies have shown that degenerative changes take place over the first 3 months post-TBI, often appearing as corpus callosum atrophy and ventricular enlargement due to white matter tissue loss. They also have confirmed the greater likelihood of frontal and temporal lesions commonly associated with such neurobehavioral deficits as memory impairment and decreased executive functioning.

Bigler also highlighted progress in the study of the pathophysiology of TBI and changes at the cellular level. In addition to white matter shear/strain effects, there is now evidence of microstructural changes, such as a breakdown of the blood–brain barrier, cellular deformation, and toxic metabolic activity, following injury. Structural and cellular damage may be further exacerbated by secondary injury from edema, hemorrhages, infection, and hypoxic/anoxic events due to brain stem or systemic injuries. Advances in the study of mechanisms of brain injury hold great promise for increasing our prognostic accuracy about potential child outcomes and for developing medical management strategies.

Noninjury-Related Characteristics

Children who sustain TBI are more likely to have preexisting academic problems and may also have had prior behavioral concerns (in this book see Farmer et al., chapter 3; Kehle, Clark, & Jenson, chapter 8; Kreutzer, Witol, & Marwitz, chapter 4; Wilkening, chapter 5). For the most part, the interaction between such preexisting problems and outcomes following TBI have not been explored. An exception to this is the research by Kreutzer et al. on the alcohol and drug use patterns of adolescents and young adults with TBI. They found that young people who were moderate to heavy alcohol users prior to TBI showed an initial drop in usage, followed by a tendency to return to preinjury alcohol use levels over time. Such results are cause for concern because alcohol use in combination with injury sequelae certainly decreases the likelihood of academic and vocational success. There is a clear need for additional research to clarify the role of preexisting risk factors in determining long-term TBI outcomes and to identify specialized treatments for these individuals.

FAMILY FACTORS

Child-related characteristics are important determinants of outcome following TBI. However, family members provide the immediate social context for children's recovery from TBI; thus, families both are affected by TBI-related changes and, in turn, affect child outcomes (Farmer & Stucky-Ropp, 1996; Rivara et al., 1993; in this book see Conoley & Sheridan, chapter 10; Wade, Taylor, Drotar, Stancin, & Yeates, chapter 7).

These transactions have only recently begun to be studied. Wade et al. described the initial phase of a prospective study investigating the effects of TBI on 96 families. They used a newly developed measure, the Family Burden of Injury Interview (FBII), as well as other measures for assessing injury impact, coping, and preinjury functioning. Families of children with severe TBI reported higher overall levels of stress and concern for their child than those of children with moderate TBI or orthopedic injuries. On average, the ratings of stress among families of children with severe injuries were only in the low to moderate range, but the variability in responses was high. Up to 25% of parents of children with severe TBI described their level of concern for their child as quite stressful or extremely stressful, a considerably higher percentage than for families of children with moderate TBI (8%) or with orthopedic problems (less than 2%).

The variable response among families of children with severe injuries may reflect the range of severity that is often captured within the "severe" category in studies of TBI (Massagli et al., 1996). Although it is consistent with conventional methodology, defining severe injury as having an initial GCS of 8 or less includes those who regain consciousness rather quickly as well as those who remain in a persistent vegetative state. Families of children with the most severe injuries (e.g., a GCS of 3 to 5) may appropriately show the greatest concern. The needs of these children and their families are virtually unknown. As the study of TBI progresses, more refined subgroups of individuals with severe injuries must be considered.

Though severity of injury is one determinant of family response, Wade et al. (chapter 7) demonstrated that family reactions to TBI are mediated by other factors as well. In their study, preexisting family problems, including chronic life stressors and maladaptive coping styles, contributed in unique ways to the prediction of injury burden, overall family ratings of the negative impact of injury, and psychological distress. Furthermore, their data suggested that family expectations may mediate distress in this early phase of recovery, as only 27% of families in the group with severe TBI indicated concern about whether their child would fully recover. This optimistic outlook is consistent with a previous study in which 80% of the families surveyed on admission to rehabilitation believed that full recovery from severe TBI was possible (Springer, Farmer, & Bouman, in press). Wade et al. found that few families expressed a need for emotional support at this phase of recovery; instead, they requested concrete assistance with financial concerns, housekeeping, and childcare.

The prospective study by Wade et al. will continue to track changes in caregiver burden and distress, social–environmental and injury-related predictors of these problems, family-identified intervention needs, and the impact of parental morbidity on child outcomes. Their comprehensive, longitudinal approach to measuring family adaption to TBI is an excellent model for studying child and family experiences and identifying family-perceived needs. Additional studies are needed to investigate the impact of TBI on siblings and extended family members and to evaluate the roles of different family members in caregiving (e.g., mothers vs. fathers). Quittner and Espelage (1996) found that parents of children with cystic fibrosis take on differing tasks in care provision and that this results in different types of role strain. Such findings in parents of children with TBI would have clear implications for treatment.

IMPACT OF LARGER ORGANIZATIONAL SYSTEMS

Children with TBI and their families are involved in transactions with larger organizational systems, including hospitals, schools, community providers, and public policy agents. Little is known about how particular characteristics of these children and their families affect service provision. In contrast, many of the chapters in this book discussed appropriate methods for professional caregivers to use to influence child outcomes, in the domains of both assessment and treatment.

Advances in Assessment

Individualized, broad-spectrum, interdisciplinary assessment has become the rule rather than the exception for understanding the nature and extent of cognitive–communicative changes associated with childhood TBI (in this book see Clark, chapter 11; D'Amato & Rothlisberg, chapter 12; Farmer et al., chapter 3; Lord-Maes & Obrzut, chapter 6). Several authors focused on the importance of defining a preinjury baseline and using new as well as more traditional standardized instruments to investigate performance in cognitive domains that are commonly affected by TBI. Such test results are essential for documenting change in functioning and indicating potential risk for academic and vocational failure (e.g., Kinsella et al., 1995).

We still lack adequate assessment instruments, particularly in the area of higher order skills such as executive functioning (e.g., initiating, planning, organizing, self-monitoring). These skills are often disrupted following TBI, due to the vulnerability of the frontal lobes (Levin et al., 1993), and are important to behavioral control, problem solving, and work production (in this book see Kehle, Clark, & Jenson, chapter 8). Recent studies have begun to supplement our knowledge about executive functioning in both normally developing and injured children (Dennis, Barnes, Donnelly, Wilkinson, & Humphreys, 1996; Levin et al., 1996), but much work remains to be done to gain a full appreciation of how these deficits affect child outcomes and how they can be most effectively assessed and treated.

Another area for further study is how to effectively use assessment information from standardized tests to create a treatment plan. There is little research available about the ecological validity of neuropsychological tests in children. That is, we have a limited database indicating how cognitive–communicative weaknesses relate to functional skills deficits in the classroom, with friends, and in other real-world settings. Clinical experience is our primary guide in this endeavor (e.g., if speed-of-processing deficits are identified, then rate of work production may be slow and length of assignments should be shortened). At present, formal cognitive assessments can be used to develop hypotheses about potential functional problems, but treatment providers must use informal assessments to evaluate the everyday impact of injury-related impairments. There are many advantages to using informal assessments as a supplement to standardized testing following TBI (in this book see Farmer et al., chapter 3), but we must continue to develop guidelines on how to conduct such assessments in a reliable and valid way (e.g., Crowley & Miles, 1991, described in in this book in Mateer et al., chapter 9).

Advances in Treatment

The addition of TBI as a special education category in the Individuals with Disabilities Education Act (IDEA; P.L. 101-476, 1990) has had far-reaching effects on children with TBI and their families (in this book see Clark, chapter 11; Silver & Oakland, chapter 13). Schools have now officially become the primary mandated provider of services to children with educationally significant changes in functioning following TBI. This shift in public policy led to a notable increase in information about the treatment of childhood TBI for educators and families (e.g., Begali, 1992; Blosser & DePompei, 1994; Goldberg, 1996; Savage & Wolcott, 1994, 1995). There has been an increased call for interdisciplinary collaboration among rehabilitation specialists, educators, and family members, and protocols for school reentry following injury have been proposed (in this book see Farmer et al., chapter 3; see also Ylvisaker et al., 1995). In chapter 13, Silver and Oakland carefully delineated steps for improving a school district's preparedness for serving children with TBI. This process of identifying service delivery models is an important part of increasing treatment options.

Although the structure for service provision shows potential for rapid improvement, the task of intervening with children remains in its early phases of development in both rehabilitation and educational settings. In the cognitive domain, Mateer et al. (chapter 9) presented an excellent example of how clinical research can extend our ability to treat deficits in attention and memory. Their chapter reviewed procedures used with adults during postacute TBI rehabilitation, studies of children with other disabilities (e.g., attention-deficit/hyperactivity disorder), and several recent studies of children with TBI. They outlined treatment strategies in three general categories: modification of the environment, direct remediation, and compensatory strategies. Research in this area must continue to define effective means of treating cognitive problems in a way that improves functioning in real-world settings. It also must identify ways to integrate cognitive remediation into traditional academic settings, where there tends to be a focus on skills development and content knowledge rather than on strategies for processing information (D'Amato & Rothlisberg, chapter 12; Ylvisaker, Szekeres, Hartwick, & Tworek, 1994).

Behavioral treatment following TBI may be the greatest long-term challenge to teachers and families. Kehle et al. (chapter 8) underscored the applicability of classic behavioral principles, as long as cognitive processing deficits are taken into account and behavioral expectations are appropriate. It can be easy to proceed too quickly to a behavioral change strategy without fully understanding the function of the behavior (Deaton, 1994). For example, refusal to do schoolwork may actually represent fatigue, an awareness of overly high expectations for work production, or self-consciousness over mistakes in front of peers. Instead of a reprimand for noncompliance, this calls for a supportive intervention in response to the child's true need (a rest break, a decrease in task expectations with subsequent shaping of successive approximations to the target behavior, or interventions designed to improve status with peers). Interdisciplinary team interactions may be particularly important when designing and implementing behavioral treatment plans, given the complex interplay between cognitivecommunicative deficits and social, emotional, and behavioral outcomes. Furthermore, pharmacological interventions still hold promise as agents for promoting behavioral regulation, particularly in combination with other forms of behavioral and cognitive remediation.

Studies of treatment efficacy are a high priority in the field of pediatric TBI. For greatest success, we must be prepared to work across disciplines and agencies, create new treatments, draw on strategies developed for children with other disabilities, and empower parents to become a central part of the treatment team. Treatment plans must be devised not only for children who return to school, but also for those who are unable to reenter traditional academic settings. Often, multiple interventions will be needed, some directed toward the child and others toward creating positive changes in the larger systems that influence child outcomes.

To illustrate the multiple factors that can influence outcome and review possible interventions, a case example will be presented. The details of the case will be discussed in terms of child, family, and larger systems factors that affect outcome over time.

Case Example

Child Factors

F.T. is a 15-year-old right-handed White boy with a history of a TBI 5 years ago. He was referred for a neuropsychological assessment by his school district because educators were unsure of how to manage F.T.'s academic and behavioral problems. F.T. had recently entered their school district as a ninth grader, and he was failing all of his classes except for a D- in science and a B+ in physical education. He had particular problems with written expression, following oral and written directions, and identifying the main idea in materials presented to him. Teachers also were concerned about his short attention span, staring spells, and poor work completion. F.T. had received special educational services under a diagnosis of learning disabilities in his previous school district. This consisted of 1 hour per day of resource room assistance to help him organize his assignments and complete his homework. Since beginning in the new school, F.T.'s attendance has been adequate, and teachers perceived him as a friendly, outgoing young man. However, they were considering a secondary educational diagnosis of behavior disorder because of the disruption caused by his impulsive and off-task behaviors.

F.T. sustained a severe TBI in an amusement park accident at the age of 10 years. He experienced full cardiopulmonary arrest at the scene of the accident and remained in a coma for 3 days. His initial Glasgow Coma Scale score was 6. A computerized tomography (CT) of the brain showed a large left temporoparietal contusion, but he had no other significant injuries. Upon transfer to acute rehabilitation 15 days postinjury, F.T. displayed a dense right-side hemiparesis and could not talk, but he could follow simple one-step commands. During rehabilitation, he showed a rapid recovery of physical mobility, self-care skills, and basic language functioning. His attention span was extremely short, his short-term memory was poor, and he was impulsive and noncompliant in therapies.

Prior to injury, F.T. was a B–C student in school. He had never been retained or received special services; however, he had participated in a psychoeducational evaluation in the second grade because he was not getting his work done in class. Results indicated above-average intellectual functioning (see Table 14.1) and average to above-average academic achievement. His mother revealed that F.T. had been physically and sexually abused for several months prior to injury, and she thought this might have contributed to his school problems.

A review of F.T.'s school and medical records indicated that he had participated in several cognitive assessments (see Table 14.1). At 2 months postinjury,

Table 14.1

Pre- and Postinjury Estimates of Intellectual Functioning in Case F.T.

	K-ABC		
	Sequential	Simultaneous	Composite
Preinjury	108	114	113
2 months postinjury	87	101	95

	WISC-III		
	Verbal	Performance	Full scale
4 years post injury	73	80	75
5 years postinjury	71	79	73

Note. K-ABC = Kaufman Assessment Battery for Children (Kaufman & Kaufman, 1983); WISC-III = Wechsler Intelligence Scale for Children (3rd. ed.; Wechsler, 1991).

his overall intellectual functioning had recovered to the average range, though he displayed marked problems with sequential processing. In contrast, 4 years after his injury, F.T. demonstrated borderline intellectual functioning.

At the time of the current assessment (5 years postinjury), F.T. underwent a single photon emission computerized tomography (SPECT) scan, which showed left temporal hypoperfusion. As shown in Table 14.1, he, again, displayed borderline intellectual abilities. Neuropsychological testing revealed significant psychological processing deficits, including moderate to severe impairments in the areas of verbal memory and learning, oral word fluency, attention, speed of processing, abstract reasoning, and problem solving. His cognitive strengths were his average to low-average visual memory and learning and his basic language and academic skills. His sensorimotor skills were variable and generally in the average range, but his right hand was consistently slower and weaker than his left. These problems were considered consistent with his history of TBI and the SPECT results.

Behaviorally, F.T. was perceived somewhat differently by his teachers and parents. The teachers and his father reported clinically significant problems with attention/concentration, work production, and noncompliance. In addition to these problems, F.T.'s mother also indicated significant concerns about social withdrawal; aggressive behaviors (arguing, fighting, mood swings, temper tantrums); and delinquent behaviors (associating with bad companions, stealing, swearing, and truancy). On a behavioral self-report measure, F.T. identified mild, but not clinically significant, problems with daydreaming and arguing, suggesting a lack of insight and self-awareness.

Family Factors

F.T.'s parents were divorced when he was 8 years old, and his father remarried prior to F.T.'s injury. His mother had full custody of F.T. and his two younger sisters, one of whom also sustained multiple injuries in the amusement park accident. According to the mother, the father had a history of alcohol abuse and domestic violence and had little contact with F.T. until the time of injury. She perceived the father's involvement at that time as related to his interest in monetary compensation from the wealthy owners of the amusement park, who were at fault for the accident. The father was barred from the hospital because he always seemed to be inebriated and was threatening in his interactions with the staff and F.T.'s mother.

Upon discharge from the rehabilitation unit, F.T. returned to a small rural community of 3,000 people, where his mother worked as an LPN. Over the next 4 years, the mother remarried twice and the family moved three times. Though she seemed to genuinely care for her son's well-being, the mother and F.T. were in constant conflict, and she reported difficulty managing his angry outbursts. On one occasion, behavioral counseling had been arranged for F.T. and his mother, but the family moved without keeping the appointment. The summer before the ninth grade, F.T. received a large cash settlement, which was placed in a trust fund for him. Around the same time, F.T. indicated a desire to live with his father and stepmother, both of whom were now steadily employed in a large city about 3 hours from the mother's home. The father reportedly was no longer drinking. At the time of the current evaluation, F.T. had been living in his father's home for 5 months.

Larger Organizational Factors

Prior to discharge from the hospital unit, rehabilitation staff met with the mother and the director of special education from F.T.'s hometown. At this discharge planning meeting, they discussed F.T.'s current cognitive and behavioral problems and provided a brief overview of the expected course of his recovery and his educational needs. Unfortunately, the rehabilitation staff and the educator were unfamiliar with the new TBI category included in the revision of IDEA. When he reentered school 6 weeks later, F.T. was classified as learning disabled and language impaired. Because of budget constraints, this small school district had been unable to hire a full-time speech–language therapist; instead, a speech–language therapist consulted weekly with the LD teacher to address F.T.'s language processing needs. At the end of the school year, the decision was made to retain F.T. in the fourth grade because he had missed so much school.

Frequent family moves made it difficult for educators to provide consistent programming for F.T. By the time he was referred 5 years postinjury, his only educational diagnosis was learning disabled, with consideration being given to an additional diagnosis of behavior disordered. Head injury was documented as a relevant factor under "Medical Concerns."

Risk and Protective Factors

F.T. certainly had multiple risk factors that could lead to a poor long-term outcome. He experienced a severe head injury with persistent cognitive and behavioral sequelae that interfered with his ability to keep up with same-age peers, as indicated by neuropsychological testing and by the decline in his IQ scores over time. He had experienced academic problems prior to his TBI that were likely associated with his history of physical and sexual abuse. His home environment was chaotic, and litigation over the TBI fueled family conflict and divisiveness. His single mother had multiple stressors, including the injury of two of her children and severe financial problems, and she did not exhibit strong behavioral management or limit-setting skills. F.T.'s recovery from TBI was affected by frequent family moves and inconsistent (and sometimes inadequate) educational services due to educators' inexperience and limited educational resources.

On the positive side, F.T.'s mother cared for and advocated for him to the best of her ability. She was generally aware of changes related to the TBI and periodically sought improved services for him. F.T.'s legal settlement provided a source of income for such services, once the case was resolved. F.T. had strengths in visual and motor functioning, as well as the ability to regulate his angry outbursts and maintain a semblance of social relationships at school. The improved stability on the paternal side of the family provided another resource for F.T.'s social and emotional needs. Finally, school personnel acted as a safety net for F.T., recognizing the extent of his problems and requesting further input from professionals familiar with brain injury.

An ecological systems model would suggest multiple points of intervention to be directed toward F.T. and members of his social environment. For example, F.T. might benefit from direct cognitive rehabilitation that included attention training and memory compensation strategies (Mateer et al., chapter 9), as well as basic problem-solving strategies. He might also show a positive response to a behavioral program having a focus on (a) antecedent structuring of the environment (e.g., breaking large tasks into smaller steps, providing written directions that could be referenced to promote recall and task completion); (b) the use of videotaping to increase self-awareness and shape on-task behaviors; and (c) frequent positive reinforcement. An evaluation for pharmacological treatment of inattentive and impulsive behaviors would also be recommended.

General and special education teachers, the school counselor, the speech–language therapist, and the family should design goals that could be implemented in multiple settings by multiple treatment providers. Work behaviors need to be targeted as a prevocational objective. Given the extent of F.T.'s verbal processing deficits, social interactions should be closely monitored to ensure that he could establish and maintain adequate friendships. Finally, educators should draw on existing public policy to specify TBI as the appropriate educational diagnosis for F.T., thus eliminating unnecessary grade retention and increasing appropriate educational programming.

In addition, the resources of the family, health care specialists, and other community agencies should be mobilized. Stability in the family system would be essential for F.T.'s continued adaptation, so family therapy and parent training should be considered. Community agencies might be able to provide job training or respite care to the mother, to reduce her overall stress level. The problem of insufficient resources could be resolved based on interagency agreements across education, health, mental health, and social services providers. A pooling of resources is often necessary to address a child's needs following TBI, but there are not always mechanisms in place for this to happen. The state government where F.T. lives had funded five TBI service coordinators to identify interagency supports, but such services were not available in F.T.'s county. Supportive models of service delivery can be extended only if there is public education and policy change.

PREVENTION

Ultimately, primary prevention is the most effective solution to the problem of childhood injury (Englander, Cleary, O'Hare, Hall, & Lehmkuhl, 1993; Peterson & Roberts, 1992). Preventing injury also requires multifaceted, systemic interventions that will have an impact on individual attitudes and behaviors, social interactions, environmental risks, and public policy. In the last several years, advances have been made in several areas. Injury prevention programs such as THINK FIRST represent campaigns to educate children and adolescents about the consequences of catastrophic injury and about behavioral strategies that will prevent or minimize injury (e.g., bike helmet and safety belt use). Families and youth have been the focus of legislated safety policies (e.g., use of infant carseats and safety belts, zero alcohol tolerance laws for minors), and consumers have been urged to purchase only safety-approved products (e.g., cribs with narrow slats to avoid anoxic injury). Legislators have increased passive, environmental forms of protection (e.g., airbags in cars, better engineering of roads and highways).

Despite this progress, many challenges to injury control efforts still exist. For example, brief school-based educational programs have improved children's attitudes and knowledge about TBI and spinal cord injuries, but they have not produced a corresponding increase in safe behaviors (Englander et al., 1993; Frank, Bouman, Cain, & Watts, 1992). Other behavioral interventions have been more successful, but they have involved more intensive and expensive individualized attention, behavioral rehearsal, and strong positive consequences for safe behaviors (Peterson & Roberts, 1992). Currently, legislated improvements in products and the environment, along with mandated behavioral safety precautions, are considered the most effective means of reducing injury risk. Unfortunately, legislated changes are often controversial and have been resisted in an effort to protect individual freedoms, as in the case of handgun control, lowered speed limits, and motorcycle helmet laws.

The solutions to these problems are complex, but there is an imperative for continued systematic program development and theory-driven research on injury prevention. Several researchers have outlined new approaches. For example, Geller et al. (1990) conceptualized a taxonomy of 24 behavioral strategies that can be tailored for use in injury prevention efforts. These range from population-wide interventions that are relatively unobtrusive and available at low cost (e.g., school-based educational programs), to individual change strategies that require intensive environmental structuring and effort (e.g., contingency management to change one person's high-risk behaviors). The idea of tailoring behavioral change strategies to individual needs is consistent with evidence that some youth are at greater risk of injury than others (Farmer & Peterson, 1995a; Kreutzer et al., chapter 4). Along a different dimension, Peterson and Brown (1994) expanded the focus of injury control efforts, highlighting the need to examine both unintentional injuries and intentional injuries due to violence, abuse, and neglect. They reviewed the traditionally separate child injury and abuse–neglect research literatures, described their many common characteristics, and identified prevention approaches suggested by this research integration. New ideas for advances in behavioral prevention strategies, combined with continued legislative and environmental interventions, can reduce injury risk and offset the high personal, social, and monetary costs of TBI and other catastrophic injuries in young people.

CONCLUSIONS

The challenge for professionals working with children who have sustained a TBI is to develop a continuum of care ranging from subacute treatment for individuals in coma to careful monitoring for late effects of injury in children with mild brain injury. We must develop effective and cost-efficient services that are accessible to all families, are age-appropriate, and are flexible enough to meet children's changing needs over time. Child outcomes must be viewed as multiply determined by social and environmental factors as well as by child characteristics. The ecological systems model presented here provides a conceptual framework for examining factors that increase the risk of poor outcomes following childhood TBI and for identifying points of intervention and prevention that can offset such risk. A systems-based approach to TBI research and program development has the potential to maximize the health and well-being of each child and family.

References

Chapter 1

Bigler, E. D. (1987). Acquired cerebral trauma: An introduction to the special series. *Journal of Learning Disabilities, 20*, 454–457.

Bigler, E. D. (Ed.). (1990). *Traumatic brain injury: Mechanisms of damage, assessment, intervention, and outcome.* Austin, TX: PRO-ED.

Galaburda, A. M. (1993). *Dyslexia and development: Neurobiological aspects of extraordinary brains.* Cambridge, MA: Harvard University Press.

Galaburda, A. M., Menard, M. T., & Rosen, G. D. (1994). Evidence for aberrant auditory anatomy in development dyslexia. *Proceedings of the National Academy of Science, 91*, 8010–8013.

Wiederholt, J. L. (1974). Historical perspectives on the education of the learning disabled. In L. Mann & D. Sabatino (Eds.), *The second review of special education* (pp. 103–152). Philadelphia: JSE Press.

Wiederholt, J. L. (1987). A preface to the special series on acquired cerebral trauma. *Journal of Learning Disabilities, 20*, 452–453.

Chapter 2

Adam, C., Baulac, M., Saint-Hilaire, J.-M., Landau, J., Granat, O., & Laplane, D. (1994). Value of magnetic resonance imaging–based measurements of hippocampal formations in patients with partial epilepsy. *Archives of Neurology, 51*, 130–138.

Adams, J., Doyle, D., Ford, I., Graham, D., & McLellan, D. (1989). Diffuse axonal injury in head injury: Definition, diagnosis, and grading. *Histopathology, 15*, 49–59.

Anderson, C., & Bigler, E. D. (1994). The role of caudate nucleus and corpus callosum atrophy in trauma-induced anterior horn dilation. *Brain Injury, 8*, 565–569.

Bigler, E. D. (1987). Acquired cerebral trauma: An introduction to the special series. *Journal of Learning Disabilities, 20*, 454–457.

Bigler, E. D. (Ed.). (1990). *Traumatic brain injury: Mechanisms of damage, assessment, intervention and outcome.* Austin, TX: PRO-ED.

Bigler, E. D. (1992). Three-dimensional image analysis of trauma-induced degenerative changes: An aid to neuropsychological assessment. Archives of Clinical Neuropsychology, 7, 449–556.

Bigler, E. D. (1994a). Neuroimaging in neuropsychology. In R. E. Kelley (Ed.), Functional neuroimaging (pp. 121–137). New York: Futura.

Bigler, E. D. (1994b). Neuroimaging and neuropsychological assessment. In C. R. Reynolds (Ed.), Cognitive assessment: A multi-disciplinary perspective (pp. 1–34). New York: Plenum.

Bigler, E. D., Blatter, D. D., Anderson, C. V., Johnson, S. C., Gale, S. D., Hopkins, R. O., & Burnett, B. (in press). Hippocampal volume in normal aging and traumatic brain injury. American Journal of Neuroradiology.

Bigler, E. D., Burr, R., Gale, S., Norman, M., Kurth, S., Blatter, D., & Abildskov, T. (1994). Day-of-injury CT scan as an index to pre-injury brain morphology. Brain Injury, 8, 231–238.

Bigler, E. D., Johnson, S. C., Anderson, C. V., Russo, A. A., Abildskov, T. J., Blatter, D. D., Gale, S. D., Ryser, D. K., MacNamara, S. E., Bailey, B.J., & Hopkins, R. O. (in press). Traumatic brain injury and memory: The role of hippocampal atrophy. Neuropsychology.

Bigler, E. D., Kurth, S., Blatter, D., & Abildskov, T. (1992). Degenerative changes in traumatic brain injury: Post-injury magnetic resonance identified ventricular expansion compared to pre-injury levels. Brain Research Bulletin, 28, 651–653.

Bigler, E. D., Kurth, S., Blatter, D., & Abildskov, T. (1993). Day-of-injury CT as an index to pre-injury brain morphology: Degree of post-injury degenerative changes identified by CT and MR neuroimaging. Brain Injury, 7, 125–134.

Bigler, E. D., & Snyder, J. (1995). Neuropsychological outcome and quantitative neuroimaging in mild brain injury. Archives of Clinical Neuropsychology, 10, 159–174.

Bigler, E. D., Yeo, R. A., & Turkheimer, E. (1989). Neuropsychological function and brain imaging. New York: Plenum Press.

Bowen, J.M., Clark, E., Bigler, E. D., Gardner, M., Nilsson, D., Gooch, J., & Pompa, J. (in press). Childhood traumatic brain injury: Neuropsychological status at the time of hospital discharge. Developmental Medicine and Child Neurology.

Courchesne, E., Yeung-Courchesne, R., & Egaas, B. (1994). Methodology in neuroanatomic measurement. Neurology, 44, 203–208.

Dixon, C. E., Lyeth, B. G., Povlischock, J. T. (1987). A fluid percussion model of experimental brain injury in the rat. Journal of Neurosurgery, 67, 110–119.

Fishman, P. S., & Mattu, A. (1993). Fate of severed cortical projection axons. Journal of Neurotrauma, 10, 457–470.

Fishman, R. A. (1992). Cerebrospinal fluid in diseases of the nervous system. Philadelphia: W. B. Saunders.

Gale, S. D., Burr, R., Bigler, E. D., & Blatter, D. D. (1993). Fornix degeneration and memory in traumatic brain injury. Brain Research Bulletin, 32, 345–349.

Gale, S. D., Johnson, S. J., Bigler, E. D., & Blatter, D. D. (1994). Traumatic brain injury and temporal horn enlargement: Correlates with tests of intelligence and memory. *Neuropsychiatry, Neuropsychology, and Behavioral Neurology, 7,* 160–165.

Gale, S. D., Johnson, S. J., Bigler, E. D., & Blatter, D. D. (1995a). Nonspecific white matter degeneration following traumatic brain injury. *Journal of the International Neuropsychological Society, 1,* 17–28.

Gale, S. D., Johnson, S. J., Bigler, E. D., & Blatter, D. D. (1995b). Trauma-induced degenerative changes in brain injury: A morphometric analysis of three patients with pre- and post-injury MR scans. *Journal of Neurotrauma, 12,* 151–158.

Hayes, R. L., & Ellison, M. D. (1989). Animal models of concussive head injury. In D. P. Becker & S. Gudeman (Eds.), *Head injury* (pp. 427–436). Philadelphia: W. B. Saunders.

Hicks, R. R., Smith, D. H., Lowenstein, D. H., Saint Marie, R., & McIntosh, T. K. (1993). Mild experimental brain injury in the rat induces cognitive deficits associated with regional neuronal loss in the hippocampus. *Journal of Neurotrauma, 10,* 405–414.

Ichise, M., Chung, D.-G., Wang, P., Wortzman, G., Gray, B. G., & Franks, W. (1994). Technetium-99m-HMPAO SPECT, CT and MRI in the evaluation of patients with chronic traumatic brain injury: A correlation with neuropsychological performance. *Journal of Nuclear Medicine, 35,* 217–226.

Johnson, S. C., Bigler, E. D., Burr, R. B., & Blatter, D. D. (1994). White matter atrophy, ventricular dilation, and intellectual functioning following traumatic brain injury. *Neuropsychology, 8,* 307–315.

Johnson, S. C., Farnworth, T., Pinkston, J. B., Bigler, E. D. & Blatter, D. D. (1994). Corpus callosum surface area across the human adult lifespan: Effect of age and gender. *Brain Research Bulletin, 35,* 373–377.

Katayama, Y., Becker, D. P., Tamura, T., & Hovda, D. A. (1990). Massive increases in extracellular potassium and the indiscriminate release of glutamate following concussive brain injury. *Journal of Neurosurgery, 73,* 889–900.

Kosslyn, S. M., Daly, P. F., McPeek, R. M., Alpert, N. M., Kennedy, D. N., & Caviness, V. S. (1993). Using locations to store shape: An indirect effect of a lesion. *Cerebral Cortex, 3,* 567–582.

Kurth, S. M., Bigler, E. D., & Blatter, D. D. (1994). Neuropsychological outcome and quantitative image analysis of acute haemorrhage in traumatic brain injury: Preliminary findings. *Brain Injury, 8,* 489–500.

Landis, D. M. D. (1994). The early reactions of non-neuronal cells to brain injury. *Annual Review of Neuroscience, 17,* 133–151.

Levin, H. S., Culhane, K. A., Fletcher, J. M., Mendelsohn, D. B., Lilly, M. A., Harward, H., Chapman, S. B., Bruce, D. A., Bertolino-Kusnerik, L., & Eisenberg, H. M. (1994). Dissociation between delayed alternation and memory after pediatric head injury: Relationship to MRI findings. *Journal of Child Neurology, 9,* 81–89.

Levin, H. S., Gary, H. E., Eisenberg, H. M., Ruff, R. M., Barth, J. T., Kreutzer, J., High, W. M., Portman, S., Foulkes, M. A., Jane, J. A., Marmarow, A., & Marshall, L. F. (1990). Neurobehavioral outcome 1 year after severe head injury: Experience of the traumatic Coma Data Bank. *Journal of Neurosurgery, 73,* 699–709.

Levin, H. S., Grafman, J., & Eisenberg, H. M. (1987). Neurobehavioral recovery from head injury. New York: Oxford University Press.

Murphy, E. J., & Horrocks, L. A. (1993). A model for compression trauma: Pressure-induced injury in cell cultures. Journal of Neurotrauma, 10, 431–444.

Neuwelt, E. A. (1989a). Implications of the blood–brain barrier and its manipulation: Vol. 1. Basic science aspects. New York: Plenum Press.

Neuwelt, E. A. (1989b). Implications of the blood–brain barrier and its manipulation: Vol. 2. Clinical aspects. New York: Plenum Press.

Povlishock, J. T. (1992). Pathobiology of traumatically induced axonal injury in animals and man. Annals of Emergency Medicine, 22, 980–986.

Povlishock, J. T. (1993, September). New approaches for assessing traumatic brain injury and repair. Paper presented at the annual meeting of the International Association for the Study of Traumatic Brain Injury, Tokyo, Japan.

Reilly, P. L., Simpson, D. A., Sprod, R., & Thomas, L. (1988). Assessing the conscious level in infants and young children: A pediatric version of the Glasgow Coma Scale. Child's Nervous System, 4, 30–33.

Salazer, A. M. (1992). Traumatic brain injury: The continuing epidemic. In A. Hachinski (Ed.), Challenges in neurology (pp. 55–67). Phildelphia: F. A. Davis.

Schmidt, R. H., & Grady, M. S. (1993). Regional patterns of blood–brain barrier breakdown following central and lateral fluid percussion injury in rodents. Journal of Neurotrauma, 10, 415–430.

Steward, O. (1989). Reorganization of neuroconnection following CNS trauma: Principles in experimental paradigm. Journal of Neurotrauma, 6, 99–152.

CHAPTER 3

Abidin, R. (1983). Parenting stress index—Manual. Charlottesville, VA: Pediatric Psychology Press.

Achenbach, T. M. (1991). Manual for the Child Behavior Checklist/4-18 and 1991 profile. Burlington: University of Vermont Department of Psychiatry.

Asarnow, R. F., Satz, P., Light, R., Lewis, R., & Neumann, E. (1991). Behavior problems and adaptive functioning in children with mild and severe closed head injury. Journal of Pediatric Psychology, 16, 543–555.

Asher, I. E. (1989). An annotated index of occupational therapy evaluation tools. Rockville, MD: The American Occupational Therapy Association.

Baker, R. S., & Epstein, A. D. (1991). Ocular motor abnormalities from head trauma. Survey of Ophthalmology, 35, 245–262.

Beery, K. E., & Buktenica, N. A. (1982). Developmental test of visual motor integration. Cleveland, OH: Modern Curriculum Press.

Begali, V. (1992). Head injury in children and adolescents: A resource and review for school and applied professionals (2nd ed.). Brandon, VT: Clinical Psychology.

Benton, A. L. (1968). Differential behavioral effects in frontal lobe disease. Neuropsychologia, 6, 53–60.

Blosser, J. L., & DePompei, R. (1994). Pediatric traumatic brain injury: Proactive intervention. San Diego, CA: Singular Publishing Group.

Braun, S. L., & Granger, C. V. (1991). A practical approach to functional assessment in pediatrics. Occupational Therapy Practice, 2, 46–51.

Bruininks, R. (1978). Bruininks-Oseretsky Test of Motor Proficiency. Circle Pines, MN: American Guidance Service.

Carney, J., & Gerring, J. (1990). Return to school following severe closed head injury: A critical phase in pediatric rehabilitation. Pediatrician, 17, 222–229.

Cobbs, L. W., Fletcher, J. M., & Levin, H. S. (1986). Neurobehavioral sequelae following head injury in children: Educational implications. Journal of Head Trauma Rehabilitation, 1, 57–65.

Colarusso, R. P., & Hammill, D. D. (1972). Motor free visual perception test. Novato, CA: Academic Therapy Publications.

Coster, W. J., Haley, S., & Baryza, M. J. (1994). Functional performance of young children after traumatic brain injury: A 6-month follow-up study. The American Journal of Occupational Therapy, 48, 211–218.

Crowley, J. A., & Miles, M. A. (1991). Cognitive remediation in pediatric head injury: A case study. Journal of Pediatric Psychology, 16, 611–627.

Deaton, A. V., & Waaland, P. (1994). Psychosocial effects of acquired brain injury. In R.C. Savage & G.F. Wolcott (Eds.), Educational dimensions of acquired brain injury (pp. 239–255). Austin, TX: PRO-ED.

DeFina, A. (1991). Portfolio assessment: Getting started. New York: Scholastic.

Delis, D. C., Kramer, J. H., Kaplan, E., & Ober, B. A. (1989). California verbal learning test: Children's version. San Antonio, TX: Psychological Corp.

Denney, D. R., & Denney, N. W. (1973). The use of classification for problem-solving: A comparison of middle and old age. Developmental Psychology, 9, 275–278.

Dennis, M. (1992). Word finding in children and adolescents with a history of brain injury. Topics in Language Disorders, 13, 66–82.

Dennis, M., & Barnes, M. A. (1990). Knowing the meaning, getting the point, bridging the gap, and carrying the message: Aspects of discourse following closed head injury in childhood and adolescence. Brain and Language, 39, 428–446.

DePaepe, J. L., & Lange, E. K. (1994). Physical assessment. In R. C. Savage & G. F. Wolcott (Eds.), Educational dimensions of acquired brain injury (pp. 345–365). Austin, TX: PRO-ED.

DePompei, R., & Blosser, J. L. (1993). Professional training and development for pediatric rehabilitation. In C.J. Durgin, N.D. Schmidt, & L.J. Fryer (Eds.), Staff development and clinical intervention in brain injury rehabilitation (pp. 229–253). Gaithersburg, MD: Aspen.

DePompei, R., & Blosser, J. L. (1994). The family as collaborator for effective school reintegration. In R. C. Savage & G. F. Wolcott (Eds.), Educational dimensions of acquired brain injury (pp. 489–506). Austin, TX: PRO-ED.

DiScala, C., Osberg, J. S., Gans, B. M., Chin, L. J., & Grant, C. C. (1991). Children with traumatic head injury: Morbidity and postacute treatment. Archives of Physical Medicine and Rehabilitation, 72, 662–666.

Epstein, N. B., Baldwin, L. M., & Bishop, D. S. (1983). The McMaster family assessment device. Journal of Marital and Family Therapy, 9, 171–180.

Ewing-Cobbs, L., Levin, H. S., Fletcher, J. M., Miner, M. E., & Eisenberg, H. M. (1990). The Children's Orientation and Amnesia Test: Relationship to severity of acute head injury and to recovery of memory. Neurosurgery, 27, 683–691.

Fay, G. C., Jaffe, K. M., Polissar, M. L., Liao, S., Rivara, J. B., & Martin, K. M. (1994). Outcome of pediatric traumatic brain injury at three years: A cohort study. Archives of Physical Medicine and Rehabilitation, 75, 733–741.

Fletcher, J. M., Ewing-Cobbs, L., Miner, M. E., Levin, H. S., & Eisenberg, H. M. (1990). Behavioral changes after closed head injury in children. Journal of Consulting and Clinical Psychology, 58, 93 98.

Folio, R., & Fewell, R. (1983). Peabody developmental scales. Allen, TX: DLM Teaching Resources.

Folstein, M. F., Folstein, S. E., & McHugh, P. R. (1975). "Mini-Mental State": A practical method for grading the cognitive state of patients for the clinician. Journal of Psychiatric Research, 12, 189–198.

Goodman, Y., Watson, D., & Burke, C. (1987). Reading miscue analysis: Alternative procedures. New York: Richard C. Owens.

Goyette, C. H., Conners, C. K., & Ulrich, R. F. (1978). Normative data on the Revised Conners Parent and Teacher Rating Scales. Journal of Abnormal Child Psychology, 6, 221–236.

Hagen, C., Malkmus, D., & Durham, P. (1981). Rancho Los Amigos: Levels of cognitive functioning. Downey, CA: Professional Staff Assoc.

Haley, S. M., Coster, W. J., & Ludlow, L. H. (1991). Pediatric functional outcome measures. Physical Medicine and Rehabilitation Clinics of North America, 2, 689–718.

Haley, S. M., Coster, W. J., Ludlow, L. H., Haltiwanger, J. T., & Andrellos, P. J. (1992). Pediatric evaluation of disability inventory. Boston: New England Medical Center Hospitals.

Hanson, S., & Clippard, D. (1992). Assessment of children with traumatic brain injury: Planning for school reentry. In S. Hanson & D. Tucker (Eds.), State of the art reviews: Physical medicine and rehabilitation (Vol. 6, pp. 483 494). Philadelphia: Hanley & Belfus.

Heaton, R. K. (1981). Wisconsin Card Sorting Test manual. Odessa, FL: Psychological Assessment Resources.

Individuals with Disabilities Education Act Amendments, 56 Fed. Reg. 41266 (1991) §160.

Iverson, G. L., Iverson, A. M., Barton, E. A., & Farmer, J. E. (1994, February). Normative data for the Children's Orientation and Amnesia Test. Poster session presented at the annual meeting of the International Neuropsychological Society, Cincinnati, OH.

Jaffe, K. M., Fay, G. C., Polissar, N. L., Martin, K. M., Shurtleff, H., Rivara, J. B., & Winn, H. R. (1992). Severity of pediatric traumatic brain injury and early neurobehavioral outcome: A cohort study. Archives of Physical Medicine and Rehabilitation, 73, 540–547.

Jaffe, K. M., Fay, G. C., Polissar, N. L., Martin, K. M., Shurtleff, H., Rivara, J. B., & Winn, H. R. (1993). Severity of pediatric traumatic brain injury and neuro-

behavioral recovery at one year—A cohort study. Archives of Physical Medicine and Rehabilitation, 74, 587–595.

Jaffe, K. M., & Hays, R. M. (1986). *Pediatric head injury: Rehabilitative medical management. Journal of Head Trauma Rehabilitation, 1, 30–40.*

Janus, P. L. (1994). *The role of school administration.* In R. C. Savage & G. F. Wolcott (Eds.), *Educational dimensions of acquired brain injury* (pp. 345–365). Austin, TX: PRO-ED.

Jones-Gotman, M., & Milner, B. (1977). *Design fluency: The inventions of nonsense drawings after focal cortical lesions. Neuropsychologia, 15, 653–674.*

Jordon, F., Murdoch, B., & Buttsworth, D. (1991). *Closed-head-injured children's performance on narrative tasks. Journal of Speech and Hearing Research, 34, 572–582.*

Jorgenson, C., Barrett, M., Huisingh, R., & Zachman, L. (1981). *The word test.* Moline, IL: Lingui Systems.

Kaufman, A. S., & Kaufman, N. L. (1985). *Kaufman test of educational achievement.* Circle Pines, MN: American Guidance Service.

Kaufman, P. M., Fletcher, J. M., Levin, H. S., Miner, M. E., & Ewing-Cobbs, L. (1993). *Attentional disturbance after pediatric closed head injury. Journal of Child Neurology, 8, 348–353.*

Klonoff, H., Clark, C., & Klonoff, P.F. (1993). *Long-term outcome of head injuries: A 23 year follow-up study of children with head injuries. Journal of Neurology, Neurosurgery, and Psychiatry, 56, 410–415.*

Knights, R. M., Ivan, L. P., Ventureyra, E. C. G., Bentivoglio, C., Stoddard, C., Winogron, W., & Bawden, H. N. (1991). *The effects of head injury in children on neuropsychological and behavioral functioning. Brain Injury, 5, 339–351.*

Kovich, K. M., & Bermann, D. E. (1988). *Head injury: A guide to functional outcomes in occupational therapy.* Rockville, MD: Aspen.

Kreutzer, J. S., Gervasio, A. H., & Camplair, P. S. (1994). *Primary caregivers' psychological status and family functioning after traumatic brain injury. Brain Injury, 8, 197–210.*

Lash, M., & Scarpino, C. (1993). *School reintegration for children with traumatic brain injuries. NeuroRehabilitation, 3, 13–25.*

Leach, L. R., Frank, R. G., Bouman, D. E., & Farmer, J. (1994). *Family functioning, depression, and social support after closed head injury. Brain Injury, 8, 599– 606.*

Lehr, E. (1990). *Psychological management of traumatic brain injuries in children and adolescents.* Rockville, MD: Aspen.

Levin, H. S., Benton, A. L., & Grossman, R. G. (1982). *Neurobehavioral consequences of closed head injury.* New York: Oxford University Press.

Levin, H. S., Culhane, K. A., Mendelsohn, D., Lilly, M. A., Bruce, D., Fletcher, J. M., Chapman, S. B., Harward, H., & Eisenberg, H. M. (1993). *Cognition in relation to magnetic resonance imaging in head-injured children and adolescents. Archives of Neurology, 50, 897–905.*

Levin, H. S., Mendelsohn, D., Lilly, M. A., Fletcher, J. M., Culhane, K. A., Chapman, S. B., Harward, H., Kusnerik, L., Bruce, D., & Eisenberg, H. M. (1994). *Tower of London performance in relation to magnetic resonance imaging following closed head injury in children. Neuropsychology, 8, 171–179.*

McCubbin, H. I., Larsen, A., & Olson, D. H. (1985). *Family crisis oriented personal evaluation scales. In D. H. Olson, H. I. McCubbin, H. Barnes, A. Larsen, M. Muxen, & M. Wilson (Eds.), Family inventories: Inventories used in a national survey of families across the life cycle. St. Paul: University of Minnesota Family Social Science.*

McKee, W. T., & Witt, J. C. (1990). *Effective teaching: A review of instructional and environmental variables. In T.B. Gutkin & C.R. Reynolds (Eds.), The handbook of school psychology (pp. 821 846). New York: Wiley.*

Miller, L. (1982). *Miller assessment for preschoolers. San Antonio, TX: Psychological Corp.*

Milner, M., Naumann, S., Literowich, W., Martin, M., Ryan, S., Sauter, W. F., Shein, G. F., & Verburg, G. (1990). *Rehabilitation engineering in pediatrics. Pediatrician, 17, 287–296.*

Moos, R. H., & Moos, B. S. (1976). *A typology of family social environments. Family Process, 15, 357–371.*

Murphy-Berman, V. A., & Wright, G. (1987). *Measures of attention. Perceptual Motor Skills, 64, 1139–1143.*

Oddy, M. (1993). *Head injury during childhood. Neuropsychological Rehabilitation, 3, 301–320.*

Papero, P. H., Prigatano, G. P., Snyder, H. M., & Johnson, D. L. (1993). *Children's adaptive behavioral competence after head injury. Neuropsychological Rehabilitation, 3, 321–340.*

Perrott, S. V., Taylor, H. G., & Montes, J. L. (1991). *Neuropsychological sequelae, familial stress, and environmental adaptation following pediatric head injury. Developmental Neuropsychology, 7, 69–86.*

Pieper, E. (1983). *A technique for discovering learning disabled adolescents' strategies for solving multiplication facts. The Pointer, 27, 40–41.*

Polissar, N. L., Fay, G. C., Jaffe, K. M., Liao, S., Martin, K. M., Shurtleff, H. A., Rivara, J. B., & Winn, H. R. (1994). *Mild pediatric traumatic brain injury: Adjusting significant levels from multiple comparisons. Brain Injury, 8, 249–264.*

Pratt, P. N., & Allen, A. S. (1989). *Occupational therapy of children (2nd ed.). St. Louis, MO: C. V. Mosby.*

Prutting, C. A., & Kirchner, D. M. (1987). *A clinical appraisal of the pragmatic aspects of language. Journal of Speech and Hearing Disorders, 52, 105–119.*

Reilly, P. L., Simpson, D. A., Sprod, R., & Thomas, L. (1988). *Assessing the conscious level in infants and young children: A pediatric version of the Glasgow Coma Scale. Child's Nervous System, 4, 30–33.*

Reitan, R. M., & Wolfson, D. (1992). *Neuropsychological evaluation of older children. South Tucson, AZ: Neuropsychology Press.*

Reschly, D. (1992). *Special education decision making and functional/behavioral assessment. In W. Stainback & S. Stainback (Eds.), Controversial issues confronting special education: Divergent perspectives (pp. 127–138). Boston: Allyn & Bacon.*

Reynolds, C. R., & Bigler, E. D. (1994). Test of memory and learning. Austin, TX: PRO-ED.

Rivara, J. B., Fay, G. C., Jaffe, K. M., Polissar, N. L., Shurtleff, H. A., & Martin, K. M. (1992). Predictors of family functioning one year following traumatic brain injury in children. Archives of Physical Medicine and Rehabilitation, 73, 899–910.

Rivara, J. B., Jaffe, K. M., Fay, G. C., Polissar, N. L., Martin, K. M., Shurtleff, H. A., & Liao, S. (1993). Family functioning and injury severity as predictors of child functioning one year following traumatic brain injury. Archives of Physical Medicine and Rehabilitation, 74, 1047–1055.

Rivara, J. B., Jaffe, K. M., Polissar, N. L., Fay, G. C., Martin, K. M., Shurtleff, H. A., & Liao, S. (1994). Family functioning and children's academic performance and behavior problems in the year following traumatic brain injury. Archives of Physical Medicine and Rehabilitation, 75, 269–279.

Russell, N. (1993). Educational considerations in traumatic brain injury: The role of the speech–language pathologist. Language, Speech, and Hearing Services in Schools, 24, 67–75.

Savage, R. C., & Wolcott, G. F. (1994). Educational dimensions of acquired brain injury. Austin, TX: PRO-ED.

Semel, E., Wiig, E. H., & Secord, W. (1987). Clinical evaluation of language fundamentals–Revised. San Antonio, TX: Psychological Corp.

Shallice, T. (1982). Specific impairments of planning. Philosophical Transactions of the Royal Society of London (Part B) 298, 199–209.

Sheslow, D., & Adams, W. (1990). Wide range assessment of memory and learning. Bloomington, DE: Jastak Associates.

Sparrow, S. S., Balla, D. A., & Cicchetti, D. E. (1984). Vineland adaptive behavior scales. Circle Pines, MN: American Guidance Service.

Story, T. B. (1991). Cognitive rehabilitation services in home and community settings. In J. S. Kreutzer & P. H. Wehman (Eds.), Cognitive rehabilitation for persons with traumatic brain injury (pp. 251–267). Baltimore: Brookes.

Teasdale, G., & Jennett, B. (1974). Assessment of coma and impaired consciousness: A practical scale. Lancet, ii, 81–84.

Trombly, C. A. (1989). Occupational therapy for physical dysfunction (3rd ed.). Baltimore: Williams & Wilkins.

Virginia Department of Education. (1992). Guidelines for educational services for students with traumatic brain injury. Richmond: Author.

Waaland, P. K., Burns, C., & Cockrell, J. (1993). Evaluation of needs of high- and low-income families following pediatric traumatic brain injury. Brain Injury, 7, 135–146.

Wechsler, D. (1991). Manual for the Wechsler Intelligence Scale for Children (3rd ed.). San Antonio, TX: Psychological Corp.

Wiig, E. H., & Secord, W. (1988). Test of language competence–Expanded edition. San Antonio, TX: Psychological Corp.

Woodcock, R. W., & Johnson, M. B. (1989). Woodcock-Johnson psycho-educational batttery–Revised (tests of achievement). Chicago: Riverside.

Worthen, B. (1993). *Critical issues that will determine the future of alternative assessment. Phi Delta Kappan, 74, 444–454.*

Ylvisaker, M. (1993). *Communication outcome in children and adolescents with traumatic brain injury. Neuropsychological Rehabilitation, 3, 367–387.*

Ylvisaker, M., Chorazy, A. J. L., Cohen, S. B., Mastrilli, J. P., Molitor, C. B., Nelson, J., Szekeres, S. F., Valko, A. S., & Jaffe, K. M. (1990). *Rehabilitative assessment following head injury in children. In M. Rosenthal, E. R. Griffith, M. R. Bond, & J. D. Miller (Eds.), Rehabilitation of the adult and child with traumatic brain injury (2nd ed., pp. 558 592). Philadelphia: F. A. Davis*

Ylvisaker, M., Hartwick, P., Ross, B., & Nussbaum, N. (1994). *Cognitive assessment. In R. C. Savage & G. F. Wolcott (Eds.), Educational dimensions of acquired brain injury (pp. 69–119). Austin, TX: PRO-ED.*

CHAPTER 4

Abrams, D., Barker, L. T., Haffey, W., & Nelson, H. (1993). *The economics of return to work for survivors of traumatic brain injury: Vocational services are worth the investment. Journal of Head Trauma Rehabilitation, 8(4), 59–76.*

Alldadi, V. (1986). *Some aspects of Methylphenidate treatment of hyperactive children. Pharmacy Alert, 16(3), 2–3.*

August, G. J., Stewart, M. A., & Holmes, C. S. (1983). *A four year follow-up study of hyperactive boys with and without conduct disorder. The British Journal of Psychiatry, 143, 192–198.*

Beck, L., Langford, W. S., MacKay, M., & Sum, G. (1975). *Childhood chemotherapy and later drug abuse and growth curve: A follow-up study of 30 adolescents. American Journal of Psychiatry, 132, 436–438.*

Brooks, D., Campsie, L., Symington, C., Beattie, A., & McKinlay, W. (1986). *The five year outcome of severe blunt head injury: A relative's view. Journal of Neurology, Neurosurgery, and Psychiatry, 49, 764–770.*

Brooks, N., Campsie, L., Symington, C., Beattie, A., & McKinlay, W. (1987). *Return to work within the first seven years of severe head injury. Brain Injury, 1, 5–19.*

Brooks, N., Symington, C., Beattie, A., Campsie, L., Bryden, J., & McKinlay, W. (1989). *Alcohol and other predictors of cognitive recovery after severe head injury. Brain Injury, 3, 235–246.*

Bruck, M. (1985). *The adult functioning of children with specific learning disabilities: A follow-up study. Advances in Applied Developmental Psychology, 1, 91–129.*

Cahalan, D., & Cisin, I. (1968a). *American drinking practices: Summary of findings from a national probability sample: I. Extent of drinking by population subgroups. Quarterly Journal of Studies on Alcohol, 29, 130–151.*

Cahalan, D., & Cisin, I. (1968b). *American drinking practices: Summary of findings from a national probability sample: II. Measurement of massed versus spaced drinking. Quarterly Journal of Studies on Alcohol, 29, 642–656.*

Clampit, M. K., & Pirkle, J. B. (1983). Stimulant medication and the hyperactive adolescent: Myths and facts. Adolescence, 18, 811–822.

Cope, N., & Hall, K. (1982). Head injury rehabilitation: Benefit of early intervention. Archives of Physical Medicine and Rehabilitation, 63, 433–437.

Corrigan, J. (1995). Substance abuse as a mediating factor in outcome from traumatic brain injury. Archives of Physical Medicine and Rehabilitation, 76, 302–309.

Dahmer, E. R., Shilling, M. A., Hamilton, B. B., Bontke, C. F., Englander, J., Kreutzer, J. S., Ragnarsson, K. T., & Rosenthal, M. (1993). A model systems database for traumatic brain injury. The Journal of Head Trauma Rehabilitation, 8(2), 12–25.

Drubach, D. A., Kelly, M. P., Winslow, B. A., & Flynn, J. P. G. (1993). Substance abuse as a factor in the causality, severity, and recurrence rate of traumatic brain injury. Maryland Medical Journal, 42, 989–993.

Engs, R. C., & Hanson, D. J. (1988). University students' drinking patterns and problems: Examining the effects of raising the purchase age. Public Health Reports, 103, 667–673.

Galbraith, S., Murray, W., Patel, A., & Knill-Jones, R. (1976). The relationship between blood alcohol and head injury and its effect on the conscious level. British Journal of Surgery, 63, 735–743.

Gittleman, R., Mannuzza, S., Shenker, R., & Bonagura, N. (1985). Hyperactive boys almost grown up. Archives of General Psychiatry, 42, 937–947.

Glow, B. A. (1989). Drugs and the disabled. In G. W. Lawson & A. W. Lawson (Eds.), Alcoholism and substance abuse in special populations (pp. 65–93). Rockville, MD: Aspen.

Gold, M. A., & Gladstein, J. (1993). Substance use among adolescents with diabetes mellitus: Preliminary findings. Journal of Adolescent Health, 14, 80–84.

Gordon, W., Mann, N., & Willer, B. (1993). Demographic and social characteristics of the traumatic brain injury model system data base. Journal of Head Trauma Rehabilitation, 8, 26–33.

Haas, J. F., Cope, D. N., & Hall, K. (1987). Premorbid prevalence of poor academic performance in severe head injury. Journal of Neurology, Neurosurgery and Psychiatry, 50, 52–56.

Hall, K. H., Karzmark, P., Stevens, M., Englander, J., O'Hare, P., & Wright, J. (1994). Family stressors in traumatic brain injury: A two year follow-up. Archives of Physical Medicine and Rehabilitation, 75, 876–884.

Hilton, M. E. (1987). Drinking patterns and drinking problems in 1984: Results from a general population survey. Alcoholism: Clinical and Experimental Research, 11, 167–175.

Kreutzer, J. S., Doherty, K. R., Harris, J. A. & Zasler, N. D. (1990). Alcohol use among persons with traumatic brain injury. Journal of Head Trauma Rehabilitation, 5, 9–20.

Kreutzer, J., Leininger, B., Doherty, K., & Waaland, P. (1987). General health and history questionnaire. Richmond: Rehabilitation Research and Training Center on Severe Traumatic Brain Injury, Medical College of Virginia.

Kreutzer, J., Wehman, P. H., Harris, J. A., Burns, C. T., & Young, H. F. (1991). Substance and crime patterns among persons with traumatic brain injury referred for supported employment. Brain Injury, 5, 177–187.

Lehmkuhl, L. D., Hall, K. M., Mann, N., & Gordon, W. A. (1993). Factors that influence costs and length of stay of persons with traumatic brain injury in acute care and inpatient rehabilitation. Journal of Head Trauma Rehabilitation, 8(2), 88–100.

Levin, H., Benton, A., & Grossman, R. G. (1982). Neurobehavioral consequences of closed head injury. New York: Oxford.

Lezak, M. D. (1995). Neuropsychological assessment (3rd ed.). New York: Oxford.

Maag, J. W., Irvin, D. M., Reid, R., & Vasa, S. (1994). Prevalence and predictors of substance use: A comparison between adolescents with and without learning disabilities. Journal of Learning Disabilities, 27, 223–234.

MacKenzie, E. J., Shapiro, S., Smith, R. T., Siegel, J. D., Moody, J., & Pitt, A. (1987). Factors influencing return to work following hospitalization for traumatic brain injury. American Journal of Public Health, 77, 329–334.

Maisto, S. A., Sobell, L. C., & Sobell, M. B. (1979). Comparison of alcoholics' self-reports of drinking behavior with reports of collateral informants. Journal of Consulting and Clinical Psychology, 47, 106–112.

Meilman, P. W., Stone, J. E., Gaylor, M. S., & Turco, J. H. (1990). Alcohol consumption by college undergraduates: Current use and 10-year trends. Journal of Studies on Alcohol, 51, 389–395.

Mills, C. J., & Noyes, H. L. (1984). Patterns and correlates of initial and subsequent drug use among adolescents. Journal of Consulting and Clinical Psychology, 52, 231–243.

Moore, D., & Polsgrove, L. (1991). Disabilities, developmental handicaps, and substance misuse: A review. International Journal of the Addictions, 26, 65–90.

Motet-Grigoras, C. N., & Schuckit, M. A. (1986). Depression and substance abuse in handicapped young men. Journal of Clinical Psychiatry, 47, 234–237.

Nath, F. P., Beastal, G., & Teasdale, G. (1986). Alcohol and traumatic brain damage. Injury, 17, 150–153.

National Institute on Drug Abuse. (1991). Drug use among youth: Findings from the 1988 National Household Survey on Drug Abuse (DHHS Publication No. ADM 91-1765). Rockville, MD: Author.

Newcomb, M. D., & Bentler, P. M. (1987). Changes in drug use from high school to young adulthood: Effects of living arrangement and current life pursuit. Journal of Applied Developmental Psychology, 8, 221–246.

O'Shanick, G. J., & Zasler, N. D. (1990). Neuropsychopharmacological approaches to traumatic brain injury. In J. S. Kreutzer & P. Wehman (Eds.), Community integration following traumatic brain injury (pp. 15–28). Baltimore: Brookes.

Ragnarsson, K. T., Thomas J. P., & Zasler N. D. (1993). Model systems of care for individuals with traumatic brain injury. Journal of Head Trauma Rehabilitation, 8(2), 1–11.

Rimel, R., Giordani, B., Barth, J., & Jane, J. (1982). Moderate head injury: Completing the clinical spectrum of brain trauma. Neurosurgery, 11, 344–351.

Robinson, T. N., Killen, J. D., Taylor, B., Telch, M. J., Bryson, S. W., Saylor, K. E., Maron, D. J., Maccoby, N., & Farquhar, J. W. (1987). Perspectives on adolescent substance use: A defined population study. Journal of the American Medical Association, 258, 2072–2076.

Ruff, R. M., Marshall, L. F., Klauber, M. R., Blunt, B. A., Grant, I., Foulkes, M. A., Eisenberg, H., Jane, J., & Marmarou, A. (1990). Alcohol abuse and neuropsychological outcome of the severely head injured. *Journal of Head Trauma Rehabilitation, 5(3),* 21–31.

Sander, A., Witol, A., & Kreutzer, J. (1996, June). Reliability of postinjury alcohol use measures: Concordance of patients' and caregivers' reports. Paper presented at the 20th annual Postgraduate Course on Rehabilitation of the Brain Injured Adult and Child, Williamsburg, Va.

Sorenson, S. B., & Kraus, J. F. (1991). Occurrence, severity and outcomes of brain injury. *Journal of Head Trauma Rehabilitation, 6(2),* 1–10.

Sparadeo, F. R. & Gill, D. (1989). Effects of prior alcohol use on head injury recovery. *Journal of Head Trauma Rehabilitation, 4(2),* 75–82.

Thomsen, I. V. (1984). Late outcome of very severe blunt head trauma: A 10–15 year second follow-up. *Journal of Neurology, Neurosurgery, & Psychiatry, 47,* 260–268.

Wisconsin Department of Health and Social Services. (1985). Alcohol use by persons with disabilities: Preliminary report. Madison, WI: State Department of Health and Social Services.

Wong, P. P., Dornan, J., Schentag, C. T., Ip, R., & Keating, A. M. (1993). Statistical profile of traumatic brain injury: A Canadian rehabilitation population. *Brain Injury, 7,* 283–294.

CHAPTER 5

Achenbach, T. M. (1991). Manual for the Child Behavior Checklist/4-18. Burlington: University of Vermont, Department of Psychiatry.

Basset S., & Slater, E. (1990). Neuropsychological function in adolescents sustaining mild closed head injury. *Journal of Pediatric Psychology, 15,* 225–236.

Bawden, H. N., Knights, R. M., & Winogron, H. W. (1985). Speeded performance following head injury in children. *Journal of Clinical and Experimental Neuropsychology, 7(1),* 39–54.

Brink, J. D., Garrett, A. L., Hale, W. R., Woo-Sam, J., & Nickel, V. L. (1970). Recovery of motor and intellectual function in children sustaining severe head injuries. *Developmental Medicine and Child Neurology, 12,* 565–571.

Brown, G., Chadwick, O., Shaffer, D., Rutter, M. C., & Traub, M. (1981). A prospective study of children with head injuries: III. Psychiatric sequelae. *Psychological Medicine, 11(1),* 63–78.

Chadwick, O., Rutter, M., Thompson, J., & Shaffer, D. (1981). Intellectual performance and reading skills after localized head injury in childhood. *Journal of Child Psychology and Psychiatry, 22,* 117–139.

Chaplin, D., Deitz, J., & Jaffe, K. (1993). Motor performance in children after traumatic brain injury. *Archives of Physical Medicine and Rehabilitation, 74,* 161–164.

Choi, S. C., Barnes, T. Y., Bullock, R., Germanson, T. A., Marmarou, A., & Young, H. F. (1994). Temporal profile of outcomes in severe head injury. Journal of Neurosurgery, 81, 119–173.

Committee on Injury Scaling. (1985). The Abbreviated injury scale. Morton Grove, IL: American Association for Automotive Medicine.

Delis, D. C., Kramer, J. H., Kaplan, E., & Ober, B. A. (1994). California verbal learning test–Children's version. San Antonio, TX: Psychological Corp.

Ellenberg, L., McComb, J. G., Siegel, S. E., & Stone, S. (1987). Factors affecting intellectual outcome in pediatric brain tumor patients. Neurosurgery, 21, 638–644.

Esparza, J., Portillo, M., Sarabia, M., Yuste, J. A., Roger, R., & Lamas, E. (1985). Outcome in children with severe head injuries. Child's Nervous System, 1, 109–114.

Ewing-Cobbs, L., Levin, H. S., Fletcher, J. M., Miner, M. E., & Eisenberg, H. M. (1990). The Children's Orientation and Amnesia Test: Relationship to severity of acute head injury and to recovery of memory. Neurosurgery, 25, 683–691.

Fay, G. G., Jaffe, K. M., Polissar, N. L., Liao, S., Rivara, J. B., & Martin, K. M. (1994). Outcome of pediatric traumatic brain injury at 3 years: A cohort study. Archives of Physical Medicine and Rehabilitation, 75, 733–741.

Fields, A. I., Coble, D. H., Pollack, M. M., Cuerdon, T. T., & Kaufman, J. (1993). Outcomes of children in a persistent vegetative state. Critical Care Medicine, 21(2), 1890–1894.

Filley, C. M., Cranberg, L. D., Alexander, M. P., & Hart, E. J. (1987). Neurobehavioral outcome after closed head injury in childhood and adolescence. Archives of Neurology, 44, 194–198.

Fletcher, J. M., & Copeland, D. R. (1988). Neurobehavioral effects of central nervous system prophylactic treatment of cancer in children. Journal of Clinical and Experimental Neuropsychology, 10(4), 495–538.

Fletcher, J. M., Ewing-Cobbs, L., Miner, M. E., Levin, H. S., & Eisenberg, H. M. (1990). Behavioral changes after closed head injury in children. Journal of Consulting and Clinical Psychology, 58(1), 93–98.

Ghajar, J., & Hariri, R. J. (1992). Management of pediatric head injury. In A. M. P. Maio (Ed.), The pediatric clinics of North America: Pediatric emergency medicine (pp. 1093–1126). Philadelphia: Saunders.

Greenspan, A. I., & MacKenzie, E. J. (1994). Functional outcome after pediatric head injury. Pediatrics, 94(4), 425–432.

Heaton, R. K., Chelune, G. J., Talley, J. L., Kay, G. G., & Curtiss, G. (1993). Wisconsin card sorting test manual, Revised and expanded. Odessa, FL: Psychological Assessment Resources.

Hofer, T. (1993). Glascow Scale relationships in pediatric and adult patients. Journal of Neuroscience Nursing, 25(4), 218–227.

Jaffe, K. M., Fay, G. C., Polissar, N. L., Martin, K. M., Shurtleff, H. A., Rivara, J. B., & Winn, H. R. (1993). Severity of pediatric traumatic brain injury and neurobehavioral outcome at 1 year—A cohort study. Archives of Physical Medicine and Rehabilitation, 74, 587–595.

Levin, H. S., Benton, A. L., & Grossman, R. G., (1982). Neurobehavioral consequences of closed head injury. New York: Oxford University Press.

Levin, H. S., Culhane, K. A., Mendelsohn, D., Lilly, M. A., Bruce, D., Fletcher, J. M., Chapman, S. B., Harward, H., & Eisenberg, H. M. (1993). Cognition in relation to magnetic resonance imaging in head-injured children and adolescents. Archives of Neurology, 50, 897–905.

Levin, H. S., Eisenberg, H. N., Wigg, N. R., & Kobayashi, K. (1982). Memory and intellectual ability after head injury in children and adolescents. Neurosurgery, 11, 668–673.

Levin, H. S., High, W. M., Ewing-Cobbs, L., Fletcher, J. M., Eisenberg, H. M., Miner, M. E., & Goldstein, F. C. (1988). Memory functioning during the first year after closed head injury in children and adolescents. Neurosurgery, 22, 1043–1052.

Levin, H. S., Mendelsohn, D., Lilly, M. A., Fletcher, J. M., Culhane, K. A., Chapman, S. B., Harward, H., Kusnerik, L., Bruce, D., & Eisenberg, H. M. (1994). Tower of London performance in relation to magnetic resonance imaging following closed head injury in children. Neuropsychology, 8(2), 171–179.

Mahoney, W. J., D'Souza, B. J., Haller, J. A., Rogers, M. C., Epstein, M. H., & Freeman, J. M. (1983). Long-term outcome of children with severe head trauma and prolonged coma. Pediatrics, 71, 756–762.

McDonald, C. M., Jaffe, K. M., Fay, G. C., Polissar, N. L., Martin, K. M., Liao, S., & Rivara, J. B. (1994). Comparison of indices of traumatic brain injury severity as predictors of neurobehavioral outcome in children. Archives of Physical Medicine and Rehabilitation, 75, 328–337.

Mendelsohn, D., Levin, H. S., Bruce, D., Lilly, M., Harward, H., Culhane, K. A., & Eisenberg, H. M. (1992). The MRI after head injury in children: Relationship to clinical features and outcome. Child's Nervous System, 8, 445–452.

Michaud, L. J., Rivara, F. P., Jaffe, K. M., Falfe, G., & Dailey, J. L. (1993). Traumatic brain injury as a risk factor for behavioral disorders in children. Archives of Physical Medicine and Rehabilitation, 74, 368–375.

Mulhern, R. K., Kovnar, E. H., Kun, L. E., Crisco, J. J., & Williams, J. M. (1988). Psychologic and neurologic function following treatment for childhood temporal lobe astrocytoma. Journal of Child Neurology, 3, 47–52.

Reitan, R. M., & Davison, L. A. (Eds.). (1974). Clinical neuropsychology: Current status and applications. Washington, DC: Winston.

Ris, M. D., & Noll, R. B. (1994). Long-term neurobehavioral outcome in pediatric brain-tumor patients: Review and methodological critique. Journal of Clinical and Experimental Neuropsychology, 16(1), 21–42.

Rivara, J. B., Jaffe, K. M., Fay, G. C., Polissar, N. L., Martin, K. M., Shurtleff, H. A., & Liao, S. (1993). Family functioning and injury severity as predictors of child functioning 1 year following traumatic brain injury. Archives of Physical Medicine and Rehabilitation, 74, 1047–1055.

Rivara, J. B., Jaffe, K. M., Polissar, N. L., Fay, G. C., Martin, K. M., Shurtleff, H. A., & Liao, S. (1994). Family functioning and children's academic performance and behavior problems in the year following traumatic brain injury. Archives of Physical Medicine and Rehabilitation, 75, 369–379.

Rossman, M. P. (1994). Acute head trauma. In F. A. Oski, C. D. DeAngelis, R. D. Feigin, J. A. McMillan, & J. B. Warshaw (Eds.), Principles and practice of pediatrics (pp. 2038–2048). Philadelphia: Lippincott.

Ruijis, M. B. M., Gabreëls, F. J. M., & Keyser, A. (1993). The relationship between neurologic trauma parameters and long-term outcome in children with closed head injury. European Journal of Pediatrics, 152, 844–847.

Ruijis, M. B. M., Gabreëls, F. J. M., & Thijssen, H. O. M. (1994). The utility of electroencephalography and cerebral computer tomography is children with mild and moderately severe closed head injuries. Neuropediatrics, 25, 73–77.

Shallice, T. (1982). Specific impairments of planning. Philosophical Transactions of the Royal Society of London, Part B, 298, 199–209.

Silber, J. H., Radcliff, J., Peckham, V., Perilongo, G., Kishnani, P., Fridman, M., Goldwein, J. W., & Meadows, A. T. (1992). Whole-brain irradiation and decline in intelligence: The influence of dose and age on IQ score. Journal of Oncology, 10, 1390–1396.

Stewart, S. M., Campbell, R. A., McCallon, D., Waller, D. A., & Andrews, W. S. (1992). Cognitive patterns in school-age children with end-stage liver disease. Journal of Developmental and Behavioral Pediatrics, 13(5), 331–338.

Teasdale, G., & Jennett, B. (1974). Assessment of coma and impaired consciousness: A practical scale. Lancet, 2, 178–180.

Walker, M. L., Storrs, B. B., Mayer, T. (1983). Factors affecting outcome in the pediatric patient with multiple trauma. Concepts in Pediatric Neurosurgery, 4, 243–252.

Wechsler, D. (1991). Wechsler intelligence scale for children–Third edition. San Antonio, TX: Psychological Corp.

Wilkening, G. N. (1989). Techniques of localization in child neuropsychology. In C. R. Reynolds & E. Fletcher-Janzen (Eds.), Handbook of clinical child neuropsychology (pp. 291–310). New York: Plenum.

Winogron, H. W., Knights, R. M., & Bawden, H. N. (1984). Neuropsychological deficits following head injury in children. Journal of Clinical Neuropsychology, 6(3), 269–286.

CHAPTER 6

Aram, D. M., & Eisele, J. A. (1994). Intellectual stability in children with unilateral brain lesions. Neuropsychologia, 32(1), 85–96.

Arffa, S., Fitzhugh-Bell, K., & Black, W. (1989). Neuropsychological profiles of children with learning disabilities and children with documented brain damage. Journal of Learning Disabilities, 22, 635–640.

Banich, M. T., Levine, S. C., Kim, H., & Huttenlocher, P. (1990). The effects of developmental factors on IQ in hemiplegic children. Neuropsychologia, 28(1), 35–47.

Bigler, E. D. (1988). Acquired cerebral trauma: Epilogue. Journal of Learning Disabilities, 21, 476–485.

Bigler, E. D. (1992). The neurobiology and neuropsychology of adult learning disorders. *Journal of Learning Disabilities, 25,* 488–506.

Bradshaw, J. L., & Nettleton, N. C. (1981). The nature of hemispheric specialization in man. *Behavioral and Brain Sciences, 4,* 51–91.

Brazzelli, B., Colombo, N., Della Sala, S., & Spinnier, H. (1994). Spared and impaired cognitive abilities after bilateral frontal damage. *Cortex, 30,* 27–51.

Chapman, S., Culhane, K. A., Levin, H. S., Harward, H., Mendelsohn, D., Ewing-Cobbs, L., Fletcher, J., & Bruce, D. (1992). Narrative discourse after closed head injury in children and adolescents. *Brain and Language, 43(1),* 42–65.

Conners, C. K. (1973). Rating scales for use in drug studies with children. *Psychopharmacology Bulletin (Special issue—Pharmacotherapy with Children),* 24–84.

Dalby, P. R., & Obrzut, J. E. (1991). Epidemiological characteristics and sequelae of closed head-injured children: A review. *Developmental Neuropsychology, 7,* 35–68.

Dobbins, C., & Russell, E. W. (1990). Left temporal brain damage pattern on the Wechsler Intelligence Scale. *Journal of Clinical Psychology, 46,* 863–868.

Donders, J. (1993). Factor structure of the WISC-R in children with traumatic brain injury. *Journal of Clinical Psychology, 49(2),* 255–260.

Eisele, J. A., & Aram, D. M. (1993). Differential effects of early hemisphere damage on lexical comprehension and production. Special Issue: Acquired childhood aphasia. *Aphasiology, 7,* 513–523.

Ewing-Cobbs, L., & Fletcher, J. M. (1990). Neuropsychological assessment of traumatic brain injury in children. In E. D. Bigler (Ed.), *Traumatic brain injury* (pp. 107–128). Austin, TX: PRO-ED.

Ewing-Cobbs, L., Fletcher, J. M., & Levin, H. S. (1986). Neurobehavioral sequelae following head injury in children: Educational implications. *Journal of Head Trauma Rehabilitation, 1,* 57–65.

Ewing-Cobbs, L., Levin, H. S., Eisenberg, H. M., & Fletcher, J. M. (1987). Language functions following closed head injury in children and adolescents. *Journal of Clinical and Experimental Neuropsychology, 9,* 575–592.

Ewing-Cobbs, J., Miner, M. E., Fletcher, J. M., & Levin, H. S. (1989). Intellectual, motor, and language sequelae following closed head injury in infants and preschoolers. *Journal of Pediatric Psychology, 14,* 531–547.

Farmer, J., & Peterson, L. (1995). Pediatric traumatic brain injury: Promoting successful school reentry. *School Psychology Review, 24,* 230–243.

Fletcher, J., & Levin, H. (1988). Neurobehavioral effects of brain injury in children. In D. K. Routh (Ed.), *Handbook of pediatric psychology* (pp. 258–295). New York: Guilford Press.

Fuerst, D. R., Fisk, J. L., & Rourke, B. P. (1989). Psychosocial functioning of learning-disabled children: Replicability of statistically derived subtypes. *Journal of Consulting and Clinical Psychology, 57,* 275–280.

Gaddes, W. H., & Edgell, D. (1994). *Learning disabilities and brain function: A neuropsychological approach* (2nd ed.). New York: Springer-Verlag.

Geschwind, N. (1979). Specialization of the human brain. *Scientific American, 24(3),* 180–199.

Goldstein, F., & Levin, H. (1991). Question-asking strategies after severe closed head injury. Brain and Cognition, 17, 23–30.

Goodyear, P., & Hynd, G. W. (1992). Attention-deficit disorder with (ADDHD) and without (ADD/WO) hyperactivity: Behavioral and neuropsychological differentiation. Journal of Clinical Child Psychology, 21, 273–305.

Hebb, D. O. (1949). Organization of behavior. New York: Wiley.

Hom, J., & Reitan, R. M. (1982). Effects of lateralized cerebral damage upon contralateral and ipsilateral sensorimotor performances. Journal of Clinical Neuropsychology, 4, 249–268.

Hooper, S. R., & Roof, K. D. (1993). Utility of the Hobby WISC-R Split Half Short Form for children and adolescents with severe head injury. Psychological Reports, 72, 371–376.

Huttenlocher, P. R. (1990). Morphometric study of human cerebral cortex development. Neuropsychologia, 28, 517–527.

Jaffee, C. C. (1982). Medical imaging. Scientific American, 70, 576–585.

John, E. R. (1986). Clinical applications of neurometrics and the brain state analyzer. Internal Medicine for the Specialist, 7, 155–191.

John, E. R., Princhep, L., Eastman, P., Friedman, J., & Kaye, H. (1983). Neurometric evaluation of cognitive dysfunctions and neurological disorders in children. Progressive Neurobiology, 21, 239–290.

Johnson, D. A. (1992). Head injured children and education: A need for greater delineation and understanding. British Journal of Educational Psychology, 62, 404–409.

Karzmark, P. (1992). Prediction of long-term cognitive outcome of brain injury with neuropsychological, severity of injury, and demographic data. Brain Injury, 6, 213–217.

Katz, L., Goldstein, G., Rudisin, S., & Bailey, D. (1993). A neuropsychological approach to the Bannatyne recategorization of the Wechsler Intelligence Scales in adults with learning disabilities. Journal of Learning Disabilities, 26, 65–72.

Kaufman, P. M., Fletcher, J. M., Levin, H. S., Miner, M. E., & Ewing-Cobbs, L. (1993). Attentional disturbance after pediatric closed head injury. Journal of Child Neurology, 8, 348–353.

Kelly, M. S., Best, C. T., & Kirk, U. (1989). Cognitive processing deficits in reading disabilities: A prefrontal cortical hypothesis. Brain and Cognition, 11, 275–293.

Kupfermann, I. (1985). Learning. In E. R. Kandel & J. C. Schwartz (Eds.), Principles of neural science (pp. 806–815). New York: Elsevier.

Lehr, E. (1990). Psychological management of traumatic brain injuries in children and adolescents. Rockville, MD: Aspen.

Levin, H. S. (1991). Pioneers in research on the behavioral sequelae of head injury. Journal of Clinical and Experimental Neuropsychology, 13(1), 133–154.

Levin, H. S., Culhane, K. A., Fletcher, J. M., Mendelsohn, E. B., Lilly, M., Harward, H., Chapman, S., Bruce, D., Kusnerik, L., & Eisenberg, H. (1994a). Disassociation between delayed alternation and memory after pediatric head injury: Relationship to MRI findings. Journal of Child Neurology, 9, 811–889.

Levin, H. S., Culhane, K. A., Mendelsohn, D., Lilly, M. A., Bruce, D., Fletcher, J. M., Chapman, S. B., Harward, H., & Eisenberg, H. M. (1993). Cognition in relation to magnetic resonance imaging in head injured children and adolescents. *Archives of Neurology, 50, 897–905.*

Levin, H. S., High, W. M., Williams, D. H., Eisenberg, H. M., Gamparo, E., Guintro, E., & Ewert, J. (1989). *Dichotic listening and manual performance in relation to magnetic resonance imaging after closed head injury. Journal of Neurology, Neurosurgery, and Psychiatry, 52, 1162–1169.*

Levin, H. S., Mendelsohn, D. G., Lilly, M. A., Fletcher, J. M., Culhane, K. A., Chapman, S. B., Harward, H., Kusnerik, L., Bruce, D., & Eisenberg, H. M. (1994b). *Tower of London performance in relation to magnetic resonance imaging following closed head injury in children. Neuropsychology, 8, 171–179.*

Lewin, W. (1968). *Rehabilitation after head injury. British Medical Journal, 1, 5–12.*

Lezak, M. D. (1988). *I.Q. RIP. Journal of Clinical and Experimental Neuropsychology, 10, 351–361.*

Martin, D. A. (1988). *Children and adolescents with traumatic brain injury: Impact on the family. Journal of Learning Disabilities, 21, 464–570.*

Martin, J. H., & Brust, J. C. (1985). *Imaging the living brain. In E. R. Kandel & J. H. Schwartz (Eds.), Principles of neural science (pp. 260–283). New York: Elsevier.*

Mattson, A. J., & Levin, H. S. (1990). *Frontal lobe dysfunction following closed head injury. Journal of Nervous and Mental Disease, 178, 282–291.*

Mattson, A. J., Levin, H. S., & Breitmeyer, B. (1994). *Visual information processing after severe closed head injury. Effects of forward and backward masking. Journal of Neurology, Neurosurgery, and Psychiatry, 57, 818–824.*

Meyers, C., & Levin, H. S. (1992). *Temporal perception following closed head injury: Relationship of orientation and attention span. Neuropsychiatry, Neuropsychology, and Behavioral Neurology, 5, 28–32.*

Murray, R., Shum, D., & McFarland, K. (1992). *Attentional deficits in head-injured children: An information processing analysis. Brain and Cognition, 18, 99–115.*

Nass, R., & Koch, D. (1987). *Temperament differences in toddlers with early unilateral right and left brain damage. Developmental Neuropsychology, 3(2), 93–99.*

Obrzut, J. E. (1987). *The elusive relationship between laterality performance and cognitive ability: A commentary. Journal of Learning Disabilities, 20, 170–171.*

Obrzut, J. E., & Hynd, G. W. (1983). *Implications of neuropsychology for learning disabilities. Journal of Learning Disabilities, 16, 532–533.*

Obrzut, J. E., & Hynd, G. W. (1987). *Cognitive dysfunction and psychoeducational assessment in individuals with acquired brain injury. Journal of Learning Disabilities, 20, 596–602.*

Obrzut, J. E., Hynd, G. W., Obrzut, A., & Pirozzolo, F. J. (1981). *Effect of directed attention on dichotic ear asymmetries in normal and learning disabled children. Developmental Psychology, 17, 118–125.*

Papanicolaou, A. C., DiScenna, A., Gillespie, L., & Aram, D. (1990). *Probe evoked potential findings following unilateral left-hemisphere lesions in children. Archives of Neurology, 47, 562–566.*

Reeder, K. P., & Logue, P. E. (1994). *The effects of traumatic brain injury on information processing. Archives of Clinical Neuropsychology, 9, 491–500.*

Reid, D., & Kelly, M. (1993). Wechsler Memory Scale–Revised in closed head injury. *Journal of Clinical Psychology, 49, 245–253.*

Reitan, R. M., & Wolfson, D. (1985). *The Halstead-Reitan Neuropsychological Test Battery: Theory and clinical interpretation. Tucson, AZ: Neuropsychological Press.*

Reitan, R. M., Wolfson, D., & Hom, J. (1992). Left cerebral dominance for bilateral simultaneous sensory stimulation. *Journal of Clinical Psychology, 48, 760–766.*

Rourke, B. P. (1987). Syndrome of nonverbal learning disabilities: The final common pathway of white-matter disease/dysfunction. *The Clinical Neuropsychologist, 1, 209–234.*

Russell, E. W., & Russell, S. L. (1993). Left temporal lobe brain damage pattern on the WAIS, addendum. *Journal of Clinical Psychology, 49, 241–242.*

Segalowitz, S. J., & Brown, D. (1991). Mild head injury as a source of developmental disabilities. *Journal of Learning Disabilities, 24, 551–559.*

Selz, M., & Reitan, R. M. (1979). Comparative test performance of normal, learning-disabled, and brain damaged older children. *Journal of Nervous and Mental Disease, 167, 298–302.*

Sherer, M., Parsons, O., Nixon, S. J., & Adams, R. (1991). Clinical validity of the Speech Sounds Perception Test and the Seashore Rhythm Test. *Journal of Clinical and Experimental Psychology, 13, 741–751.*

Sherer, M., Scott, J., Parsons, O. A., & Adams, R. L. (1994). Relative sensitivity of the WAIS-R, subtests and the selected HRNB measures to the effects of brain damage. *Archives of Clinical Neuropsychology, 9, 427–436.*

Shue, K. L., & Douglas, V. I. (1992). Attention deficit hyperactivity disorder and the frontal lobe syndrome. *Brain and Cognition, 20, 104–124.*

Spreen, O. (1989). The relationship between learning disability, emotional disorders, and neuropsychology: Some results and observations. *Journal of Clinical and Experimental Neuropsychology, 11, 117–140.*

Stiles, J., & Nass, R. (1991). Spatial grouping ability in young children with congenital right or left hemisphere brain injury. *Brain and Cognition, 15, 201–222.*

Szekeres, S. F., & Meserve, N. F. (1994). Collaboration intervention in schools after traumatic brain injury. *Topics in Language Disorders, 15(1), 21–36.*

Thal, D. J., Marchman, V. A., Stiles, J., Aram, D., Trachner, D., Nass, R., & Bates, E. (1991). Early lexical development in children with focal brain injury. *Brain and Language, 40, 491–527.*

Thompson, N. M., Francis, D. J., Steubing, K. K., & Fletcher, J. M. (1994). Motor, visual spatial, and somatosensory skills after closed head injury in children and adolescents: A study of change. *Neuropsychology, 8, 333–342.*

Verduyn, W. H., Hilt, J., Roberts, M. A., & Roberts, R. J. (1992). Multiple partial seizure-like symptoms following minor closed head injury. *Brain Injury, 6(3), 245–260.*

Vikki, J., & Holst, P. (1989). Speed–accuracy optimization in acquisition of figures after focal cerebral lesion. *Cortex, 25, 363–369.*

Villa, G., Gainotti, G., DeBonis, C., & Marra, C. (1990). Double disassociation between temporal and spatial pattern processing in patients with frontal and parietal damage. *Cortex, 26, 399–407.*

Wechsler, D. (1974). *Wechsler intelligence scale for children–Revised. San Antonio, TX: Psychological Corp.*

Wechsler, D. (1981). *Wechsler adult intelligence scale–Revised.* San Antonio, TX: Psychological Corp.

Wechsler, D. (1987). *Wechsler Memory Scale–Revised manual.* San Antonio, TX: Psychological Corp.

Williams, D. L., Gridley, B. E., & Fitzhugh-Bell, K. (1992). Cluster analysis of children and adolescents with brain damage and learning disabilities using neuropsychological, psychoeducational, and sociobehavioral variables. *Journal of Learning Disabilities, 25,* 290–299.

Wilson, J. T., Teasdale, G. M., Hadley, D. M., Wiedmann, K. D., & Lang, D. (1994). Post traumatic amnesia: Still a valuable yardstick. *Journal of Neurology, Neurosurgery, and Psychiatry, 57,* 198–201.

Wood, R. L. (1989). Attention disorders in brain injury rehabilitation. *Journal of Learning Disabilities, 21,* 327–332.

Ylvisaker, M., & Feeney, T. J. (1994). Communication and behavior: Collaboration between speech–language pathologists and behavioral psychologists. *Topics in Language Disorders, 15,* 37–54.

Ylvisaker, M., Kolpan, K. I., & Rosenthal, M. (1994). Collaboration in preparing for personal injury suits after TBI. *Topics in Language Disorders, 15,* 1–20.

CHAPTER 7

Boll, R. (1983). Minor head injury in children—Out of sight, but not out of mind. *Journal of Clinical Child Psychology, 12,* 74–80.

Brooks, D. N. (1991). The head-injury family. *Journal of Clinical and Experimental Neuropsychology, 13,* 155–188.

Brown, G., Chadwick, O., Schaffer, P. Rutter, M., & Traub, M. (1981). A prospective study of children with head injuries: III. Psychiatric sequelae. *Psychological Medicine, 11,* 63–78.

Byles, J., Byrne, C., Boyle, M. H., & Oxford, O. R. (1988). Ontario Child Health Study: Reliability and validity of the General Functioning subscale of the McMaster Family Assessment Device. *Family Process, 27,* 97–104.

Carver, C., Scheier, M., & Weintraub, J. (1989). Assessing coping strategies: A theoretically based approach. *Journal of Personality and Social Psychology, 56,* 267–283.

Derogatis, L., & Melisaratos, N. (1983). The Brief Symptom Inventory: An introductory report. *Psychological Medicine, 13,* 595–605.

Derogatis, L. R., & Spencer, P. M. (1982). Administration and procedures: BSI manual-I. Baltimore: Clinical Psychometric Research.

Drotar, S., Taylor, H. G., Wade, S. L., Stancin, T., Schatschneider, C., & Yeates, K. O. (1996). The Family Burden of Injury Interview: Reliability and validity studies. Unpublished manuscript.

Fletcher, J., Ewing-Cobbs, L., Miner, M., Levin, H., & Eisenberg, H. (1990). Behavioral changes after closed head injury in children. *Journal of Consulting and Clinical Psychology, 58,* 93–98.

Fletcher, J., & Levin, H. (1988). Neurobehavioral effects of brain injury in children. In D. Routh (Ed.), Handbook of pediatric psychology (pp. 258–295). New York: Guilford.

Goldstein, F., & Levin, H. (1987). Epidemiology of pediatric closed head injury: Incidence, clinic characteristics, and risk factors. Journal of Learning Disabilities, 20, 518–525.

Hack, M., Taylor, H. G. Klein, N., Eiben, R., Schatschneider, C., & Mercuri-Minich, N. (1994). School-age outcomes in children with birth weights under 750g. The New England Journal of Medicine, 331, 753–759.

Harris, B., Schwaitzberg, S., Seman, T., & Herman, C. (1989). The hidden morbidity of pediatric trauma. Journal of Pediatric Surgery, 24, 103–106.

Jennett, B., & Bond, M. (1975). Assessment of outcome after severe brain damage. Lancet, 1, 480–487.

Levin, H., Benton, A., & Grossman, R. (1982). Neurobehavioral consequences of closed head injury. New York: Oxford University Press.

Livingston, M. G., & Brooks, D. N. (1988). The burden on families of the brain injured: A review. Journal of Head Trauma Rehabilitation, 3, 6–15.

Mayer, T., Matlack, M., Johnson, D., & Walker, M. (1980). The Modified Injury Severity Scale in pediatric multiple trauma patients. Journal of Pediatric Surgery, 15, 719–726.

Miller, I. W., Bishop, D. S., Epstein, N. B., & Keitner, G. I. (1985). The McMaster Family Assessment Device: Reliability and validity. Journal of Marital and Family Therapy, 11, 345–356.

Moos, R. H., Fenn, C. B., Billings, A. G., & Moos, B. I. (1989). Assessing life stressors and social resources: Applications to alcoholic patients. Journal of Substance Abuse, 1, 135–152.

Oddy, M., Humphrey, M., & Uttley, D. (1978). Stresses upon the relatives of head-injured patients. British Journal of Psychiatry, 133, 507–513.

Perrott, S., Taylor, H., & Montes, J. (1991). Neuropsychological sequela, family stress, and environmental adaptation following pediatric head injury. Developmental Neuropsychology, 7, 69–86.

Rivara, J. B. (1994). Family functioning following pediatric traumatic brain injury. Pediatric Annals, 23, 38–43.

Rivara, J., Fay, G., Jaffe, K., Polissar, N., Shurtleff, H., & Martin, K. (1992). Predictors of family functioning one year following traumatic brain injury in children. Archives of Physical Medicine and Rehabilitation, 73, 899–910.

Rolland, J. S. (1987). Chronic illness and the life cycle: A conceptual framework. Family Process, 26, 203–221.

Rutter, M. (1981). Psychological sequelae of brain damage in children. American Journal of Psychiatry, 138, 1533–1534.

Rutter, M., Chadwick, O., & Shaffer, D. (1983). Head injury. In M. Rutter (Ed.), Developmental neuropsychiatry (pp. 83–111). New York: Guilford.

Stein, R. E. K., & Jessop, D. T. (1985). PACTS papers/AECOM: Tables documenting the psychometric properties of a measure of the impact of chronic illness on a family. Bronx, NY: Department of Pediatrics, Albert Einstein College of Medicine.

Taylor, H. G., Drotar, D., Wade, S., Yates, K., Stancin, T., & Klein, S. (in press). Recovery from traumatic brain injury in children: The importance of the family. In S. Broman & M. E. Michael (Eds.), Traumatic brain injury in children. Cambridge, England: Oxford University Press.

Waaland, P., & Kreutzer, J. (1988). Family response to childhood traumatic brain injury. Journal of Head Trauma Rehabilitation, 3, 51–63.

Wade, S., Drotar, D., Taylor, H. G., & Stancin, T. (1995). Assessing the effects of traumatic brain injury (TBI) on family functioning: Conceptual and methodological issues. Journal of Pediatric Psychology, 20, 737–753.

CHAPTER 8

Asarnow, R. F., Satz, P., Light, R., & Lewis, R. (1991). Behavior problems and adaptive functioning in children with mild and severe closed head injury. Journal of Pediatric Psychology, 16, 543–555.

Bandura, A. (1986). Social foundations of thought and action: A social-cognitive theory. Englewood Cliffs, NJ: Prentice-Hall.

Begali, V. (1992). Head injury in children and adolescents: A resource and review for school and allied professionals. Brandon, VT: Clinical Psychology Publishing.

Bijur, P. E., Haslum, M., & Golding, J. (1990). Cognitive and behavioral sequelae of mild head injury in children. Pediatrics, 86, 337–344.

Brown, G. W., Chadwick, O., Shaffer, D., Rutter, M., & Traub, M. (1981). A prospective study of children with head injuries: 3. Psychiatric sequelae. Psychological Medicine, 11, 63–78.

Capruso, D., & Levin, H. S. (1992). Cognitive impairment following closed head injury. Neurology Clinics, 10, 879–893.

Casey, R., Ludwig, S., & McCormick, M. C. (1986). Morbidity following minor head trauma in children. Pediatrics, 78, 497–502.

Clark, E., Baker, B. K., Gardner, M. K., Pompa, J. L., & Tait, F. V. (1990). Effectiveness of stimulant drug treatment for attention problems. School Psychology International, 11, 227–234.

Cope, D. N. (1987). Psychopharmacologic considerations in the treatment of traumatic brain injury. Journal of Head Trauma Rehabilitation, 2, 2–5.

Dalby, P. R., & Obrzut, J. E. (1991). Epidemiologic characteristics and sequelae of closed head–injured children and adolescents: A review. Developmental Neuropsychology, 7(1), 35–68.

Deaton, A. V. (1994). Changing the behaviors of students with acquired brain injuries. In R. C. Savage & G. F. Wolcott (Eds.), Educational dimensions of acquired brain injury (pp. 257–276). Austin, TX: PRO-ED.

Dempster, F. N. (1988). The spacing effect: A case study in the failure to apply the results of psychological research. American Psychologist, 43, 627–634.

Di Scala, C., Osberg, J. S., Gans, B. M., Chin, L. J., & Grant, C. C. (1991). Children with traumatic head injury: Morbidity and postacute treatment. Archives of Physical Medicine and Rehabilitation, 72, 662–666.

Donders, J. (1992). Premorbid behavioral and psychosocial adjustment of children with traumatic brain injury. Journal of Abnormal Child Psychology, 20, 233–246.

Fay, G. C, Jaffe, K. M., Polissar, N. L., Liao, S., Martin, K. M., Shurtleff, H. A., Rivara, J. M., & Winn, H. R. (1994). Mild pediatric traumatic brain injury: A cohort study. Archives of Physical Medicine and Rehabilitation, 74, 895–901.

Fletcher, J. M., Ewing-Cobbs, L., Miner, M. E., Levin, H. S., & Eisenberg, H. M. (1993). Behavioral changes after closed head injury in children. Journal of Consulting and Clinical Psychology, 58, 93–98.

Foxx, R. M., & Shapiro, S. T. (1978). The time-out ribbon: A non-exclusionary time-out procedure. Journal of Applied Behavior Analysis, 11, 125–136.

Franzen, M. D., & Lovell, M. R. (1987). Behavioral treatments of aggressive sequelae of brain injury. Psychiatric Annals, 17, 389–396.

Glenn, M. B. (1987a). A pharmacological approach to aggressive and disruptive behaviors after traumatic brain injury: Part 1. Journal of Head Trauma Rehabilitation, 2, 71–73.

Glenn, M. B. (1987b). A pharmacological approach to aggressive and disruptive behaviors after traumatic brain injury: Part 2. Journal of Head Trauma Rehabilitation, 2, 80–81.

Greenspan, A. I. & MacKenzie, E. J. (1994). Functional outcome after pediatric head injury. Pediatrics, 94, 425–432.

Haas, J. F., & Cope, N. (1985). Neuropharmacologic management of behavior sequelae in head injury: A case report. Archives in Physical Medicine Rehabilitation, 66, 472–474.

Heller, M. S., & White, M. A. (1975). Rates of approval and disapproval to higher and lower ability classes. Journal of Educational Psychology, 67, 769–800.

Jaffe, K. M., Fay, G. C., Polissar, N. L., Martin, K. M., Shurtleff, H., Rivara, J. B., & Winn, H. R. (1993). Severity of pediatric traumatic brain injury and early neurobehavioral outcome: A cohort study. Archives of Physical Medicine and Rehabilitation, 73, 540–547.

Kehle, T. J., Clark, E., Jenson, W. R., & Wampold, B. E. (1986). Effectiveness of self-observation with behavior disordered elementary school children. School Psychology Review, 15, 289–295.

Kehle, T. J., & Gonzales, F. (1991). Self-modeling for emotional and social concerns of childhood. In P. W. Dowrick (Ed.), A practical guide to video in the behavioral sciences (pp. 221–252). New York: Wiley.

Kehle, T. J., Jenson, W. R., & Clark, E. (1992). Teacher acceptance of psychological interventions: An allegiance to intuition? School Psychology International, 13, 307–312.

Kehle, T. J., Sutilla, H., & Visnic, M. (1994, March). Augmentation of self-modeling with behavioral strategies: Case study of an intentional enuretic and electively mute child. Paper presented at the annual meeting of the National Association of School Psychologists, Seattle, WA.

Knights, R. M., Ivan, L. P., Ventureyra, E. C., Bentivoglio, C., Stoddart, C., Winogron, W., & Bawden, H. N. (1991). The effects of head injury in children on neuropsychological and behavioural functioning. Brain Injury, 5, 339–351.

Levin, H. S. (1987). Neurobehavioral sequelae of head injury. In P. R. Cooper (Ed.), Head injury (2nd ed.). Baltimore: Williams and Wilkins.

Malec, J. (1984). Training the brain-injured client in behavioral self-management skills. In B. A. Edelstein & E. T. Couture (Eds.), Behavioral assessment and rehabilitation of the traumatically brain damaged (pp. 121–150). New York: Plenum.

Mapou, R. L. (1992). Neuropathology and neuropsychology of behavioral disturbance following traumatic brain injury. In C. L. Long & L. K. Ross (Eds.), Handbook of head trauma: Acute care to recovery (pp. 75–90). New York: Plenum.

McAllister, T. W. (1992). Neuropsychiatric sequelae of head injuries. Psychiatric Clinics of North America, 15, 522–534.

McKinlay, W. W., Brooks, M. R., Bond, M. R., Martinage, D. P., & Marshall, M. M. (1981). The short term outcome of severe blunt head injury as reported by relatives of the injured patients. Journal of Neurology, Neurosurgery and Psychiatry, 48, 527–533.

Michaud, L. J., Duhaime, A., & Batshaw, M. L. (1993). Traumatic brain injury in children. Pediatric Clinics of North America, 40, 553–565.

Michaud, L. J., Rivara, F. P., Jaffe, K. M., Fay, G., & Dailey, J. L. (1993). Traumatic brain injury as a risk factor for behavioral disorders in children. Archives of Physical Medicine Rehabilitation, 74, 368–375.

Reavis, H. K., Jenson, W. R., Kukic, S. J., & Morgan, D. P. (1993). Utah's BEST project: Behavioral and educational strategies for teachers. Salt Lake City: Utah State Office of Education.

Rhode, G., Jenson, W. R., & Reavis, H. K. (1993). The tough kid book: Practical classroom management strategies. Longmont, CO: Sopris West.

Rose, M. J. (1988). The place of drugs in the management of behavior disorders after traumatic brain injury. Journal of Head Trauma Rehabilitation, 3, 7–13.

Rosenthal, M., & Bond, M. R. (1990). Behavioral and psychiatric sequelae. In M. Rosenthal, M. Bond, E. R. Griffith, & J. D. Miller (Eds.), Rehabilitation of the adult and child with traumatic brain injury (pp. 179–192). Philadelphia: Davis.

Shutte, R. C., & Hopkins, B. L. (1970). The effects of teacher attention on following instructions in a kindergarten class. Journal of Applied Behavior Analysis, 3, 117–122.

Siassi, I. (1982). Lithium treatment of impulsive behavior in children. Journal of Clinical Psychiatry, 45, 482–484.

Silver, J. M., & Yudofsky, S. C. (1987). Aggressive behavior in patients with neuropsychiatric disorders. Psychiatric Annals, 17, 367–370.

Thomas, D. A., Becker, W. C., & Armstrong, M. (1968). Production and elimination of disruptive classroom behavior by systematically varying teachers' behavior. Journal of Applied Behavior Analysis, 1, 35–45.

Tompkins, C. A., Holland, A. L., Ratcliff, G., & Costello, A. J. (1990). Predicting cognitive recovery from closed head injury in children and adolescents. Brain and Cognition, 13(1), 86–97.

Van Houten, R., & Doley, D. M. (1983). Are social reprimands effective? In S. Axelrod & J. Apsche (Eds.), The effects of punishment on human behavior (pp. 45–70). New York: Academic Press.

Van Houten, R., Nau, P., MacKenzie-Keating, D., Sameoto, D., & Calavecchie, B. (1982). An analysis of some variables influencing the effectiveness of reprimands. Journal of Applied Behavior Analysis, 15, 65–83.

White, M. A. (1975). Natural rates of teacher approval and disapproval in the classroom. Journal of Applied Behavior Analysis, 8, 367–372.

Wood, R. L. (1987). Brain injury rehabilitation: A neurobehavioral approach. Rockville, MD: Aspen.

Yudofsky, S. C., Silver, J. M., & Schneider, S. E. (1987). Pharmacological treatment of aggression. Psychiatric Annals, 17, 397–404.

CHAPTER 9

Abikoff, H. (1987). An evaluation of cognitive behavior therapy for hyperactive children. In B. B. Lahey & A. E. Kazdin (Eds.), Advances in clinical child psychiatry (Vol. 10, pp. 171–216). New York: Plenum.

Abikoff, H. (1991). Cognitive training in ADHD children: Less to it than meets the eye. Journal of Learning Disabilities, 24, 205–209.

Baddeley, A. D. (1992). Implicit memory and errorless learning: A link between cognitive theory and neuropsychological rehabilitation? In L. R. Squire & N. Butters (Eds.) Neuropsychology of memory (2nd ed., pp. 309–314). New York: Guilford Press.

Barkley, R. A. (1988). Attention. In M. G. Tramontana & S. R. Hooper (Eds.), Assessment issues in child neuropsychology (pp. 145–176). New York: Plenum.

Barkley, R. A., Copeland, A. P., and Sivage, C. (1980). A self-control classroom for hyperactive children. Journal of Autism and Developmental Disorders, 10, 75–89.

Barth, J. T., Gideon, D. A., Sciara, A. D., Halsey, P. H., & Anchor, K. N. (1986). Forensic aspects of mild head trauma. Journal of Head Trauma Rehabilitation, 1, 62–70.

Beers, S. R. (1992). Cognitive effects of mild head injury in children and adolescents. Neuropsychology Review, 3(4), 281–320.

Ben-Yishay, Y., Piasetsky, E. B., & Rattock, J. (1987). A systematic method for amelioratirig disorders in basic attention. In M. J. Meyer, A. L. Benton, & L. Diller (Eds.), Neuropsycholcgical rehabilitation (pp. 165–181). Edinburgh: Churchill Livingstone.

Bigler, E. D. (1987). Acquired cerebral trauma: Behavioral, neuropsychiatric, psychoeducational assessment, and cognitive retraining issues. Journal of Learning Disabilities, 20, 579–580.

Binder, L. M. (1986). Persisting symptoms after mild head injury: A review of the postconcussive syndrome. Journal of Clinical and Experimental Neuropsychology, 8, 323–346.

Boll, T. J., & Barth, J. T. (1981). Neuropsychology of brain damage in children. In S. B. Filskov & T. J. Barth (Eds.), Handbook of clinical neuropsychology (Vol. 1, pp. 418–452). New York: Wiley.

Borkowski, J. G., Peck, V. A., Reid, M. K., & Kurtz, B. E. (1983). Impulsivity and strategy transfer: Metamemory as mediator. Child Development, 54, 459–473.

Brady, H. V., & Richnian, L. C. (1994). Visual versus verbal mnemonic training effects on memory-deficient and language-deficient subgroups of children with reading disability. Developmental Neuropsychology, 10, 335–347.

Brickenkamp, R. (1981). Test d2: Concentration–Endurance Test: Manual (5th ed.). Gottigen, Germany: Verlag für Psychologie.

Brooks, D. N., & Baddeley, A. D. (1976). What can amnesic patients learn? Neuropsychalogia, 14, 111–122.

Case, R. (1992). The role of the frontal lobes in the regulation of cognitive development. Brain and Cognition, 20, 51–73.

Case, R., Kurland, D. M., & Goldberg, J. (1982). Operational efficiency and the growth of short-term memory span. Journal of Experimental Child Psychology, 33, 386–404.

Cermak, L. S. (1975). Imagery as an aid to retrieval for Korsakoff patients. Cortex 11, 163–169.

Charness, N., Milberg, W., & Alexander, M. P. (1988). Teaching an amnesic a complex cognitive skill. Brain and Cognition, 8, 253–272.

Cobb, D. E., & Evans, J. R. (1981). The use of biofeedback techniques with school-aged children exhibiting behavioral and/or learning problems. Journal of Abnormal Child Psychology, 9(2), 251–281.

Cohen, N. J., & Squire, L. R. (1980). Preserved learning and retention of pattern-analyzing skill in amnesia: Dissociation of "knowing how" and "knowing that." Science, 210, 207–209.

Colvin, G. (1990). Procedures for preventing serious acting-out behavior in the classroom. Direct Instruction Newsletter, 9, 27–30.

Crovitz, H. F. (1979). Memory retraining in brain-damaged patients: The airplane list. Cortex, 15, 131–134.

Crowley, J. A., & Miles, M. A. (1991). Cognitive remediation in pediatric head injury: A case study. Journal of Pediatric Psychology, 16, 611–627.

Dalby, P. R., & Obrzut, H. E. (1991). Epidemiological characteristics and sequelae of closed head-injured children and adolescents: A review. Developmental Neuropsychology, 7(1), 35–68.

Dennis, M. (1988). Language and the young damaged brain. In T. Boll & B. K. Bryant (Eds.), Clinical neuropsychology and brain function: Research, measurement, and practice (Vol. 7, pp. 87–123). Washington, DC: American Psychological Association.

Dennis, M., Barnes, M. A., Donnelly, R. E., Wilkinson, M., & Humphreys, R. P. (1996). Appraising and managing knowledge: Metacognitive skills after childhood head injury. Developmental Neuropshycology, 12(1), 77–103.

Diller, L., Ben-Yishay, Y., Gerstman, L. J., Goodkin, R., Gordon, W., & Weinberg, J. (1974). Studies of cognition and rehabilitation in hemiplegia. New York: NYU Medical Center.

Donders, J. (1993). Memory functioning after traumatic brain injury in children. Brain Injury, 7, 431–437.

Engelmann, S. E., & Carnine, D. (1982). Corrective mathematics. Chicago: Science Research Associates.

Ericsson, K. A., & Chase, W. G., (1982). Exceptional memory. American Scientist, 70, 607–615.

Eslinger, P. J., & Grattan, L. M. (1991). Perspective on the developmental consequences of early frontal lobe damage: Introduction. Developmental Neuropsychology, 7, 257–260.

Ewing-Cobbs, L., Fletcher, J. M., & Levin, H. S. (1985). Neuropsychological sequelae following pediatric head injury. In M. Ylvisaker (Ed.), Head injury rehabilitation: Children and adolescents (pp. 71–89). San Diego: College-Hill.

Fay, G. C., Jaffe, K. M., Nayak, L. P., Shequan, L., J'May, B., & Martin, K. (1994). Outcome of pediatric traumatic brain injury at three years: A cohort study. Archives of Psychical Medicine and Rehabilitation, 75, 733–741.

Flavell, J. H., Miller, P. H., & Miller, S. A. (1993) Cognitive development (3rd ed.). Englewood Cliffs, NJ: Prentice-Hall.

Fletcher, J. M., Ewing-Cobbs, L., McLaughlin, E. J., & Levin, H. S. (1985). Cognitive and psychosocial sequelae of head injury in children: Implications for assessment and management. In B. F. Brooks (Ed.), The injured child (pp. 30–39). Austin: University of Texas Press.

Fletcher, J. M., Ewing-Cobbs, L., Miner, M. E., Levin, H. S., & Eisenberg, H. M. (1990). Behavioral changes after closed head injury in children. Journal of Consulting and Clinical Psychology, 58(1), 93–98.

Franzen, M. D., & Haut, M. W. (1991). The psychological treatment of memory impairment: A review of empirical studies. Neuropsychology Review, 2, 29–63.

Fussey, I., & Giles, G. M. (1988). Rehabilitation of the severely brain injured adult: A practical approach. London: Croom Helm.

Garner, R., & Alexander, P. A. (1989). Metacognition: Answered and unanswered questions. Educational Psychologist, 24(2), 143–158.

Ghatala, E. S., Levin, J. R., Pressley, M., & Goodwin, D. (1986). A componential analysis of the effects of derived and supplied-utility information on children's strategy selections. Journal of Experimental Child Psychology, 41, 76–92.

Gianutsos, R., & Gianutsos, J. (1979). Rehabilitating the verbal recall of brain-damaged patients by mnemonic training: An experiental demonstration using single case methodology. Journal of Clinical Neuropsychology, 1, 117–135.

Glang, A., Singer, G., Cooley, E., & Tish, N. (1992). Tailoring direct instruction techniques for use with elementary students with brain injury. Journal of Head Trauma Rehabilitation, 7(4), 93–108.

Glisky, E. L. (1992). Computer-assisted instruction for patients with traumatic brain injury: Teaching of domain-specific knowledge. Journal of Head Trauma Rehabilitation, 7(3), 1–12.

Glisky, E. L., & Schacter, D. L. (1986). Remediation of organic disorders: Current status and future perspectives. Journal of Head Trauma Rehabilitation, 1, 54–63.

Glisky, E. L., & Schacter, D. L. (1987). Acquisition of domain-specific knowledge in organic amnesia: Training for computer-related work. Neuropsychologia, 25, 893–906.

Glisky, E. L., & Schacter, D. L. (1988). Long-term retention of computer learning by patients with memory disorders. Neuropsychologia, 26, 173–178.

Glisky, E. L., & Schacter, D. L. (1989). Extending the limits of complex learning in organic amnesia: Computer training in a vocational domain. Neuropsychologia, 27, 107–120.

Glisky, E. L., Schacter, D. L., & Tulving, E. (1986a). Computer learning by memory-impaired patients: Acquisition and retention of complex knowledge. Neuropsychologia, 24, 313–328.

Glisky, E. L., Schacter, D. L., & Tulving, E. (1986b). Learning and retention of computer-related vocabulary in amnesic patients: Method of vanishing cues. Journal of Clinical and Experimental Neuropsychology, 8, 292–312.

Goldstein, F. G., & Levin, H. S. (1987). Epidemiology of pediatric closed head injury: Incidence, clinical characteristics and risk factors. Journal of Learning Disabilities, 20, 518–525.

Gordon, M., Thomason, D., Cooper, S., & Ivers, C. L. (1991). Nonmedical treatment of ADHD/hyperactivity: The attention training system. Journal of School Psychology, 29, 151–159.

Graf, P., & Schacter, D. L. (1985). Implicit and explicit memory for new associations in normal and amnesic patients. Journal of Experimental Psychology: Learning, Memory and Cognition, 11, 501–518.

Grattan, L. M., & Eslinger, P. J. (1992). Long term psychological consequences of childhood frontal lobe lesion in patient DR. Brain and Cognition, 20, 185–195.

Gray, J. M., & Robertson, I. (1989). Remediation of attentional difficulties following brain injury: Three experimental single case studies. Brain Injury, 3, 163–170.

Gray, J. M., Robertson, I., Pentland, B., & Anderson, S. (1992). Microcomputer-based attentional retraining after brain damage: A randomized group controlled trial. Neuropsychological Rehabilitation, 2, 97–115.

Gulbrandsen, G. B. (1984). Neuropsychological sequelae of light head injuries in older children 6 months after trauma. Journal of Clinical Neuropsychology, 6, 257–268.

Harris, J. E. (1992). Ways to help memory. In B. Wilson & N. Moffat (Eds.), Clinical management of memory problems (2nd ed., pp. 59–85). London: Aspen.

Johnson, D. A., Roethig-Johnston, K., & Middleton, J. (1988). Development and induction of an attentional test for head-injured children—I. Information processing capacity in a normal sample. Journal of Child Psychology and Psychiatry, 29, 199–208.

Kail, R., & Bisanz, J. (1982). Information processing and cognitive development. In H. Reese (Ed.), Advances in child development and behavior (Vol. 17, pp. 45–81). New York: Academic Press.

Kaufmann, P. M., Fletcher, J. M., Levin, H. S., & Miner, M. E. (1993). Attentional disturbance after pediatric closed head injury. Journal of Child Neurology, 8, 348–353.

Kendall, P. C., & Braswell, L. (1993). Cognitive–behavioral therapy for impulsive children. New York: Guilford.

Kendall, P. C., & Panichelli-Mindel, S. M. (1995). Cognitive behavioral treatments. Journal of Abnormal Child Psychology, 34(1), 107–124.

Kennard, M. A., (1942). Cortical reorganization of motor function. Archives of Neurology and Psychology, 48, 227–240.

Kerns, K. A., Thomson, J., & Youngman, P. (1993, March). Development of a compensatory memory system for an adolescent. Paper presented at the Pediatric Brain Injury Conference, Vancouver, British Columbia.

Klonoff, H., Clark, C., & Klonoff, P. S. (1993). Long-term outcome of head injuries: A 23 year follow up study of children with head injuries. Journal of Neurology, Neurosurgery and Psychiatry, 56(4), 410–415.

Knights, R. M., Ivan, L. P., Ventureyra, E. C. G., Bentivoglio, C., Stoddardt, C., Winogron, W., & Bawden, H. N. (1991). The effects of head injury in children on neuropsychological and behavioral functioning. Brain Injury, 5, 339–351.

Lee, S. W. (1991). Biofeedback as a treatment for child hyperactivity: A critical review of the literature. Psychological Reports, 68(1), 163–192.

Levin, H. S., Benton, A. L., & Grossman, R. G. (1982). Neurobehavioral consequences of closed head injury. New York: Oxford University Press.

Levin, H. S., Cuihâne, K. A., Mendelsohn, D., Lilly, M. A., Bruce, D., Fletcher, J. M., Chapman, S. B., Harward, H., & Eisenberg, H. M. (1993). Cognition in relation to magnetic resonance imaging in head-injured children and adolescents. Archives of Neurology, 50, 897–905.

Levin, H. S., Ewing-Cobbs, L., & Benton, A. L. (1984). Age and recovery from brain damage: A review of clinical studies. In S. W. Scheff (Ed.), Aging and recovery of function in the central nervous system (pp. 169–205). New York: Plenum.

Levin, H. S., High, W., Ewing-Cobbs, L., Fletcher, J. M., Eisenberg, H. M., Miner, M. E., & Goldstein, F. (1988). Memory functioning during the first year after closed head injury in children and adolescents. Neurosurgery, 22, 1043–1052.

Loper, A. B. (1982). Metacognitive training to correct academic deficiency. Topics in Learning & Learning Disabilities, 2, 61–68.

Lubar, J. F. (1991). Discourse on the development of EEG diagnostics and biofeedback for attention-deficit/hyperactivity disorders. Biofeedback and Self-Regulation, 16(3), 201–225.

Lubar, J. O., & Lubar, J. F. (1984). Electroencephalographic biofeedback of SMR and beta for treatment of attention deficit disorders in a clinical setting. Biofeedback and Self-Regulation, 9, 1–23.

Mateer, C. A. (1992). Systems of care for post-concussive syndrome. In L. J. Horn & N. D. Zasler (Eds.), Rehabilitation of post-concussive disorders (pp. 143–160). Philadelphia: Henley & Belius.

Mateer, C. A., & Sohlberg, M. M. (1988). A paradigm shift in memory rehabilitation. In H. Whitaker (Ed.), Neuropsychological studies of nonfocal brain injury: Dementia and closed head injury (pp. 204–219). New York: Springer-Verlag.

Mateer, C. A., Sohlberg, M. M., & Youngman, P. (1990). The management of acquired attention and memory disorders following mild closed head injury. In R. Wood (Ed.), Cognitive rehabilitation in perspective (pp. 68–96). London: Taylor & Francis.

Mateer, C. A., & Williams, D. (1991). Effects of frontal lobe injury in childhood. Developmental Neuropsychology, 7(2), 359–376.

McCarney, S. B. (1989). Attention deficit disorders evaluation scale. Columbia, MI: Hawthorne Educational Services.

Mullin, L. L., & Lange, U. A. (1984). Does the ability of kindergarten children to retain auditory and visual stimuli improve with training? Language, Speech and Hearing Services in Schools, 15(3), 210–215.

Niemann, H., Ruff, R. M., & Baser, C. A. (1990). Computer-assisted attention retraining in head injured individuals: A controlled efficacy study of an outpatient program. Journal of Consulting and Clinical Psychology, 58, 811–817.

O'Connor, M., & Cermak, L. S. (1987). Rehabilitation of organic memory disorders. In M. J. Meier, A. L. Benton, & L. Diller (Eds.), Neuropsychological rehabilitation (pp. 260–279). New York: Guilford.

Prigatano, G. P. (1991). Disturbances in self-awareness of deficit after traumatic brain injury. In G. P. Prigatano & D. L. Schacter (Eds.), Awareness of deficit after brain injury (pp. 111–126). New York: Oxford University Press.

Prigatano, G. P., O'Brien, K. P., & Klonoff, P. S. (1993). Neuropsychological rehabilitation of young adults who suffer brain injury in childhood: Clinical observations. Neuropsychological Rehabilitation, 3, 411–421.

Reid, M. K., & Borkowski, J. G. (1987). Causal attributions of hyperactive children: Implications for teaching strategies and self control. Journal of Educational Psychology, 79, 296–307.

Rutter, M. (1981). Psychological sequelae of brain damage in children. American Journal of Psychiatry, 183, 1533–1542.

Schinitter-Edgecombe, M., Fahy, J. F., Whelan, J. P., & Long, C. J. (1995). Memory remediation after severe closed head injury: Notebook training versus supportive therapy. Journal of Clinical and Consulting Psychology, 63, 484–489.

Schretlin, D., Bobholz, J. H., & Brandt, J. (in press). Development and psychometric properties of the Brief Test of Attention. The Clinical Neuropsychologist.

Semrud-Clikeman, M., Teeter, P. A., Parle, N., & Connor, R. T. (1995, April) Innovative approaches for working with children with ADHD. Paper presented at the annual conference of the American Educational Research Association, San Francisco, CA.

Sidman, M., & Stoddard, L. T. (1967). The effectiveness of fading in programming in simultaneous form discrimination for retarded children. Journal of Experimental Analysis of Behavior, 10, 3–15.

Sivak, M., Hill, C. S., Henson, D. L., Butler, B. P., Silber, S. M., & Olson, P. (1984). Improved driving performance following perceptual retraining in persons with brain damage. Archives of Physical Medicine and Rehabilitation, 65, 163–167.

Sohlberg, M. M., & Mateer, C. A. (1987). Effectiveness of an attention training program. Journal of Clinical and Experimental Neuropsychology, 19, 117–130.

Sohlberg, M. M., & Mateer, C. A. (1989a). Introduction to cognitive rehabilitation: Theory and practice. New York: Guilford.

Sohlberg, M. M., & Mateer, C. A. (1989b). Training use of compensatory memory books: A three stage behavioral approach. Journal of Clinical and Experimental Neuropsychology, 11, 871–891.

Squire, L. R. (1987). Memory and brain. New York: Oxford University Press.

Sturm, W., Hartje, W., Orgass, B., & Willmes, K. (1993). Computer-assisted rehabilitation of attention impairments. In F. Stachowiak (Ed.), Developments in the assessment and rehabilitation of brain-damaged patients (pp. 126–151). Tubingen, Germany: Narr.

Tansey, M. A. (1985). Brainwave signatures: An index reflective of the brain's functional neuroanatomy: Further findings on the effect of EEG sensorimotor rhythm biofeedback training on the neurologic precursors of learning disabilities. International Journal of Psychophysiology, 3, 85–99.

Tansey, M. A. (1990). Righting the rhythms of reason: EEG biofeedback training as a therapeutic modality in a clinical office setting. Medical Psychotherapy, 3, 57–68.

Telzrow, C. F. (1987). Management of academic and educational problems in head injury. Journal of Learning Disabilities, 20, 57–68

Terrace, H. S. (1963). Discrimination learning with and without "errors." Journal of Experimental Analysis of Behavior, 6, 1–27.

Thompson, N. M., Francis, D. J., Stuebing, K. K., Fletcher, J. M., Ewing-Cobbs, L., Miner, M. E., Levin, H. S., & Eisenberg, H. M., (1994). Motor, visual-spatial, and somatasensory skills after closed head injury in children and adolescents: A study of change. Neuropsychology, 8(3), 333–342.

Thomson, J. (1995). Rehabilitation of high school–aged individuals with traumatic brain injury through utilization of an attention training program. Journal of the International Neuropsychological Society, 1, 149.

Thomson, J. B., & Kerns, K. A. (in press). Cognitive rehabilitation of the child with mild traumatic brain injury. In S. Raskin & C. A. Mateer (Eds.), Neuropsychological management of mild traumatic brain injury. New York: Oxford University Press.

Touchette, P. E. (1968). The effects of graduated stimulus change on the acquisition of a simple discrimination in severely retarded boys. Journal of Experimental Analysis of Behavior, 11, 39–48.

Unsal, A., & Segalowitz, S. J. (1985). Sources of P300 attenuation after head injury: Single-trial amplitude, latency jitter, and EEG power. Psychophysiology, 32, 249–256.

Van Zomeren, A. H., & Brouwer, W. H. (1994). Clinical neuropsychology of attention. New York: Oxford University Press.

Wang, A. Y., & Richarde, R. S. (1987). Development of memory-monitoring and self-efficacy in children. Psychological Reports, 60, 647–658.

Warrington, E. K, & Weinskrantz, L. (1968). New method of testing long-term retention with special reference to amnesic patients. Nature, 217, 972–974.

Warrington, E. K., & Weinskrantz, L. (1974). The effect of prior learning on subsequent retention in amnesic patents. Neuropsychologia, 12, 419–428.

White, W. A. T. (1988). A meta-analysis of the effects of direct instruction in special education. Education and Treatment of Children, 11, 364–374.

Williams, D. J. (1989). A process-specific training program in the treatment of attention deficits in children. Unpublished doctoral dissertation, University of Washington.

Wilson, B. (1982). Success and failure in memory training following a cerebral vascular accident. Cortex, 18, 581–594.

Wilson, B. (1987). Rehabilitation of memory. New York: Guilford.

Wilson, B. A., Baddeley, A., Evans, J., & Shiel, A. (1994). Errorless learning in the rehabilitation of memory impaired people. Neuropsychological Rehabilitation, 4, 307–326.

Wilson, B. A., & Evans, J. J. (1996). Error-free learning in the rehabilitation of people with memory impairments. Journal of Head Trauma Rehabilitation, 11, 54–64.

Wood, R. L., & Fussey, I. (1987). *Computer-assisted cognitive retraining: A controlled study. International Disability Studies, 9, 149–153.*

Ylsivaker, M. (1985). *Head injury rehabilitation: Children and adolescents. San Diego: College-Hill.*

Zimmerman, B. J. (1990). *Self-regulated learning and academic achievement: An overview. Educational Psychologist, 25(1), 3–17.*

CHAPTER 10

Allen, K., Linn, R. T., Gutierrez, H., & Willer, B. S. (1994). *Family burden following traumatic brain injury. Rehabilitation Psychology, 39, 30–48.*

Asarnow, R. F., Lewis, R., & Neumann, E. (1991). *Behavior problems and adaptive functioning in children with mild and severe closed head injury. Journal of Pediatric Psychology, 16, 545–555.*

Barry, P., & O'Leary, J. (1989). *Roles of the psychologist on a traumatic brain injury rehabilitation team. Rehabilitation Psychology, 34(2), 83–90.*

Ben-Yishay, Y., & Prigatano, G. P. (1990). *Cognitive rehabilitation. In M. Rosenthal, M. R. Bond, J. D. Miller, & E. R. Griffith (Eds.). Rehabilitation of the adult and child with traumatic brain injury (2nd ed., pp. 393–409). Philadelphia: Davis.*

Bigler, E. E. (1989). *Behavioural and cognitive changes in traumatic brain injury: A spouse's perspective. Brain Injury, 3, 73–78.*

Black, P., Jeffries, J. J., Blumer, D., Wellner, A., & Walker, A. E. (1969). *The posttraumatic syndrome in children. In A. E. Walker, E. E. Caveness, & M. Critchley (Eds.), The late effects of head injury (pp. 187–201). Springfield, IL: Thomas.*

Bond, M. R. (1983). *Effects on the family system. In M. Rosenthal, E. R. Griffith, & M. R. Bond (Eds.), Rehabilitation of the head injured adult (pp. 209–217). Philadelphia: F. A. Davis.*

Bragg, R. M., Klockars, A. J., & Berninger, V. W. (1992). *Comparison of families with and without adolescents with traumatic brain injury. Journal of Head Trauma Rehabilitation, 7(3), 94–108.*

Breslau, N. (1982). *Siblings of disabled children: Birth order and age-spacing effects. Journal of Abnormal Child Psychology, 10, 85–96.*

Breslau, N. (1983). *The psychological study of chronically ill and disabled children: Are healthy siblings appropriate controls? Journal of Abnormal Child Psychology, 11, 379–391.*

Brooks, D. N. (1984). *Head injury and the family. In D. N. Brooks (Ed.), Closed head injury: Psychological, social and family consequences (pp. 123–147). Cambridge, England: Oxford University Press.*

Brooks, D. N. (1991a). *The head-injured family. Journal of Clinical Experimental Neuropsychology, 13, 155–188.*

Brooks, D. N. (1991b). *The effectiveness of post-acute rehabilitation. Brain Injury, 1, 5–19.*

Brooks, D. N., Campsie, L., Symington, C., Beattie, A., & McKinlay, W. (1986). *The Five-year outcome of severe blunt head injury: A relative's view. Journal of Neurology, Neurosurgery, and Psychiatry, 49, 764–800.*

Brooks, D. N., Campsie, L., Symington, C., Beattie, A., & McKinlay, W. (1987). The effects of severe-head injury on patient and relatives within seven years of injury. Journal of Head Trauma Rehabilitation, 2(2), 1–13.

Brooks, D. N., & McKinlay, W. (1983). Personality and behavioral changes after severe blunt head injury: A relative's view. Journal of Neurology, Neurosurgery, and Psychiatry, 46, 336–344.

Chadwick, O. (1985). Psychological sequelae of head injury in children. Developmental Medicine and Child Neurology, 27, 69–79.

Chinitz, S. P. (1981). A sibling group for brothers and sisters of handicapped children. Children Today, 15, 21–23.

DePompei, R., & Zarski, J. J. (1989). Families, head injury, and cognitive-communicative impairments: Issues for family counseling. Topics in Language Disorders, 9, 78–89.

Dyson, L., Edgar, E., & Crnic, K. (1989). Psychological predictors of adjustment by siblings of developmentally disabled children. American Journal of Mental Retardation, 94, 292–302.

Eiben, C. F., Anderson, T. P., Lockman, L., Matthews, D. J., Dryjia, R., Martin, J., Burrill, C., Gottesman, N., O'Brian, P., & Witte, L. (1984). Functional outcome of closed head injury in children and young adults. Archives of Physical Medicine Rehabilitation, 65, 168–170.

Ferrari, M. (1984). Chronic iliness: Psychosocial effects on siblings—I. Chronically ill boys. Journal of Child Psychology and Psychiatry, 25, 459–476.

Fletcher, J. M., Ewing-Cobbs, L., Miner, M. E., Levin, H. S., & Eisenberg, H. M. (1990). Behavioral changes after closed head injury in children. Journal of Consulting and Clinical Psychology, 58, 93–98.

Frankowski, R. F. (1985). Head injury mortality in urban populations and its relation to the injured child. In B. F. Brooks (Ed.), The injured child (pp. 20–29). Austin: University of Texas Press.

Gardner, R. A. (1973). The family book about minimal brain dysfunction. New York: Jason Aronson.

Goldstein, F. C., & Levin, H. S. (1987). Epidemiology of pediatric head injury: Incidence, clinical characteristics, and risk factors. Journal of Learning Disabilities, 20, 518–525.

Hall, K. M., Karzmark, P., Stevens, M., Englander, J., O'Hare, P., & Wright, J. (1994). Family stressors in traumatic brain injury: A two year follow-up. Archives of Physical Medicine and Rehabilitation, 75, 876–884.

Harvey, D. H. P., & Greenway, A. P. (1984). The self concept of physically handicapped children and their non-handicapped siblings: An empirical investigation. Journal of Child Psychology and Psychiatry, 25, 273–284.

Jackson, A., & Haverkamp, D. E. (1991). Family response to traumatic brain injury. Counseling Psychology Quarterly, 4, 355–356.

Kaplan, S. P. (1988). Adaptation following serious brain injury: An assessment after one year. Journal of Applied Rehabilitation Counseling, 19(3), 3–7.

Katz, R. T., & Deluca, J. (1992). Sequelae of minor traumatic brain injury. American Family Physician, 46, 1491–1498.

Kratochwill, T. R., & Bergan, J. R. (1990). Behavioral consultation in applied settings: An individual guide. New York: Plenum.

Kreutzer, J. S., Marwitz, J. H., & Kepler, K. (1992). Traumatic brain injury: Family response and outcome. Archives of Physical Medicine and Rehabilitation, 73, 771–778.

Lavigne, J. V., & Ryan, M. (1979). Psychologic adjustment of siblings of children with chronic illness. Pediatrics, 63, 616–622.

Leaf, L. E. (1993). Traumatic brain injury: Affecting family recovery. Brain Injury, 7, 543–546.

Lehr, E. (1990). Psyclzological management of traumatic brain injuries in children and adults. Rockville, MD: Aspen.

Lezak, M. D. (1978). Living with a characterologically altered brain injured patient. Journal of Clinical Psychiatry, 39, 592–598.

Lezak, M. D. (1986). Psychological implications of traumatic brain damage for the patient's family. Rehabilitation Psychology, 31, 241–250.

Lezak, M. D. (1988). Brain damage is a family affair. Journal of Clinical and Experimental Neuropsychology, 10, 111–123.

Livingston, M. G., & Brooks, D. N. (1988). The burden on families of the brain injured: A review. Journal of Head Trauma Rehabilitation, 2(4), 6–15.

Livingston, M. G., Brooks, D. N., & Bond, M. R. (1985a). Three months after severe head injury: Psychiatric and social impact on relatives. Journal of Neurology, Neurosurgery, and Psychiatry, 48, 870–875.

Livingston, M. G., Brooks, D. N., & Bond, M. R. (1985b). Patient outcome in the year following severe head injury and relatives' psychiatric and social functioning. Journal of Neurology, Neurosurgery, and Psychiatry, 48, 527–533.

Martin, D. A. (1988). Children and adolescents with traumatic brain injury: Impact on the family. Journal of Learning Disabilities, 21, 464–470.

Mauss-Clum, N., & Ryan, M. (1981). Brain injury and the family. Journal of Neurosurgical Nurses, 13, 165–169.

McGuire, T. L., & Rothenberg, M. B. (1986). Behavioral and psychosocial sequelae of pediatric brain injury. Journal of Head Trauma Rehabilitation, 1(4), 16.

Miller, L. (1993). Family therapy of brain injury: Syndromes, strategies, and solutions. The American Journal of Family Therapy, 21, 111–121.

National Head Injury Foundation. (1985). An educator's manual: What educators need to know about students with traumatic brain injury. Framingham, MA: Author.

Orsillo, S. M., McCaffrey, R. J., & Fisher, J. M. (1993). Siblings of head-injured individuals: A population at risk. Journal of Head Trauma Rehabilitation, 8, 102–115.

Panting, A., & Mercy, P. (1972). The long term rehabilitation of severe head injuries with particular reference to the need for social and medical support for the patient's family. Rehabilitation, 38, 33–37.

Parke, R. D. (1986). Fathers, families, and support systems: Their role in the development of at-risk and retarded infants and children. In J. J. Gallagher & P. M. Vietze (Eds.), Families of handicapped persons: Research, programs, and policy issues (pp. 101–113). Baltimore: Brookes.

Rivara, J. B., Fay, G. C., Jaffe, K. M., Pollissar, N. L., Shurtleff, H. A., & Martin, K. M. (1992). Predictors of family functioning one year following traumatic brain injury in children. *Archives of Physical Medicine and Rehabilitation, 73,* 899–910.

Rivara, J. B., Jaffe, K. M., Fay, G. C., Pollissar, N. L., Martin, K. M., Shurtleff, H. A., & Liao, S. (1993). Family functioning and injury severity as predictors of child functioning one year following traumatic brain injury. *Archives of Physical Medicine and Rehabilitation, 74,* 1047–1055.

Romano, M. D. (1974). Family response to traumatic head injury. *Scandinavian Journal of Rehabilitation Medicine, 6,* 1–5.

Rosenthal, M., & Muir, C. A. (1983). Methods of family intervention. In M. Rosenthal, E. R. Griffith, & M. R. Bond (Eds.), *Rehabilitation of the head injured adult* (pp. 407–419). Philadelphia: F. A. Davis.

Rosenthal, M., & Young, T. (1988). Effective family intervention after traumatic brain injury: Theory and practice. *Journal of Head Trauma Rehabilitation, 3,* 42–50.

Sheridan, S. M., & Kratochwill, T. R. (1992). Behavioral parent–teacher consultation: Conceptual and research considerations. *Journal of School Psychology, 30,* 117–139.

Sheridan, S. M., Kratochwill, T. R., & Bergan, J. R. (1996). *Conjoint behavioral consultation: A procedural manual.* New York: Plenum.

Simeonsson, R. J., & Bailey, D. B. (1986). Siblings of handicapped children. In J. J. Gallagher & P. M. Vietze (Eds.), *Families of handicapped persons: Research, programs, and policy issues* (pp. 67–77). Baltimore: Brookes.

Slater, E. J., & Rubenstein, E. (1987). Family coping with trauma in adolescents. *Psychiatric Annals, 17,* 786–794.

Taylor, S. C. (1980). The effect of chronic childhood illnesses upon well siblings. *Maternal–Child Nursing Journal, 9,* 109–116.

Testani-Dufour, L., Chappel-Aiken, L., & Gueldner, S. (1992). Traumatic brain injury: A family experience. *Journal of Neuroscience Nursing, 24,* 317–323.

Waaland, P. K. (1990). Family response to childhood brain injury. In J. S. Kreutzer & P. H. Wehman (Eds.), *Community integration following traumatic brain injury* (pp. 224–247). Baltimore: Brookes.

Waaland, P. K., & Kreutzer, J. S. (1988). Family response to childhood traumatic brain injury. *Journal of Head Trauma Rehabilitation, 3(4),* 51–63.

Zarski, J. J., DePompei, R., & Zook, A. (1988). Traumatic head injury: Dimensions of family responsivity. *Journal of Head Trauma Rehabilitation, 3(4),* 31–41.

Zarksi, J. J., Hall, D. E., & DePompei, R. (1987). Closed head injury patients: A family therapy approach to the rehabilitation process. *American Journal of Family Therapy, 15(1),* 62–68.

CHAPTER 11

Anderson, N. (1995). *Perceptions of school-based professionals regarding traumatic brain injury.* Unpublished master's thesis, University of Utah, Salt Lake City.

Baer, R. (1992). One year follow-up of Utah students exiting special education in 1990–92. (Available from Mountain Plains Regional Resource Center, 178 N. Research Parkway, Suite 112, Logan, UT 84321)

Begali, V. (1992). Head injury in children and adolescents. Brandon, VT: Clinical Psychology.

Bijur, P. E., Haslum, M., & Golding, J. (1990). Cognitive and behavioral sequelae of mild head injury in children. Pediatrics, 86, 337–344.

Blosser, J. L., & DePompei, R. (1989). The head-injured student returns to school: Recognizing and treating deficits. Topics in Language Disorders, 9(2), 67–77.

Blosser, J. L., & DePompei, R. (1991). Preparing education professionals for meeting the needs of students with traumatic brain injury. Journal of Head Trauma Rehabilitation, 6(1), 73–82.

Carney, J., & Gerring, J. (1990). Return to school following severe closed head injury: A critical phase in pediatric rehabilitation. Pediatrician, 17, 222–229.

Chadwick, O., Rutter, M., Brown, G., Shaffer, D., & Traub, M. (1981). A prospective study of children with head injuries: II. Cognitive sequelae. Psychological Medicine, 11(1), 49–61.

Costeff, H., Groswasser, Z., & Goldstein, R. (1990). Long-term follow-up review of 31 children with severe closed head trauma. Journal of Neurosurgery, 73, 684–687.

DePompei, R., & Blosser, J. L. (1991). Families of children with traumatic brain injury as advocates in school reentry. Neuro-Rehabilitation, 1, 29–37.

DiScala, C., Osberg, J. S., Gans, B. M., Chin, L. J., & Grant, C. C. (1991). Children with traumatic head injury: Morbidity and postacute treatment. Archives of Physical Medicine & Rehabilitation, 72, 662–666.

Ewing-Cobbs, L., Levin, H. S., Eisenberg, H. M., & Fletcher, J. M. (1987). Language functions following closed-head injury in children and adolescents. Journal of Clinical and Experimental Neuropsychology, 9, 575–592.

Fay, G. C., Jaffe, K. M., Polissar, N. L., Liao, S., Rivara, J. B., & Martin, K. M. (1994). Outcome of pediatric traumatic brain injury at three years: A cohort study. Archives of Physical Medicine & Rehabilitation, 75, 733–741.

Filley, C. M., Cranberg, L. D., Alexander, M. P., & Hart, E. J. (1987). Neurobehavioral outcome after closed head injury in childhood and adolescence. Archives of Neurology, 44, 194–198.

Golden, C. J., Puisch, A. D., & Hammeke, T. A. (1985). Luria-Nebraska neuropsychological battery: Forms I and II manual. Los Angeles: Western Psychological Corp.

Goldstein, F. C., & Levin, H. S. (1985). Intellectual and academic outcome following closed head injury in children and adolescents: Research strategies and empirical findings. Developmental Neuropsychology, 1, 195–214.

Greenspan, A. L., & MacKenzie, E. J. (1994). Functional outcome after pediatric head injury. Pediatrics, 94(2), 425–432.

Jaffe, K. M., Fay, G. C., Polissar, N. L., Martin, K. M., Shurtleff, H. A., Rivara, J. B., & Winn, H. R. (1993). Severity of pediatric traumatic brain injury and neurobehavioral recovery at one year—A cohort study. Archives of Physical Medicine & Rehabilitation, 74, 587–595.

Katsiyannis, A., & Conderman, G. (1994). Serving individuals with traumatic brain injury. Remedial and Special Education, 15, 319–325.

Klonoff, H., Clark, C., & Klonoff, P. (1993). Long-term outcome of head injuries: A 23 year follow up of children with head injuries. Journal of Neurology, Neurosurgery and Psychiatry, 56, 410–415.

Knight, R. M., Ivan, L. P., Ventureyra, E. C., Bentivoglio, C., Stoddart, C., Winogron, W., & Bawden, H. N. (1991). The effects of head injury in children on neuropsychological and behavioral functioning. Brain Injury, 5, 339–351.

Kraus, J. F., Fife, D., & Cox P. (1986). Incidence, severity and external causes of pediatric brain injury. American Journal of Diseases of Children, 140, 687–693.

Kraus, J. F., Rock, A., & Hemyarai, P. (1990). Brain injuries among infants, children, adolescents and young adults. American Journal of Diseases of Children, 144, 684–691.

Lanser, J. B., Jennekens-Schinkel, A., & Peters, A.C. (1988). Headache after closed head injury in children. Headache, 176–179.

Lash, M. (1994, Summer). Families and students get caught between medical and educational systems. (Available from Research and Training Center in Rehabilitation and Childhood Trauma, 750 Washington St., #75K-R, Boston, MA 02111)

Levin, H. S., Benton, A., & Grossman, R. G. (1982). Neurobehavioral consequences of closed head injury. New York: Oxford University Press.

Long, C. J., & Ross, L. K. (1992). Handbook of head trauma. New York: Plenum.

Max, W., MacKenzie, E. J., & Rice, D. P. (1991). Head injuries: Costs and consequences. Journal of Head Trauma Rehabilitation, 6, 76–87.

Michaud, L. J., Duhaime, A., & Gatshaw, M. L. (1993). Traumatic brain injury in children. Pediatric Clinics of North America, 40, 553–565.

Michaud, L. J., Rivara, F. P., & Grady, M. S. (1992). Predictors of survival and severity of disability after severe brain injury in children. Neurosurgery, 31, 254–264.

Michaud, L. J., Rivara, F. P., Jaffe, K. M., Fay, G., & Dailey, J. L. (1993). Traumatic brain injury as a risk factor for behavioral disorders in children. Archives of Physical Medicine and Rehabilitation, 74, 368–375.

Mira, M. P., Meck, N. E., & Tyler, J. S. (1988). School psychologists' knowledge of traumatic head injury: Implications for training. Diagnostique, 13, 174–180.

Mira, M. P., & Tyler, J. S. (1991). Students with traumatic brain injury: Making the transition from hospital to school. Focus on Exceptional Children, 23(5), 1–12.

Morgan, D. P., & Jenson, W. R. (1988). Teaching behaviorally disordered students: Preferred practices. Columbus, OH: Merrill.

Murphy, L. L., Close-Conoley, J., & Impara, J. C. (1994). Tests in print (Vol. 4). Lincoln: University of Nebraska Press.

Papas, B. (1993). Managing aggression: New strategies for the hospital setting. Headlines, 4(2), 2–8.

Reitan, R. M., & Wolfson, D. (1993). The Halstead-Reitan neuropsychological test battery. Tucson, AZ: Reitan Neuropsychology Lab.

Reynolds, C. R., & Bigler, E. D. (1994). Tests of memory and learning. Austin, TX: PRO-ED.

Rutter, M. (1981). Psychological sequelae of brain damage in children. American Journal of Psychiatry, 138, 1533–1544.

Savage, R. (1985). A survey of traumatically brain injured children within school-based special education programs. Rutland, VT: Head Injury/Stroke Independence Project.

Savage, R. (1991). Identification, classification and placement issues for students with traumatic brain injuries. Journal of Head Trauma Rehabilitation, 6(1), 1–9.

Savage, R. C., & Wolcott, G. F. (1988). An educator's manual: What educators need to know about students with traumatic brain injury. Southborough, MA: National Head Injury Foundation.

Savage, R. C., & Wolcott, G. F. (1994). Educational dimensions of acquired brain injury. Austin, TX: PRO-ED.

Thompson, N. M., Francis, D. J., Stuebing, K. K., Fletcher, J. M., Ewing-Cobbs, L., Miner, M. E., Levin, H. S., & Eisenberg, H. M. (1994). Motor, visual-spatial and somatosensory skills after closed head injury in children and adolescents: A study of change. Neuropsychology, 8(3), 333–342.

Thomsen, I. (1984). Late outcome of very severe blunt head trauma: A 10–15 year second follow-up. Journal of Neurology, Neurosurgery and Psychiatry, 47, 260–268.

Utah State Office of Education (USOE). (1993). Guidelines for serving students with traumatic brain injuries. Salt Lake City: USOE.

Winogron, H. W., Knight, R. M., & Bawden, H. N. (1984). Neuropsychological deficits following head injury in children. Journal of Clinical Neuropsychology, 6, 269–286.

Ylvisaker, M. (1986). Language and communication disorders following pediatric head injury. Journal of Head Trauma Rehabilitation, 1(4), 48–56.

Ylvisaker, M., Hartwick, P., & Stevens, M. (1991). School reentry following head injury: Managing the transition from hospital to school. Journal of Head Trauma Rehabilitation, 6, 10–22.

Ylvisaker, M., & Weinstein, M. (1989). Recovery of oral feeding after pediatric head injury. Journal of Head Trauma Rehabilitation, 4, 51–63.

Zasler, N. D., & Kreutzer, J. S. (1991). Families of children with traumatic brain injury as advocates in school reentry. Neuro-Rehabilitation, 1, 29–37.

CHAPTER 12

Adams, L., Carl, C. A., Covino, M. E., Filbin, J., Knapp, J., Rich, J. P., Warfield, M. A., & Yenowine, W. (1991). Guidelines paper: Traumatic brain injuries. Denver: Colorado Department of Education, Special Education Services Unit.

Begali, V. (1994). The role of the school psychologist. In R. C. Savage & G. F. Wolcott (Eds.), Educational dimensions of acquired brain injury (pp. 453–474). Austin, TX: PRO-ED.

Bigler, E. D. (Ed.). (1990a). Traumatic brain injury: Mechanisms of damage, assessment, intervention, and outcome. Austin, TX: PRO-ED.

Bigler, E. D. (1990b). Neuropathology of traumatic brain injury. In E. D. Bigler (Ed.), Traumatic brain injury: Mechanisms of damage, assessment, intervention, and outcome. Austin, TX: PRO-ED.

Bigler, E. D., & Nussbaum, N. L. (1989). Child neuropsychology in the private med-icalpractice. In C. R. Reynolds & E. Fletcher-Janzen (Eds.), Handbook of clinical child neuropsychology (pp. 557–572). New York: Plenum.

Blosser, J. L., & DePompei, R. (1991). Preparing education professionals for meeting the needs of students with traumatic brain injury. Journal of Head Trauma Rehabilitation, 6(1), 73–82.

Blosser, J. I., & DePompei, R. (1994). Creating an effective classroom environment. In R. C. Savage & G. F. Wolcott (Eds.), Educational dimensions of acquired brain injury (pp. 413–452). Austin, TX: PRO-ED.

Bruce, D. A. (1990). Scope of the problem—early assessment and management. In M. Rosenthal, E. R. Griffith, M. R. Bond, & J. D. Miller (Eds.), Rehabilitation of the adult and child with traumatic brain injury (2nd ed., pp. 521-538). Philadelphia: Davis.

Code of Federal Regulations 34. (July, 1993). Parts 300 to 399. Education. Washington, DC: Office of the Federal Register National Archives and Records Administration.

Cohen, S. B. (1986). Educational reintegration and programming for children with head injuries. Journal of Head Trauma Rehabilitation, 1(4), 22–29.

Crisp, R. (1992). Awareness of deficit after traumatic brain injury: A literature review. The Australian Therapy Journal, 39, 15–21.

D'Amato, R. C. (1990). A neuropsychological approach to school psychology. School Psychology Quarterly, 5, 141–160.

D'Amato, R. C. (1991, March). Mary had a little impairment: What neuropsychology can offer school psychology. Paper presented at the annual meeting of the National Association of School Psychologists, Dallas, TX.

D'Amato, R. C., & Dean, R. S. (1987). Psychological assessment reports, individual edu-cational plans and daily lesson plans: Are they related? Professional School Psychology, 2, 93–101.

D'Amato, R. C., & Rothlisberg, B. A. (Eds.). (1992). Psychological perspectives on interven-tion: A case study approach to prescriptions for change. White Plains, NY: Longman.

D'Amato, R. C., Rothlisberg, B. A., & Rhodes, R. L. (in press). Utilizing aneuropsycho-logical paradigm for understanding common educational and psychological tests. In C. R. Reynolds & E. Fletcher-Janzen (Eds.), Handbook of clinical child neuropsy-chology (2nd ed.). New York: Plenum.

Dean, R. S., & Gray, J. W. (1990). Traditional approaches to neuropsychological assessment. In C. R. Reynolds & R. W. Kamphaus (Eds.), Handbook of psycho-logical and educational assessment of children: Intelligence and achievement (pp. 371–388). New York: Guilford.

Deaton, A. V. (1990). Behavioral change strategies for children and adolescents with traumatic brain injury. In E. D. Bigler (Ed.), Traumatic brain injury (pp. 231–249). Austin, TX: PRO-ED.

Dennis, M. (1992). Word finding in children and adolescents with a history of brain injury. Topics in Language Disorders, 13, 66–82.

Ewing-Cobbs, L., Fletcher, J. M., & Levin, H. S. (1986). Neurobehavioral sequelae fol-lowing head injury in children: Educational implications. Journal of Head Trauma Rehabilitation, 1(4), 57–65.

Federal Register. (1975). Education for All Handicapped Children Act; Public Law 94-142.

Federal Register. (October 1990). Individuals with Disabilities Education Act (IDEA— P.L. 101-476).

Fletcher, J. M., & Taylor, H. G. (1984). Neuropsychological approaches to children: Towards a developmental neuropsychology. Journal of Clinical Neuropsychology, 6, 39–56.

Gaddes, W. H., & Edgell, D. (1994). Learning disabilities and brain function (3rd ed.). New York: Springer-Verlag.

Gray, J. W., & Dean, R. S. (1989). Approaches to the cognitive rehabilitation of children with neuropsychological impairment. In C. R. Reynolds & E. Fletcher-Janzen (Eds.), Handbook of clinical child neuropsychology (pp. 397–408). New York: Plenum.

Haley, S. M., Cioffi, M. I., Lewis, J. E., & Baryza, M. J. (1990). Motor dysfunction in children and adolescents after traumatic brain injury. Journal of Head Trauma Rehabilitation, 5(4), 77–90.

Hammill, D. D. (1991). Detroit tests of learning aptitude: Examiner's manual (3rd ed.). Austin, TX: PRO-ED.

Harrington, D. E. (1990). Educational strategies. In M. Rosenthal, E. R. Griffith, M. R. Bond, & J. D. Miller (Eds.), Rehabilitation of the adult and child with traumatic brain injury (2nd ed., pp. 476–492). Philadelphia: Davis.

Hartlage, L. C., & Telzrow, C. F. (1983). The neuropsychological bases of educational intervention. Journal of Learning Disabilities, 16, 521–528.

Hill, R. B., Baldo, A. J., & D'Amato, R. C. (1994). The interaction of teacher personality and student behavior on special education referral decisions. Manuscript submitted for publication.

Hynd, G. W., & Willis, W. G. (1988). Pediatric neuropsychology. New York: Grune & Stratton.

Jaffe, K. M., Brink, J. D., Hays, R. M., & Chorazy, A. J. L. (1990). Specific problems associated with pediatric head injury. In M. Rosenthal, E. R. Griffith, M. R. Bond, & J. D. Miller (Eds.), Rehabilitation of the adult and child with traumatic brain injury (2nd ed., pp. 539–557). Philadelphia: Davis.

Kaufman, A. S. (1979a). Cerebral specialization and intelligence testing. Journal of Research and Development in Education, 12, 96–107.

Kaufman, A. S. (1979b). Intelligent testing with the WISC-R. New York: Wiley.

Kaufman, A. S. (1990). Assessing adolescent and adult intelligence. Boston: Allyn & Bacon.

Lehr, E. (1990). Psychological management of traumatic brain injuries in children and adolescents. Rockville, MD: Aspen.

Leu, P. W., & D'Amato, R. C. (1994, March). Right child, wrong teacher: Using an ecological assessment for intervention. Paper presented at the annual meeting of the National Association of School Psychologists, Seattle, WA.

Lezak, M. D. (1983). Neuropsychological assessment (2nd ed.). New York: Oxford University Press.

Los Amigos Research and Educational Institute. (1990). Rancho Los Amigos scale of cognitive functioning. Downey, CA: Rancho Los Amigos Medical Center.

Medical Economics Data. (1993). The PDR family guide to prescription drugs. Montvale, NJ: Author.

Merrell, K. W. (1994). Assessment of behavioral, social, and emotional problems: Direct and objective methods for use with children and adolescents. White Plains, NY: Longman.

Posthill, S. M., & Roffman, A. J. (1991). The impact of a transitional training program for young adults with learning disabilities. Journal of Learning Disabilities, 24, 619–629.

Prigatano, G. P. (1990). Recovery and cognitive retraining after cognitive brain injury. In E. D. Bigler (Ed.), Traumatic brain injury (pp. 273–295). Austin, TX: PRO-ED.

Reiff, H. B., & deFur, S. (1992). Transition for youths with learning disabilities: A focus on developing independence. Learning Disability Quarterly, 15, 237–249.

Reynolds, C. R., & Fletcher-Janzen, E. (Eds.). (1989). Handbook of clinical child neuropsychology. New York: Plenum.

Rojewski, J. W. (1992). Key components of model transition services for students with learning disabilities. Learning Disability Quarterly, 15, 135–150.

Rosen, C. D., & Gerring, J. P. (1986). Head trauma: Educational reintegration. San Diego: College-Hill.

Russell, N. K. (1993). Educational considerations in traumatic brain injury: The role of the speech–language pathologist. Language, Speech, and Hearing Services in Schools, 24, 67–75.

Rutter, M. (Ed.) (1983). Developmental neuropsychiatry. New York: Guilford.

Sachs, P. R. (1991). Treating families of brain-injury survivors. New York: Springer-Verlag.

Sachs, P. R., & Redd, C. A. (1993). The Americans with Disabilities Act and individuals with neurological impairments. Rehabilitation Psychology, 38, 87–101.

Sattler, J. M. (1992). Assessment of children (3rd ed., rev.). San Diego: Sattler.

Savage, R. C. (1987). Educational issues for the head-injured adolescent and young adult. Journal of Head Trauma Rehabilitation, 2(1), 1–10.

Savage, R. C., & Wolcott, G. F. (Eds.). (1994). Educational dimensions of acquired brain injury. Austin, TX: PRO-ED.

Scuccimarra, D. J., & Speece, D. L. (1990). Employment outcomes and social integration of students with mild handicaps: The quality of life two years after high school. Journal of Learning Disabilities, 23, 213–219.

Soar, R. S., & Soar, R. M. (1979). Emotional climate and management. In P. L. Peterson & H. J. Walberg (Eds.), Research on teaching: Concepts, findings, and implications (pp. 271–307). New York: Plenum.

Taylor, H. G. (1987). Childhood sequelae of early neurological disorders: A contemporary perspective. Developmental Neuropsychology, 3, 153–164.

Teasdale, G., & Jennett, B. (1974). Assessment of coma and impaired consciousness: A practical scale. Lancet, 2, 81–84.

Telzrow, C. F. (1985). The science and speculation of rehabilitation in developmental neuropsychological disorders. In L. C. Hartlage & C. F. Telzrow (Eds.), The neuropsychology of individual differences: A developmental perspective (pp. 271–307). New York: Plenum.

Telzrow, C. F. (1990). Management of academic and educational problems in traumatic brain injury. In E. D. Bigler (Ed.), Traumatic brain injury (pp. 251–272). Austin, TX: PRO-ED.

Utah TBI Task Force. (1994). Utah traumatic brain injuries training for school personnel: Trainers' manual. Salt Lake City: Utah State Office of Education.

Waaland, P. K., & Kreutzer, J. S. (1988). Family response to childhood traumatic brain injury. Journal of Head Trauma Rehabilitation, 3(4), 51–63.

Wedding, D., Horton, A. M., & Webster, J. S. (Eds.). (1986). Handbook of clinical and behavioral neuropsychology. New York: Springer-Verlag.

Whitten, J. C., D'Amato, R. C., & Chittooran, M. M. (1992). A neuropsychological approach to intervention. In R. C. D'Amato & B. A. Rothlisberg (Eds.), Psychological perspectives on intervention: A case study approach to prescriptions for change (pp. 112–136). White Plains, NY: Longman.

Ylvisaker, M., Chorazy, A. J. L., Cohen, S. B., Mastrilli, J. P., Molitor, C. B., Nelson, J., Szekeres, S. F., Valko, A. S., & Jaffe, K. M. (1990). In M. Rosenthal, E. R. Griffith, M. R. Bond, & J. D. Miller (Eds.), Rehabilitation of the adult and child with traumatic brain injury (2nd ed., pp. 521–538). Philadelphia: Davis.

CHAPTER 13

Alves, W., Macciocchi, S. N., & Barth, J. T. (1993). Postconcussive symptoms after uncomplicated mild head injury. Journal of Head Trauma Rehabilitation, 8, 48–59.

Barth, J. T., Alves, W. M., Ryan, T. V., Macciocchi, S. N., Rimel, R. W., Jane, J. A., & Nelson, W. E. (1989). In H. S. Levin, H. M. Eisenberg, & A. L. Benton (Eds.), Mild head injury (pp. 257–275). New York: Oxford University Press.

Barth, J. T., Macciocchi, S. N., Giordani, B., Rimel, R., Jane, J. A., & Boll, T. J. (1983). Neuropsychological sequelae of minor head injury. Neurosurgery, 13, 529–533.

Bassett, S. S., & Slater, E. J. (1990). Neuropsychological function in adolescents sustaining mild closed head injury. Journal of Pediatric Psychology, 15, 225–236.

Bijur, P. E., Haslum, M., & Golding, J. (1990). Cognitive and behavioral sequelae of mild head injury in children. Pediatrics, 86, 337–344.

Boll, T. J. (1983). Minor head injury in children: Out of sight but not out of mind. Journal of Clinical Child Psychology, 12, 74–80.

Boll, T. J., & Barth, J. (1983). Mild head injury. Psychiatric Developments 3, 263–275.

Chapman, S. B., Culhane, K. A., Levin, H. S., Harward, H., Mendelsohn, D., Ewing-Cobbs, L., Fletcher, J. M., & Bruce, D. (1992). Narrative discourse after closed head injury in children and adolescents. Brain and Language, 43, 42–65.

Creswell, W., Newman, I., & Anderson, C. (1985). School health practice. St. Louis, MO: Times Mirror/Mosby.

DePompei, R., & Blosser, J. (1987). Strategies for helping head-injured children successfully return to school. Language, Speech, and Hearing Services in Schools, 18, 292–300.

DePompei, R., & Blosser, J. L. (1993). Professional training and development for pediatric rehabilitation. In C. J. Durgin, N. D. Schmidt, & L. J. Fryer (Eds.), Staff development and clinical intervention in brain injury rehabilitation (pp. 229–256). Gaithersburg, MD: Aspen.

Donders, J. (1993). Memory functioning after traumatic brain injury in children. Brain Injury, 7, 431–437.

Eisenberg, H. M., & Levin, H. S. (1989). Computed tomography and magnetic resonance imaging in mild to moderate head injury. In H. S. Levin, H. M. Eisenberg, & A. L. Benton (Eds.), Mild head injury (pp. 133–141). New York: Oxford University Press.

Ewing-Cobbs, L., Levin, H. S., Eisenberg, H. M., & Fletcher, J. M. (1987). Language functions following closed-head injury in children and adolescents. Journal of Clinical and Experimental Neuropsychology, 9, 575–592.

Farmer, T. (1992). Legal foundations: What is Section 504 and why did Congress enact it? Austin, TX: First Statewide Training Institute for Section 504 Coordinators and Hearing Officers.

Fay, G. C., Jaffe, K. M., Polissar, N. L., Liao, S., Martin, K. M., Shurtleff, H. A., Rivara, J. B., & Winn, H. R. (1993). Mild pediatric traumatic brain injury: A cohort study. Archives of Physical Medicine and Rehabilitation, 74, 895–901.

Fay, G. C., Jaffe, K. M., Polissar, N. L., Liao, S., Rivara, J. B., & Martin, K. M. (1994). Outcome of pediatric traumatic brain injury at 3 years: A cohort study. Archives of Physical Medicine and Rehabilitation, 75, 733–741.

Fletcher, J. M., Ewing-Cobbs, L., Miner, M. E., Levin, H. S., & Eisenberg, H. M. (1990). Journal of Consulting and Clinical Psychology, 58, 93–98.

Goldstein, F. C., & Levin, H. S. (1990). Epidemiology of traumatic brain injury: Incidence, clinical characteristics, and risk factors. In E. D. Bigler (Ed.), Traumatic brain injury: Mechanisms of damage, assessment, intervention, and outcome (pp. 51–67). Austin, TX: PRO-ED.

Gronwall, D. (1989). Cumulative and persisting effects of concussion on attention and cognition. In H. S. Levin, H. M. Eisenberg, & A. L. Benton (Eds.), Mild head injury (pp. 153–162). New York: Oxford University Press.

Hammond, M. D. (1995, March 17). Re-integrating TBI children into the classroom. Occupational Therapy Forum, 10, 2–3.

Individuals with Disabilities Education Act of 1990, 20 U.S.C. §§1401–1461.

Kaufmann, P. M., Fletcher, J. M., Levin, H. S., Miner, M. E., & Ewing-Cobbs, L. (1993). Attentional disturbance after pediatric closed head injury. Journal of Child Neurology, 8, 348–353.

Kraus, J. F., Fife, D., Cox, P., Ramstein, K., & Conroy, C. (1986). Incidence, severity, and external causes of pediatric brain injury. American Journal of Diseases of Children, 140, 687–693.

Levin, H. S., & Benton, A. L. (1986). Developmental and acquired dyscalculia in children. In I. Flehmig & L. Stern (Eds.), Child development and learning behavior (pp. 317–322). Stuttgart, Germany: Gustav Fisher.

Levin, H. S., & Eisenberg, H. M. (1979). Neuropsychological outcome of closed head injury in children and adolescents. Child's Brain, 5, 281–292.

Levin, H. S., Ewing-Cobbs, L., & Fletcher, J. M. (1989). Neurobehavioral outcome of mild head injury in children. In H. S. Levin, H. M. Eisenberg, & A. L. Benton (Eds.), Mild head injury (pp. 189–213). New York: Oxford University Press.

Levin, H. S., High, W. M., Ewing-Cobbs, L., Fletcher, J. M., Eisenberg, H. M., Miner, M. E., & Goldstein, F. C. (1988). Memory functioning during the first year after closed head injury in children and adolescents. Neurosurgery, 22, 1043–1052.

Levin, H. S., Mattis, S., Ruff, R. M., Eisenberg, H. M., Marshall, L. F., Tabaddor, K., High, W. M., & Frankowski, R. F. (1987). Neurobehavioral outcome following minor head injury: A three-center study. Journal of Neurosurgery, 66, 234–243.

Oakland, T. (1994). Psychoeducational evaluations under Section 504. Texas Psychologist, 45, 9–12.

Oakland, T., & Stavinoha, P. (1992, August). Neuropsychological assessment and intervention: Roles for school psychology. Paper presented at the American Psychological Association's annual convention, Toronto, Canada.

Papero, P. H., Prigatano, G. P., Snyder, H. M., & Johnson, D. L. (1993). Children's adaptive behavioral competence after head injury. Neuropsychological Rehabilitation, 3, 321–340.

Reitan, R. M., & Wolfson, D. (1994). A selective and critical review of neuropsychological deficits and the frontal lobes. Neuropsychology Review, 4, 161–198.

Rehabilitation Act of 1973, 29 U.S.C. §974(a).

Rhodes, R. L., Hofen, B., Karren, K., & Rollins, L. M. (1981). Elementary school health. Boston: Allyn & Bacon.

Ruff, R. M., Levin, H. S., Mattis, S., High, W. M., Marshall, L. F., Eisenberg, H. M., & Tabaddor, K. (1989). Recovery of memory after mild head injury: A three-center study. In H. S. Levin, H. M. Eisenberg, & A. L. Benton (Eds.), Mild head injury (pp. 176–188). New York: Oxford University Press.

Russell, N. K. (1993). Educational considerations in traumatic brain injury: The role of the speech–language pathologist. Language, Speech, and Hearing Services in Schools, 24, 67–75.

Savage, R. C. (1985). A survey of traumatic brain injured children within school-based education programs. Rutland, VT: Head Injury/Stroke Independence Project.

Savage, R. C., & Carter, R. (1984). Re-entry: The head injured student returns to school. Cognitive Rehabilitation, 2, 28–33.

Stahl, C. (1995, February 27). Undetected mild head injury can wreck lives. Advance for Occupational Therapists, 11, 13.

Teasdale, G., & Jennett, B. (1974). Assessment of coma and impaired consciousness: A practical scale. Lancet, 2, 81–84.

Telzrow, K. (1987). Management of academic and educational problems in head injury. Journal of Learning Disabilities, 20, 536–545.

Webb, R. B., & Sherman, R. R. (1989). Schooling and society. New York: Macmillan.

Wechsler, D. (1974). Wechsler intelligence scale for children–Revised. San Antonio, TX: Psychological Corp.

CHAPTER 14

Begali, V. (1992). Head injury in children and adolescents: A resource and review for school and applied professionals (2nd ed.). Brandon, VT: Clinical Psychology Publishing.

Blosser, J. L., & DePompei, R. (1994). Pediatric traumatic brain injury: Proactive intervention. San Diego: Singular Publishing.

Deaton, A. (1994). Changing the behaviors of students with acquired brain injuries. In R. C. Savage & G. F. Wolcott (Eds.), Educational dimensions of acquired brain injury (pp. 257–275). Austin, TX: PRO-ED.

Dennis, M., Barnes, M. A., Donnelly, R. E., Wilkinson, M., & Humphreys, R. P. (1996). Appraising and managing knowledge: Metacognitive skills after childhood head injury. Developmental Neuropsychology, 12, 77–103.

Englander, J., Cleary, S., O'Hare, P., Hall, K. M., & Lehmkuhl, D. L. (1993). Implementing and evaluating injury prevention programs in the traumatic brain injury model systems of care. Journal of Head Trauma Rehabilitation, 8, 101–113.

Farmer, J. E., & Peterson, L. (1995a). Injury risk factors in children with attention deficit hyperactivity disorder. Health Psychology, 14, 325–332.

Farmer, J. E., & Peterson, L. (1995b). Pediatric traumatic brain injury: Promoting successful school reentry. School Psychology Review, 24, 230–243.

Farmer, J. E., & Stucky-Ropp, R. (1996). Family transactions and traumatic brain injury. In H. H. Stonnington & B. Uzzell (Eds.), Recovery after traumatic brain injury (pp. 275–288). Mahwah, NJ: Erlbaum.

Frank, R. G., Bouman, D. E., Cain, E., & Watts, C. (1992). Primary prevention of catastrophic injury. American Psychologist, 47, 1045–1049.

Geller, E. S., Berry, T. D., Ludwig, T. D., Evans, R. E., Gilmore, M. R., & Clarke, S. W. (1990). A conceptual framework for developing and evaluating behavior change strategies for injury control. Health Education Research, 5, 125–137.

Goldberg, A. L. (1996). Acquired brain injury in childhood and adolescence: A team and family guide to educational program development and implementation. Springfield, IL: Charles C. Thomas.

Kaufman, A., & Kaufman, N. (1983). Kaufman assessment battery for children. Circle Pines, MN: American Guidance Service.

Kazak, A. E., Segal-Andrews, A. M., & Johnson, K. (1995). Pediatric psychology research and practice: A family/systems approach. In M. C. Roberts (Ed.), Handbook of pediatric psychology (2nd ed., pp. 84–104). New York: Guilford.

Kinsella, G., Prior, M., Sawyer, M., Murtagh, D., Eisenmajer, R., Anderson, V., Bryan, D., & King, G. (1995). Neuropsychological deficit and academic performance in children and adolescents following traumatic brain injury. Journal of Pediatric Psychology, 20, 753–767.

Levin, H. S., Culhane, K. A., Mendelsohn, D., Lilly, M. A., Bruce, D., Fletcher, J. M., Chapman, S. B., Harward, H., & Eisenberg, H. M. (1993). Cognition in relation to magnetic resonance imaging in head-injured children and adolescents. Archives of Neurology, 50, 897–905.

Levin, H. S., Fletcher, J. M., Kufera, J. A., Harward, H., Lilly, M. A., Mendelsohn, D., Bruce, D., & Eisenberg, H. M. (1996). Dimensions of cognition measured by the Tower of London and other cognitive tasks in head-injured children and adolescents. Developmental Neuropsychology, 12, 17–34.

Massagli, T. L., Jaffe, K. M., Fay, G. C., Polissar, N. L., Liao, S., & Rivara, J. B. (1996). Neurobehavioral sequelae of severe pediatric traumatic brain injury: A cohort study. Archives of Physical Medicine and Rehabilitation, 77, 223–231.

Mullins, L. L., Gillman, J., & Harbeck, C. (1992). *Multiple level interventions in pediatric psychology settings: A behavioral-systems perspective.* In A. M. LaGreca, L. J. Siegel, & C. E. Walker (Eds.), *Stress and coping in child health* (pp. 377–399). New York: Guilford.

Peterson, L., & Brown, D. (1994). Integrating child injury and abuse–neglect research: Common histories, etiologies, and solutions. *Psychological Bulletin, 116,* 293–315.

Peterson, L., & Roberts, M. C. (1992). Complacency, misdirection, and effective prevention of children's injuries. *American Psychologist, 47,* 1040–1044.

Quittner, A. L., & Espelage, D. L. (1996, August). *Parental caregiving for children: Role strain and marital satisfaction.* Paper presented at the annual meeting of the American Psychological Association, Toronto, Canada.

Rivara, J. B., Jaffe, K. M., Fay, G. C., Polissar, N. L., Martin, K. M., Shurtleff, H. A., & Liao, S. (1993). Family functioning and injury severity as predictors of child functioning one year following traumatic brain injury. *Archives of Physical Medicine and Rehabilitation, 74,* 1047–1055.

Savage, R. C., & Wolcott, G. F. (1994). *Educational dimensions of acquired brain injury.* Austin, TX: PRO-ED.

Savage, R. C., & Wolcott, G. F. (Eds.). (1995). *An educator's manual: What educators need to know about students with brain injury.* Washington, DC: Brain Injury Association.

Springer, J. A., Farmer, J. E., & Bouman, D. E. (in press). Misconceptions about traumatic brain injury among relatives of rehabilitation patients. *Journal of Head Trauma Rehabilitation.*

Taylor, H. G., & Fletcher, J. M. (1995). Editorial: Progress in pediatric neuropsychology. *Journal of Pediatric Psychology, 20,* 695–701.

Wallendar, J. L., & Thompson, R. J. (1995). Psychosocial adjustment of children with chronic physical conditions. In M. C. Roberts (Ed.), *Handbook of pediatric psychology* (2nd ed., pp. 124–141). New York: Guilford.

Wechsler, D. (1991). *Wechsler intelligence scale for children.* (3rd ed.). San Antonio, TX: Psychological Corp.

Ylvisaker, M., Feeney, T., Maher-Maxwell, N., Meserve, N., Geary, P. J., & DeLorenzo, J. P. (1995). School reentry following severe traumatic brain injury: Guidelines for educational planning. *Journal of Head Trauma Rehabilitation, 10,* 25–41.

Ylvisaker, M., Szekeres, S. F., Hartwick, P., & Tworek, P. (1994). Cognitive intervention. In R. C. Savage & G. F. Wolcott (Eds.), *Educational dimensions of acquired brain injury* (pp. 121–184). Austin, TX: PRO-ED.

Contributors

Erin D. Bigler, professor, psychology, Brigham Young University

Elaine Clark, associate professor and director, School Psychology Program, University of Utah

Dana S. Clippard, doctoral student, special education, University of Missouri–Columbia

Jane C. Conoley, associate dean for research, University of Nebraska–Lincoln Teacher's College

Rik Carl D'Amato, professor, school psychology, and director of the Clinical Neuropsychology Laboratory, University of Northern Colorado

Dennis Drotar, professor, psychiatry and pediatrics, Case Western Reserve University School of Medicine, and professor and director of research training, pediatric psychology, Department of Psychology, Case Western Reserve University School of Medicine

Karen L. Eso, master's candidate, clinical neuropsychology, University of Victoria, Canada

Janet E. Farmer, assistant professor, physical medicine and rehabilitation, University of Missouri–Columbia School of Medicine

William R. Jenson, professor and chair, Department of Educational Psychology, University of Utah

Thomas J. Kehle, professor and director, School Psychology Program, University of Connecticut

Kimberly A. Kerns, assistant professor, psychology, University of Victoria, Canada

Jeffrey S. Kreutzer, professor, Department of Physical Medicine and Rehabilitation and Division of Neurological Surgery, Department of Surgery, Medical College of Virginia

Janiece Lord-Maes, adjunct assistant professor, school psychology, University of Arizona

Yvette Luehr-Wiemann, speech–language pathologist, St. John's Mercy Medical Center, St. Louis

Jennifer Harris Marwitz, research coordinator, Department of Physical Medicine and Rehabilitation, Medical College of Virginia

Catherine A. Mateer, professor, psychology, and director of clinical training, University of Victoria, Canada

Thomas Oakland, professor and chair, Department of Foundations of Education, University of Florida

John E. Obrzut, professor, school psychology, University of Arizona

Stephanie Owings, senior occupational therapist, Rusk Outpatient BRIDGE program, Columbia, Missouri

Barbara A. Rothlisberg, associate professor, educational psychology, and director of the MA/EdS Program in School Psychology, Ball State University

Susan M. Sheridan, associate professor, Department of Educational Psychology, University of Utah

Cheryl H. Silver, assistant professor, Department of Rehabilitation Science and Division of Psychology, Department of Psychiatry, University of Texas Southwestern Medical Center

Terry Stancin, assistant professor, pediatrics, Case Western Reserve University School of Medicine, and staff psychologist, Metro-Health Medical Center, Cleveland

H. Gerry Taylor, associate professor, pediatrics, Case Western Reserve University School of Medicine, and director, pediatric psychology, Rainbow Children's Hospital

Shari L. Wade, adjunct assistant professor, pediatrics, Case Western Reserve University School of Medicine

Greta N. Wilkening, associate professor, pediatrics and neurology, University of Colorado Health Sciences Center, The Children's Hospital

Adrienne D. Witol, neuropsychology postdoctoral fellow

Edward Wright, assistant professor, and director of pediatric rehabilitation, University of Missouri–Columbia School of Medicine

Keith Owen Yeates, assistant professor, pediatrics, The Ohio State University, and director of pediatric neuropsychology, Columbus Children's Hospital

Author Index

Abidin, R. 54
Abikoff, H. 166
Abildskov, T. 13, 16, 19, 20, 21, 22, 26
Abrams, D. 63
Achenbach, T. M. 54, 94
Adams, J. 11
Adams, L. 217, 219, 222, 228, 232, 233, 235
Adams, R. 110
Adams, W. 43
Alexander, M. P. 91, 172, 194, 196
Alexander, P. A. 67
Alldadi, V. 66
Allen, A. S. 50
Allen, K. 178, 180, 182
Alpert N. M. 29
Alves, W. 240, 243
Anchor, K. N. 155
Anderson, C. V. 13, 21, 26, 254
Anderson, N. 192
Anderson, S. 160
Anderson, T. P. 177
Anderson, V. 266
Andrellos, P. J. 53
Andrews, W. S. 85
Aram, D. M. 108
Arffa, S. 105, 106
Armstrong, M. 145
Asarnow, R. F. 53, 54, 137, 183
Asher, I. E. 51
August, G. J. 66

Baddeley, A. D. 172, 173
Baer, R. 204
Bailey, B. J. 13

Bailey, D. 102, 181
Baker, B. K. 149
Baker, R. S. 50
Baldo, A. J. 231
Baldwin, L. M. 54
Balla, D. A. 53
Bandura, A. 146
Banich, M. T. 111
Barker, L. T. 63
Barkley, R. A. 160, 166
Barnes, M. A. 45, 167, 266
Barnes, T. Y. 83, 86
Barrett, M. 48
Barry, P. 179
Barth, J. T. 64, 154, 155, 239, 243
Barton, E. A. 42
Baryza, M. J. 52, 215, 222
Baser, C. A. 160, 162
Bassett, S. S. 89, 241, 242
Bates, E. 108
Batshaw, M. L. 135, 150
Bawden, H. N. 53, 54, 55, 138, 154, 196, 199
Beastal, G. 77
Beattie, A. 64, 70, 178, 179
Beck, L. 66
Becker, D. P. 13
Becker, W. C. 145
Beers, S. R. 154, 155
Beery, K. E. 51
Begali, V. 35, 36, 41, 54, 141, 194, 217, 232, 267
Bentivoglio, C. 53, 54, 55, 138, 154, 199
Bentler, P. M. 66

Subject Index